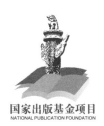

National Key Book Publishing Planning Project of the 13th Five-Year Plan

"十三五"国家重点图书出版规划项目

International Clinical Medicine Series Based on the Belt and Road Initiative

"一带一路"背景下国际化临床医学丛书

国家出版基金项目
NATIONAL PUBLICATION FOUNDATION

Emergency Medicine

急诊医学

Chief Editor　Zhu Changju　Zhang Mao　Gao Yanxia
主编　　　　朱长举　　　张 茂　　高艳霞

U0339684

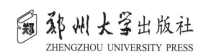

郑州大学出版社
ZHENGZHOU UNIVERSITY PRESS

图书在版编目(CIP)数据

急诊医学 = Emergency Medicine：英文／朱长举，张茂，高艳霞主编. — 郑州：郑州大学出版社，2020. 12

("一带一路"背景下国际化临床医学丛书)

ISBN 978-7-5645-6472-8

Ⅰ. ①急…　Ⅱ. ①朱…②张…③高…　Ⅲ. ①急诊 - 临床医学 - 英文　Ⅳ. ①R459.7

中国版本图书馆 CIP 数据核字(2019)第 131186 号

急诊医学 = Emergency Medicine：英文

项目负责人	孙保营　杨秦予	策 划 编 辑	李龙传
责 任 编 辑	陈文静	装 帧 设 计	苏永生
责 任 校 对	张彦勤	责 任 监 制	凌　青　李瑞卿

出版发行	郑州大学出版社有限公司	地　　址	郑州市大学路 40 号(450052)
出 版 人	孙保营	网　　址	http://www.zzup.cn
经　　销	全国新华书店	发行电话	0371-66966070
印　　刷	河南文华印务有限公司		
开　　本	850 mm×1 168 mm　1／16		
印　　张	21.75	字　　数	832 千字
版　　次	2020 年 12 月第 1 版	印　　次	2020 年 12 月第 1 次印刷

书　　号	ISBN 978-7-5645-6472-8	定　　价	129.00 元

Staff of Expert Steering Committee

Chairmen

Zhong Shizhen   Li Sijin   Lü Chuanzhu

Vice Chairmen

Bai Yuting   Chen Xu   Cui Wen   Huang Gang   Huang Yuanhua
Jiang Zhisheng   Li Yumin   Liu Zhangsuo   Luo Baojun   Lü Yi
Tang Shiying

Committee Member

An Dongping	Bai Xiaochun	Cao Shanying	Chen Jun	Chen Yijiu
Chen Zhesheng	Chen Zhihong	Chen Zhiqiao	Ding Yueming	Du Hua
Duan Zhongping	Guan Chengnong	Huang Xufeng	Jian Jie	Jiang Yaochuan
Jiao Xiaomin	Li Cairui	Li Guoxin	Li Guoming	Li Jiabin
Li Ling	Li Zhijie	Liu Hongmin	Liu Huifan	Liu Kangdong
Song Weiqun	Tang Chunzhi	Wang Huamin	Wang Huixin	Wang Jiahong
Wang Jiangang	Wang Wenjun	Wang Yuan	Wei Jia	Wen Xiaojun
Wu Jun	Wu Weidong	Wu Xuedong	Xie Xieju	Xue Qing
Yan Wenhai	Yan Xinming	Yang Donghua	Yu Feng	Yu Xiyong
Zhang Lirong	Zhang Mao	Zhang Ming	Zhang Yu'an	Zhang Junjian
Zhao Song	Zhao Yumin	Zheng Weiyang	Zhu Lin	

专家指导委员会

主 任 委 员

钟世镇　李思进　吕传柱

副主任委员（以姓氏汉语拼音为序）

白育庭　陈　旭　崔　文　黄　钢　黄元华　姜志胜

李玉民　刘章锁　雒保军　吕　毅　唐世英

委　　　员（以姓氏汉语拼音为序）

安东平　白晓春　曹山鹰　陈　君　陈忆九　陈哲生

陈志宏　陈志桥　丁跃明　杜　华　段钟平　官成浓

黄旭枫　简　洁　蒋尧传　焦小民　李才锐　李国新

李果明　李家斌　李　玲　李志杰　刘宏民　刘会范

刘康栋　宋为群　唐纯志　王华民　王慧欣　王家宏

王建刚　王文军　王　渊　韦　嘉　温小军　吴　军

吴卫东　吴学东　谢协驹　薛　青　鄢文海　闫新明

杨冬华　余　峰　余细勇　张莉蓉　张　茂　张　明

张玉安　章军建　赵　松　赵玉敏　郑维扬　朱　林

Staff of Editor Steering Committee

Chairmen

Cao Xuetao   Liang Guiyou   Wu Jiliang

Vice Chairmen

Chen Pingyan	Chen Yuguo	Huang Wenhua	Li Yaming	Wang Heng
Xu Zuojun	Yao Ke	Yao Libo	Yu Xuezhong	Zhao Xiaodong

Committee Member

Cao Hong	Chen Guangjie	Chen Kuisheng	Chen Xiaolan	Dong Hongmei
Du Jian	Du Ying	Fei Xiaowen	Gao Jianbo	Gao Yu
Guan Ying	Guo Xiuhua	Han Liping	Han Xingmin	He Fanggang
He Wei	Huang Yan	Huang Yong	Jiang Haishan	Jin Chengyun
Jin Qing	Jin Runming	Li Lin	Li Ling	Li Mincai
Li Naichang	Li Qiuming	Li Wei	Li Xiaodan	Li Youhui
Liang Li	Lin Jun	Liu Fen	Liu Hong	Liu Hui
Lu Jing	Lü Bin	Lü Quanjun	Ma Qingyong	Ma Wang
Mei Wuxuan	Nie Dongfeng	Peng Biwen	Peng Hongjuan	Qiu Xinguang
Song Chuanjun	Tan Dongfeng	Tu Jiancheng	Wang Lin	Wang Huijun
Wang Peng	Wang Rongfu	Wang Shusen	Wang Chongjian	Xia Chaoming
Xiao Zheman	Xie Xiaodong	Xu Falin	Xu Xia	Xu Jitian
Xue Fuzhong	Yang Aimin	Yang Xuesong	Yi Lan	Yin Kai
Yu Zujiang	Yu Hong	Yue Baohong	Zeng Qingbing	Zhang Hui
Zhang Lin	Zhang Lu	Zhang Yanru	Zhao Dong	Zhao Hongshan
Zhao Wen	Zheng Yanfang	Zhou Huaiyu	Zhu Changju	Zhu Lifang

编审委员会

Editorial Staff

Shi Junxia	The First Affiliated Hospital of Henan University
Wang Lin	The First Affiliated Hospital of Guangzhou University of Chinese Medicine
Wang Nan	The First Affiliated Hospital of Zhengzhou University
Wang Qianmei	Air Force Military Medical University Xijing Hospital
Xu Zhigao	The First Affiliated Hospital of Zhengzhou University
Yao Dongqi	The Second Hospital of Hebei Medical University
Yin Wen	Air Force Military Medical University Xijing Hospital
Zeng Mei	Qilu Hospital of Shandong University
Zhang Junqiang	The Second Hospital of Lanzhou University
Zhang Rui	The First Affiliated Hospital of Zhengzhou University
Zhang Yao	The Second Hospital of Lanzhou University

作者名单

主　审

于学忠　　中国医学科学院北京协和医院

陈玉国　　山东大学齐鲁医院

吕传柱　　海南医学院

主　编

朱长举　　郑州大学第一附属医院

张　茂　　浙江大学医学院附属第二医院

高艳霞　　郑州大学第一附属医院

副主编

李　毅　　中国医学科学院北京协和医院

朱志强　　郑州大学第一附属医院

李铁刚　　中国医科大学附属盛京医院

杨宇霞　　郑州大学第一附属医院

张国秀　　河南科技大学第一附属医院

穆　琼　　贵州医科大学附属医院

编　委（以姓氏汉语拼音排序）

曹　彦　　湖南省人民医院

陈海鸣　　南昌大学第一附属医院

邓　颖　　哈尔滨医科大学附属第二医院

高玉雷　　天津医科大学总医院

菅向东　　山东大学齐鲁医院

李　楠　　大连医科大学附属第一医院

李培武　　兰州大学第二医院

李小刚　　中南大学湘雅医院

刘丽平　　兰州大学第一临床学院

石金河　　新乡医学院

时俊霞　河南大学第一附属医院

王　林　广州中医药大学第一附属医院

王　楠　郑州大学第一附属医院

王倩梅　空军军医大学西京医院

徐志高　郑州大学第一附属医院

姚冬奇　河北医科大学第二医院

尹　文　空军军医大学西京医院

曾　梅　山东大学齐鲁医院

张军强　兰州大学第二医院

张　瑞　郑州大学第一附属医院

张　瑶　兰州大学第二医院

Preface

At the Second Belt and Road Summit Forum on International Cooperation in 2019 and the Seventy–third World Health Assembly in 2020, General Secretary Xi Jinping stated the importance for promoting the construction of the "Belt and Road" and jointly build a community for human health. Countries and regions along the "Belt and Road" have a large number of overseas Chinese communities, and shared close geographic proximity, similarities in culture, disease profiles and medical habits. They also shared a profound mass base with ample space for cooperation and exchange in Clinical Medicine. The publication of the International Clinical Medicine series for clinical researchers, medical teachers and students in countries along the "Belt and Road" is a concrete measure to promote the exchange of Chinese and foreign medical science and technology with mutual appreciation and reciprocity.

Zhengzhou University Press coordinated more than 600 medical experts from over 160 renowned medical research institutes, medical schools and clinical hospitals across China. It produced this set of medical tools in English to serve the needs for the construction of the "Belt and Road". It comprehensively coversaspects in the theoretical framework and clinical practicesin Clinical Medicine, including basic science, multiple clinical specialities and social medicine. It reflects the latest academic and technological developments, and the international frontiers of academic advancements in Clinical Medicine. It shared with the world China's latest diagnosis and therapeutic approaches, clinical techniques, and experiences in prescription and medication. It has an important role in disseminating contemporary Chinese medical science and technology innovations, demonstrating the achievements of modern China's economic and social development, and promoting the unique charm of Chinese culture to the world.

The series is the first set of medical tools written in English by Chinese medical experts to serve the needs of the "Belt and Road" construction. It systematically and comprehensively reflects the Chinese characteristics in Clinical Medicine. Also, it presents a landmark achievement in the implementation of the "Belt and Road" initiative in promoting exchanges in medical science and technology. This series is theoretical in nature, with each volume built on the mainlines in traditional disciplines but at the same time introducing contemporary theories that guide clinical practices, diagnosis and treatment methods, echoing the latest research findings in Clinical Medicine.

As the disciplines in Clinical Medicine rapidly advances, different views on knowledge, inclusiveness, and medical ethics may arise. We hope this work will facilitate the exchange of ideas, build common ground while allowing differences, and contribute to the building of a community for human health in a broad spectrum of disciplines and research focuses.

Nick Lemoine

Foreign Academician of the Chinese Academy of Engineering

Dean, Academy of Medical Sciences of Zhengzhou University

Director, Barts Cancer Institute, London, UK

6th August, 2020

Foreword

Emergency medicine is aspecialty that consists of nearly all aspects of medicine. Emergency medicine is a recognized board certified medical specialty, which has its own numerous subspecialies. Nowadays, emergency medicine is developing rapidly. The clinical, teaching and scientific research of emergency medicine have made great progress. As we all know, emergency medicine has entered the "3.0 era", targeting the precise diagnosis and treatment.

We have compiled this book to update the current new ideas and knowledge on the basis of the latest emergency evidence. Moreover, at present, there are few textbooks for undergraduate students to teach, so we write this book to make up the margin.

The chapters are presented by organ-system (i. e. , cardiovascular emergencies, pulmonary emergencies, and gastrointestinal emergencies), as well as special topics (i. e. , environmental emergencies, trauma, toxicology). The common emergency diseases and conditions encountered in ED are elaborated in this book, ranging from epidemiology, etiology, principle, clinical feature, differential diagnose, to emergency room management of disease. In addition, it covers procedures in ER, such as cardiopulmonary resuscitation (CPR), emergency ultrasound, mechanical ventilation and others.

Although this edition is primarily designed for the study of foreign medical students, we hope it is also available for Chinese emergency physicians, intensivists, and emergency nurses.

This book has been written for more than one year. In compiling the book, we receive assistance from many sources, and acknowledge those people for their invaluable support. The authors of this book are all experienced doctors working in emergency department for a long time. They come from large teaching hospitals or medical centers. They have rich experience in clinical, scientific research, teaching and book writing. Thank them for spending much time out of their busy schedule and their family to write this book.

Authors

Contents

Section 1　General Theory

Section 2　Intensive Situation

Section 3   Cardiac Emergencies

Section 4 Surgical Emergencies

Section 5   Disaster Medicine

Section 1

General Theory

Chapter 1

Characteristics of Emergency Medicine

Emergency medicine is recognized as an independent secondary discipline in clinical medicine in most countries in the world. Emergency medicine mainly studies the occurrence and development of trauma and sudden medical problems. The subjects are patients with trauma and sudden medical problems. Main contents of the study: translocation, diagnosis, initial evaluation, stability, diagnosis, treatment and preventive decision-making as well as emergency medical teaching and management. The research fields include: pre-hospital (on-site first aid), emergency department (emergency treatment), critical care unit (resuscitation of critically ill patients, initial assessment and stability), emergency preparedness for disaster medicine, treatment and prevention of poisoning. Emergency medicine is a very distinctive medical discipline. The level of emergency medicine reflects the general of clinical medicine in a hospital or even a country to a certain extent.

1.1 Development of emergency medicine

The history of emergency medicine development is relatively short. Before the emergency medicine becomes an independent discipline, each clinical discipline has its own emergency department to carry out emergency treatment for their specialist. But with the progress of medical science and the rapid development of global urbanization and the rapid increase in the demand for emergency medicine, the pattern has been found to be unable to adapt to the increasing needs of health care. Therefore, under the support of the government, the emergency medical service system (emergency medical service system, EMSS) and the first aid network are becoming more and more complete. The department of emergency medical treatment in the hospital has also developed under the support of the government and the hospital, forming its own characteristic theory, teaching and management system as well as the unique operating mode. Against this background, emergency medicine was born as an independent secondary clinical discipline. In 1979, international recognition of emergency medicine was recognized as the 23rd specialty in the field of medicine.

1. 2 Difference between emergency medicine and other secondary clinical disciplines

With the progress of medical science, the deepening of people's understanding, the development of clinical diagnosis and treatment technology, and the more and more specialized branch departments, the existing medical models are becoming more and more unable to meet the needs of the people. At present, medical specialties are based on the various systems of the human, but on the contrary, many patients often have dysfunction of multiple systems. The model ignores the integrity of the human, the state lacks the knowledge to diagnose and deal with the whole body's function state, which leads to serious consequences.

Under such circumstances, the emergence of emergency medicine is undoubtedly refreshing. Emergency medicine is not based on the traditional disciplines, but to provide timely emergency medical rescue service. The scope of emergency medicine is not confined to the hospital, but covers the areas of pre-hospital first aid, disaster medicine, hospital emergency and treatment. This system is also called the emergency medical service system.

Traditional disciplines are confined to the hospital, and have not yet formed a perfect service from pre-hospital to hospital. Emergency medicine not only absorbs the essence of modern medicine, but also overcomes the shortcomings of the traditional disciplines. At the same time, emergency medicine attaches great importance to timeliness, early recognition and early intervention, and finds and judges the hidden dangers of life safety in the first time.

After more than thirty years of development, emergency medicine has grown into a new medical specialty with its own distinctive professional characteristics, which are intersecting from professional knowledge, thinking, diagnosis and treatment technology with other traditional specialties. Emergency medicine is not a "marginal subject", nor is it so-called "multidisciplinary". In any way, emergency medicine is one of the mainstream department in the field of clinical medicine, but it is undeniable that emergency medicine is still a new subject. In order to serve better, there are many problems that need further research and discussion, and many aspects need to be further improved. However, emergency medicine is undoubtedly one of the most promising and promising disciplines.

1.3 The urgency of time in Emergency medicine

Whether it is pre-hospital first aid, disaster site emergency medical rescue and hospital emergency, emergency medical services are all the patients and wounded who are in urgent need of medical help, and all kinds of emergency, dangerous, heavy patients and injured people have a "golden time", and the "golden time" is given the necessary treatment and can be reduced to the maximum. The low mortality rate of patients and wounded patients is the key to successful rescue.

For emergency medicine, "time is life". In order to meet the special requirements of "time" in emergency medicine, it requires that the organization and layout of the department of emergency medicine are reasonable, open all day, management science, rescue instrument in place, and the rescue procedure is concise on the basis of scientific and reasonable, so as to facilitate operation and practice. All the emergency medical workers have the concept of the time window of various emergency treatment, basic knowledge to master, rescue, skilful and responsive, able to seize the "prime time" and improve the success rate of the rescue.

1.4   Particularity of thinking and clinical decision-making in emergency medicine

Emergency medicine involves a wide range of fields, far more than other clinical medical specialties. Emergency physicians often face a large number of clinical diagnosis and treatment problems on duty, requiring emergency physicians to make reasonable disposal in case of limited data and unidentified etiological diagnosis. The clinical decision-making ability and emergency thinking of the emergency specialist is especially important.

The emergency medicine emphasizes the understanding of the pathophysiology in the patient, the status of the function of the organs and the relationship between the functions of the organs, and grasp the most likely and most serious problems at present. At the same time, we should pay attention to the cause of acute aggravation and adopt the shortest and most effective measures at the shortest time in order to gain time and opportunity for further specialist treatment.

In order to meet the special clinical thinking and clinical decision-making model of emergency medicine, the emergency medical department must train all the emergency medical workers to be good at finding the essence from the phenomenon, and do not pass any clues in the clinical work, and find the most dangerous factors.

Emergency medicine is closely related to pre-hospital care and public health emergencies. In recent years, public health emergencies have become more and more intense. There are both man-made and natural disasters, of course, more serious infectious diseases, food and occupational poisoning events. For these public health emergencies, pre-hospital first aid and emergency medical rescue is indispensable for emergency medical treatment. So emergency medical practitioners should be prepared at any time. Emergency medicine and public health emergencies are closely related. Emergency physicians should have a strong ability to identify and deal with emergency public health emergencies, improve the ability to treat emergency public health patients and prevent the epidemic and spread of major infectious diseases.

Although emergency medicine is a new subject, but it is a major subject of clinical medicine. Although after more than thirty years of development, emergency medicine has preliminarily shown its own unique clinical specialty, but it still in the process of growing up. This requires us to fully understand the position of emergency medicine in clinical medicine, formulate relevant access system, specialist training system, welfare treatment system and so on, and promote the development of emergency medicine.

Zhu Changju

Chapter 2

Pre-hospital Emergency Treatment

Pre-hospital emergency treatment is an important part of the emergency medical service system. It is also the basis of the hospital emergency treatment. It is not the whole process of dealing with the disease, but focus on the acute stage of treatment. Accurate, reasonable and fast pre-hospital care measures play an important role in saving patients' lives, reducing disability rate and mortality.

Pre-hospital care is characterized by strong sociality, time urgency, various diseases and poor environmental conditions for emergency treatment.

2.1 The basic principles of pre-hospital first aid

Ensure the safety of the field. When the first aid personnel arrive at the scene, they should first ensure their own safety and start treatment under the condition of excluding or avoiding danger. For example, when the accident scene arrives on the highway, the ambulance should stop in front of the accident car so as not to be followed by the rear end of the car. When the electric shock scene is reached, it should be confirmed that the electric has been turned off to avoid contact with the charged body.

Recovery priority. In case of heart beat, respiratory arrest and fracture, the cardiopulmonary resuscitation should be made by cardiopulmonary resuscitation, until the heart and breath are restored, and the basic life signs tend to be stable, and then the fracture is fixed.

Facing life critical patients, we should first strive for time to rescue at the scene, and strive to stabilize the situation and then transport. In the process of transfer, we can not stop rescuing and coordinate the steps.

When encountering a large number of sick and wounded patients, there are many people in the scene, we should be co-ordinated, do a tight and orderly division of labor and cooperation.

2.2 Pre-hospital emergency allocation

Pre-hospital care requires not only ambulances, but also certain first-aid equipment and medicines. First aid personnel should be standby, emergency equipment and medicines are well prepared, first aid bags or first aid boxes should be regularly checked, maintained, registered, and taken it to the site whenever necessary.

At present, most of the pre-hospital emergency organizations in China are staffed by ambulances. There are generally two types of ambulances, general and critical care. The general ambulance consists of 1 first aid physician, 1 nurse and 1 driver, the critical care vehicle is composed of at least 1-2 specialist first aid physicians, 1-2 nurses and 1 driver, and 1 stretcher can be added when necessary.

All kinds of first aid drugs can be prepared for 3-5 branches according to the needs. More than 6-10 first aid drugs can be prepared. They are packed in boxes and marked outside the box.

2.3　Implementation of pre-hospital first aid

The purpose of pre-hospital first aid is to rescue life and safe transport. Medical staff must master the basic procedures of pre-hospital first aid and basic life rescue technology, so as to make the first aid quick, accurate, effective and safe.

2.4　The importance of pre-hospital first aid

When many people are injured or poisoned at the same time, in order to make the light and serious wounded who need first aid to get their needs and improve the treatment efficiency, it is necessary to carry out the examination according to the possibility of tight pursuit and rescue. The technical personnel who have been trained, experienced and highly organized, should classify according to the principle of danger, micro and minor injury.

2.5　Judgement and evaluation spot inspection of the wounded individual in the field

The on-site diagnosis of patients is based on the decision to give priority to first aid. Therefore, it should be evaluated according to the injuries of the wounded, and the general requirement should be completed in a short time (1-2 minutes) for those who are extremely painful or critically ill, and the others should have a different physical examination according to the condition, symptoms and signs. It is difficult to develop a unified assessment procedure for acute and serious injuries, but the common purpose of the assessment is to find out the problems that can endanger the patient's life in a short time.

2.5.1　A (airway)

Examine patients airway, in order to find out if there is any throat blockage, oral foreign bodies or secretions. At this point, the mandible should be lifted first to lift up the base of the tongue, remove foreign bodies, remove secretions and accumulate blood.

2.5.2　B (breathing)

To observe the patient's respiration, pay attention to it frequency and amplitude, and consider whether the respiratory exchange volume is enough.

2.5.3   C (circulation)

Circulatory check whether the pulse frequency of patients is regular and powerful, whether the heart sounds are loud or not, and blood pressure. In particular, prompt cardiac arrest should be quickly determined so as to start cardiopulmonary resuscitation immediately.

2.5.4   D (decision)

Decides to quickly assess the basic situation of the patient and determine what emergency measures are needed, based on the preliminary examination of the respiration and circulation.

2.5.5   E (examination)

Inspection will undergo further examination after the above basic examination.

In order to prevent missed diagnosis and misdiagnosis of vital signs, it is advocated to adopt "CRASH-PLAN" methods: C (circulation, heart and circulatory system), R (respiration, chest and respiratory system), A (abdomen, abdominal viscera), S (spine, spinal, craniocerebral), H (head, pelvis), P (limbs, limbs)), A (arteries, peripheral artery), N (nerves, peripheral nerve).

The assessment should be quick and soft, with different emphasis on the assessment of different causes, which depends on the experience and choice of the evaluator, but it must not delay the rescue and delivery time. The first aid mark and first aid area division to the field injured patien.

(1) In the scene first aid, the color pen or the glue cloth is used to mark the patient's striking position to show the condition and number.

1) Red: indicating the serious condition, endangering life.

2) Yellow: indicating that the disease is serious, but it has not endanger the life.

3) Green: the degree of injury is light.

4) Black: express the patient has died.

5) Blue: it can be added with the above colors, indicating that the sick have been dyed, including radioactive contamination and infectious diseases.

(2) When a large number of patients at the scene, the most simple and effective first aid should be divided into the following four areas, so as to facilitate the orderly rescue.

1) The area of the sufferer: the area of the wounded and the patient, the classified label is hung in this area, and the necessary rescue work is provided.

2) The emergency area: the critically ill patients used to receive red and yellow signs, and to do further work, such as the resuscitation of shock, breathing, cardiac arrest.

3) Lighter patients.

4) Taiping district: parked dead.

After preliminary judgment, emergency personnel should immediately implement rescue measures for patients, including artificial respiration, cardiac press, cardiac shock defibrillation, ECG monitoring, endotracheal intubation, pneumothorax decompression, hemostasis, fracture fixation, etc. The implementation of these rescue measures can be interspersed in the process of assessment and physical examination. Due to the limitation of the site conditions, patients should be transferred to the hospital emergency department as soon as possible with the patient's condition permissible.

Zhu Changju

Section 2

Intensive Situation

Chapter 3

Sepsis

3.1 Introduction

Sepsis is a potentially life-threatening complication of an infection, which occurs when chemicals released into the bloodstream to fight the infection trigger inflammatory responses throughout the body. This inflammation can trigger a cascade of changes that can damage multiple organ systems even organ failure. If sepsis progresses to septic shock, blood pressure drops dramatically, which may lead to death.

3.2 Epidemiology

Sepsis, as a complication of some infectious diseases, involves generalized organ dysfunction and leads to relatively high mortality. Its early diagnosis can be difficult, and the prevention of mortality remains problematic. Sepsis is usually nosocomial if it occurrs ≥3 days after hospitalization and community-acquired if onset is in <3 days. Sepsis is in 58% of adult and 43% of children. Respiratory tract infection is the most common pre-sepsis diagnosis, but *Escherichia coli* in adults, *Klebsiella* spp. in children ≥1 year of age, and *Enterococcus* spp. in infants age <1 year are the most common strains isolated in blood. An etiologic agent is not found in 33% of patients, and the mortality is about 25%.

3.3 Pathophysiology

Typically, a bacterial pathogen enters a sterile site in which resident cells can detect the invader and initiate the host response. The host response is initiated when innate immune cells, particularly macrophages, recognize and bind to microbial components. Binding immune cell surface receptors to microbial components initiates a series of steps that result in the phagocytosis of invading bacteria, bacterial killing, and phagocytosis of debris from injured tissue. These processes are associated with the production and release of a range of proinflammatory cytokines by macrophages, leading to the recruitment of additional inflammatory cells, such as leukocytes. This response is highly regulated by a mixture of pro-inflammatory and anti-inflammatory mediators. When a limited number of bacteria invade, the local host responses are generally sufficient to clear the pathogens. The end result is normally tissue repair and healing.

Despite a clear understanding of the inflammatory and coagulation mechanisms triggered during the early stage of severe sepsis, not much is known about the cellular aspects underlying the mechanisms that ultimately lead to organ dysfunction and death. Widespread cellular injury may occur when the immune response spreads beyond the site of infection causing sepsis. Cellular injury is the precursor to organ dysfunction. The precise mechanism of cellular injury is not understood, but proposed mechanisms include tissue ischemia, cytopathic injury, and an altered rate of apoptosis. The mechanism of organ failure in sepsis may relate to decreased oxygen utilization associated with mitochondrial dysfunction rather than or in addition to poor oxygen delivery to tissues. The cellular injury, accompanied by the release of pro-inflammatory and anti-inflammatory mediators, often progresses to organ dysfunction. No organ system is protected from the consequences of sepsis. They are most commonly involved include the circulation, lung, gastrointestinal tract, kidney, and nervous system.

3.4 Diagnosis

3.4.1 Susceptible populations, causes and clinical presentation

Sepsis usually occurs among those populations with the age of more than 65 years old. In addition, those living with compromised immune systems—such as HIV patients, cancer patients, or patients awaiting organ transplant can also be at increased risk of sepsis. Likewise, antibiotic-resistant bacteria can also result in sepsis prone infections.

Currently, sepsis can be led by any type of infection—bacterial, viral or fungal, and the most likely varieties include pneumonia, abdominal infection, kidney infection and bloodstream infection.

Until now, sepsis is usually viewed as a type of infection that occurs in three stages. Sepsis is the mildest stage of the infection. Progression to severe sepsis occurs in the second stage. And septic shock occurs in the final stage. The patients with sepsis in the first, or mild stage, typically exhibit an accelerated heart rate (higher than 90 beats/min), quickened breathing rate (exceeding 20 breaths/min), as well as a diagnosed infection (typically of the kidneys, blood, lungs or abdomen). However, a patient in septic shock will also display extremely decreased blood pressure and be unable to respond to fluid replacement. Sepsis is a progressive syndrome that starts mild, leads to severe sepsis, and then septic shock. This means that worsening sepsis can cause thrombopoiesis, severely restricting blood flow to the vital organs—including lungs, kidneys, heart, and brain—and causing organ failure.

3.4.2 Laboratory test and radiographic examination

Recommended tests include a complete blood count with differential, basic metabolic panel, measurement of lactate and liver enzyme levels, coagulation studies, and urinalysis. Suspected respiratory infections should be evaluated using chest radiography and arterial blood gas testing to assess hypoxemia and acid-base abnormalities. If disseminated intravascular coagulation is suspected, fibrin degradation products, d-dimer levels, and fibrinogen levels should be measured. Several biologic markers of sepsis such as C-reactive protein, procalcitonin, activated partial thromboplastin time, and interleukin-6 may have diagnostic and prognostic implications. Blood cultures (two peripheral and from each indwelling catheter), urine culture, stool culture (for diarrhea or recent antibiotic use), sputum culture, and skin and soft tissue culture should be conducted. However, blood culture results are negative in 50% -65% of patients with sepsis. Cerebrospinal, joint, pleural, and peritoneal fluid should be evaluated as clinically indicated.

Echocardiography is recommended to diagnose endocarditis, and should be performed in patients with a heart murmur or suspected intravenous drug use. Evaluation for pulmonary embolus requires chest computed tomography (CT) or ventilation-perfusion scanning, and suspected abdominal or pelvic infection requires abdominal and pelvic CT. Evaluation of renal abscess or complicated pyelonephritis often requires renal ultrasonography or CT. Head CT should be considered for patients presenting with altered mental status to rule out intracranial hemorrhage, abscess, or malignancy.

3.5 Key points of diagnosis

(1) Systemic inflammatory response syndrome often occur due to a variety of severe clinical insults, and the response is manifested by 2 or more of the following conditions: ①body temperature >38 ℃ or <36 ℃; ②heart rate >90 beats/min; ③respiratory rate >20 breaths/min or $PaCO_2$ <32 mmHg; ④white blood cell count >12×10^9/L or <4×10^9/L.

(2) Sepsis. The above mentioned systemic inflammatory response syndrome in combination with infection.

(3) Severe sepsis. Sepsis with evidence of acute organ dysfunction (hypotension, lactic acidosis, reduced urine output, reduced PaO_2/FiO_2 ratio, raised creatinine or bilirubin, thrombocytopenia, raised international normalized ratio, acute alteration in mental status and so on).

(4) Septic shock. Sepsis with persistent hypotension after fluid resuscitation.

3.6 Differential diagnosis

Syndromes that mimic sepsis include hypovolemia, acute blood loss, acute pulmonary embolism, acute myocardial infarction, acute pancreatitis, transfusion reaction, diabetic ketoacidosis, and adrenal insufficiency.

3.7 Management

Early management of sepsis requires respiratory stabilization. Supplemental oxygen should be given to all patients. Mechanical ventilation is recommended when supplemental oxygen fails to improve oxygenation, when respiratory failure is imminent, or when the airway can not be protected. Perfusion is assessed after respiratory stabilization. Hypotension signifies inadequate tissue perfusion. Clinical signs of hypoperfusion include cold or clammy skin, altered mental status, oliguria or anuria, and lactic acidosis.

After initial respiratory stabilization, treatment consists of fluid resuscitation, vasopressor therapy, infection identification and control, prompt antibiotic administration, and the removal or drainage of the infection source (Figure 3-1).

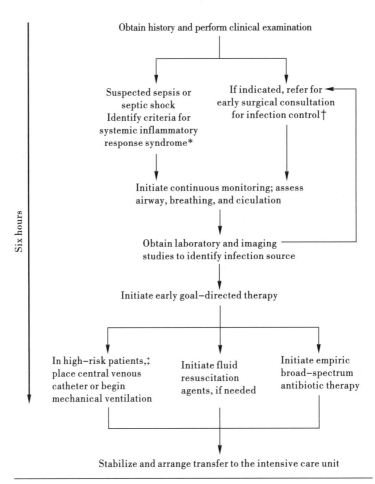

Six hours

Obtain history and perform clinical examination

Suspected sepsis or septic shock
Identify criteria for systemic inflammatory response syndrome*

If indicated, refer for early surgical consultation for infection control†

Initiate continuous monitoring; assess airway, breathing, and ciculation

Obtain laboratory and imaging studies to identify infection source

Initiate early goal–directed therapy

In high–risk patients,‡ place central venous catheter or begin mechanical ventilation

Initiate fluid resuscitation agents, if needed

Initiate empiric broad–spectrum antibiotic therapy

Stabilize and arrange transfer to the intensive care unit

*— Two out of four criteria must be present to identify systemic inflammatory response syndrome: fever, tachycardia, tachypnea, and leukocytosis or leukopenia

†—Surgical intercention required for intra–abdominal perforation, obstruction, abscess, or necrotizing infection. Infectd devices usually require removal

‡—High–risk patients have systolic blood pressure < 90 mmHg after 20–40 mL per kg volume challenge or lactate level > 36 mg / dL (4 mmol/L)

Figure 3–1   Algorithm for the management of sepsis. This process should be completed within a six–hour time frame

Zhang Mao

Chapter 4

Shock

4.1 Introduction

Shock is defined as the inadequate delivery of oxygen to tissues causing cellular dysfunction and injury. It can be classified mainly into four categories: hypovolemic, distributive, obstructive, and cardiogenic. Rapid recognition of the patient in shock and the prompt management to correct shock are the critical skills for clinicians.

4.2 Epidemiology

Hypovolemic shock, the most common type, results from loss of circulating blood or its components. Loss of circulating volume can be due to decreased whole blood and/or interstitial fluid. While the incidence of hypovolemic shock from extracellular fluid loss is difficult to quantify, it is known that hemorrhagic shock is primarily caused by trauma.

Septic shock is the most common type of distributive shock presented in the emergency department. It's critical to remember that nearly half of septic patients who present with certain degree of end−organ damage will have cryptic shock, meaning that they have inadequate tissue perfusion despite normal arterial pressure. Anaphylaxis, the second leading etiology of distributive shock, can occur at any age regardless of prior history.

Cardiogenic shock (CS) results from failure of the pump function. The incidence of CS is in decline which can be attributed to increased use of primary percutaneous coronary intervention (PCI) for acute myocardial infarction. However, approximately 5%–8% of ST segment elevated myocardial infarction (STEMI) and 2%–3% of non−ST−segment elevation myocardial infarction (NON−STEMI) cases can result in CS.

Obstructive shock occurs when circulatory flow is mechanically inhibited, mostly results from tension pneumothorax or cardiac tamponade. The prevalence of pericardial effusions in the overall population is unknown.

4.3　Pathophysiology

Shock exists when the delivery of oxygen and metabolic substrates to tissues is insufficient to maintain normal metabolism. This implies an imbalance between substrate delivery and requirements at the cellular level. Tissue hypoperfusion is associated with activated cardiovascular and neuroendocrine reactions responsible for compensating for and reversing inadequate tissue perfusion. The pathophysiologic sequelae may be due to either the direct effects of inadequate tissue perfusion on cellular and tissue function or the body's adaptive responses producing undesirable consequences. The consequences of shock may vary from minimal physiologic disturbance with complete recovery to profound circulatory disturbance, organ dysfunction, and even death.

4.3.1　Hypovolemic shock

Hypovolemic shock results from depletion of intravascular volume. As a response, the body compensates with increased sympathetic tone, resulting in increased heart rate, increased cardiac contractility, and peripheral vasoconstriction. The first changes in vital signs seen in hypovolemic shock include an increase in diastolic blood pressure with narrowed pulse pressure. As volume status continues to decrease, systolic blood pressure drops, oxygen delivery to vital organs is unable to meet their oxygen demand. Thus, cells shift from aerobic metabolism to anaerobic metabolism, resulting in lactic acidosis. As sympathetic drive increases, blood flow is mobilized from visceral organ and skin to the heart and brain. This propagates tissue ischemia and worsens lactic acidosis. If it is not corrected, there will be worsening hemodynamic compromise and, eventually, death.

4.3.2　Distributive shock

Inflammatory mediators play a major role in the development of distributive shock. Inflammatory cytokines released in sepsis and toxic shock syndrome induce systemic vasodilation and capillary leak, as well as cardiomyopathy. The systemic release of histamine in anaphylaxis results in similar effects. Interactions between catecholamines and adrenergic receptors in blood vessels are crucial in other causes of distributive shock. Both norepinephrine and epinephrine stimulate α_1 receptors on arterioles to cause vasoconstriction and regulate blood pressure. In the case of neurogenic shock, the sympathetic nervous system is compromised, which leads to reduced catecholamine delivery to these receptors.

4.3.3　Obstructive shock

In most cases, tension pneumothorax is caused by traumatic injury, such as a rib fracture or penetrating injury that causes damage to the lung or chest. It results in increased pressure in the pleural space, collapsing major blood vessels that return blood to the heart. Pneumothorax can also be a complication of certain procedures such as lung biopsy, placement of central venous catheter, thoracotomy, or it can occur spontaneously.

There is physiologic amount of fluid surrounding the heart within the pericardium. When the volume of fluid increase quickly, the chambers of the heart are compressed, and tamponade physiology develops rapidly with much smaller volumes. Under this pressure, the chambers of the heart are unable to relax leading to decreased venous return, filling, or cardiac output. Slow growing effusion, such as those due to autoimmune disease or neoplasms, allows for stretching of the pericardium, and effusion can become quite large before leading to tamponade physiology.

4.3.4   Cardiogenic shock

The pathophysiology of CS is complex and not fully understood. Myocardial ischemia causes derangement of left ventricular systole and diastole, resulting in profound depression of myocardial contractility. This, in turn, leads to a potentially catastrophic and vicious spiral of reduced cardiac output and low blood pressure perpetuating further coronary ischemia and impairment of contractility. Several physiologic compensatory processes ensue. These include activation of the sympathetic system leading to peripheral vasoconstriction which may improve coronary perfusion at the cost of increased afterload, and tachycardia which increases myocardial oxygen demand and subsequently worsens myocardial ischemia.

4.4   Diagnosis

The diagnosis is generally based on a combination of symptoms, physical and auxiliary examination.

4.4.1   Hypovolemic shock

For patients with hemorrhagic shock, a history of trauma or recent surgery is present. For hypovolemic shock due to fluid losses, medical history and physical check should attempt be included to identify possible sources where extracellular fluid loss, such as gastrointestinal tract, kidney, skin, or third-space. Symptoms of hypovolemic shock can be associated with volume depletion, electrolyte imbalance, or acid-base disorder that accompany hypovolemic shock. Patients with volume depletion may complain of thirst, muscle cramps, and/or orthostatic hypotension. Severe hypovolemic shock can result in mesenteric and coronary ischemia that can cause abdominal or chest pain. Agitation, lethargy, or confusion may result from insufficient cerebral perfusion.

Many laboratory test results can be abnormal in hypovolemic shock. Patients can have increased blood urea nitrogen and serum creatinine as a result of prerenal kidney dysfunction. Hypernatremia or hyponatremia can happen, as can hyperkalemia or hypokalemia. Lactic acidosis can be a result from anaerobic metabolism. The status of acid-base balance can be variable as patients with large digestive tract losses can be alkalotic. In cases of hemorrhagic shock, hematocrit and hemoglobin can be severely decreased.

4.4.2   Septic shock

In 2016, the Third International Consensus Definition for Sepsis and Septic Shock (Sepsis-3) defined sepsis as life-threatening organ dysfunction resulting from dysregulated host responses to infection, and defined septic shock as a subset of sepsis in which underlying circulatory, cellular, and metabolic abnormalities are profound enough to substantially increase the risk of mortality. More specifically, septic shock is described as a clinically defined subset of sepsis cases, wherein, despite adequate fluid resuscitation, patients have hypotension requiring vasopressors to maintain a mean arterial blood pressure above 65 mmHg and have an elevated serum lactate concentration of more than 2 mmol/L. The Sequential Organ Failure Assessment (SOFA) score is used to codify the degree of organ dysfunction.

4.4.3   Obstructive shock

On examination, breath sounds may be diminished and percussion hyperresonant on the affected side.

Some traumatic pneumothoraxes are associated with subcutaneous emphysema. Pneumothorax may be difficult to diagnose from physical exam. However, it is essential to make the diagnosis of tension pneumothorax on physical exam. Beck's triad of distended neck veins, distant heart sounds and hypotension help in making this diagnosis. A late finding associated with tension pneumothorax includes tracheal deviation away from the affected side. Chest radiography, ultrasonography, or CT can be used for diagnosis, although diagnosis from a chest X-ray is more common. Radiographic findings of 2.5 cm air space are equivalent to a 30% pneumothorax. Occult pneumothoraxes may be diagnosed by CT but are usually clinically insignificant. The extended focused abdominal sonography for trauma (e-FAST) exam has been a more recent diagnostic tool for pneumothorax.

The diagnosis of cardiac tamponade can be made based on history and physical exam findings. ECG may be helpful, especially if it shows low voltages or electrical alternans, which is the classic ECG finding in cardiac tamponade due to the swinging of the heart within the pericardium that is filled with fluid. This is a rare ECG finding, and most commonly the ECG finding of cardiac tamponade is sinus tachycardia. A chest X-ray may show an enlarged heart and may strongly suggest pericardial effusion if a prior chest radiograph with a normal cardiac silhouette is available for comparison. CT chest can also determine pericardial effusion.

Echocardiography is the best imaging modality to use at the bedside. Echocardiography can not only confirm there is a pericardial effusion, but also determine its size, and whether it is causing compromise of cardiac function. The medical literature is replete with studies that show clinicians (e. g. , emergency physician) with limited training using point-of-care echo can perform focused echocardiograms to answer specific questions such as whether there is a significant pericardial effusion.

4.4.4 Cardiogenic shock

Rapid identification of the patient with pump failure and effectively corrective actions are essential in preventing further decrease in cardiac output. If increased myocardial oxygen needs can not be met, there will be progressive and unremitting cardiac dysfunction. Blunt injury to the heart is rarely severe enough to induce pump failure, but manifestations of shock in the setting of a patient at risk should raise one's index of suspicion. Evidence of blunt thoracic injury such as sternal fracture, multiple rib fractures, tenderness or hematomas in the chest wall or precordial area, or a history of a direct precordial impact identifies a patient at increased risk for a blunt cardiac injury. Elderly patients with known preexisting cardiac disease are at increased risk of suffering injury-related cardiac complications including cardiac failure.

4.5　Management

4.5.1 Hypovolemic shock

For patients in hypovolemic shock due to fluid losses, the exact fluid deficit can not be determined. Therefore, it is prudent to start with 2 liters of isotonic electrolyte solution infused rapidly as an attempt to quickly restore tissue perfusion. Fluid repletion can be monitored by measuring blood pressure, urine output, mental status, and peripheral edema. Multiple modalities exist for measuring fluid responsiveness such as ultrasound, central venous pressure monitoring, and pulse pressure fluctuation as described above. In general, for hypovolemic shock, vasopressors should not be used because they may worsen tissue perfusion. Electrolyte fluid resuscitation is preferred over colloid solutions for severe volume. The type of electrolyte solution used to resuscitate the patient can be individualized based on the biochemical indicators, estimated volume of resuscitation, acid/base status of the patient, and physician or institutional preferences. Isotonic saline is hyperchloremic relative to blood plasma, and resuscitation with large amounts can lead to a hyperchloremic metabolic acidosis. There are some other isotonic fluids with lower chloride concentrations, such as lactated Ringer's solution or Plasma-Lyte. These solutions are often referred to as buffered or balanced electrolyte solution. Some evidences suggested that patients who need large volume resuscitation may have a less renal injury with restrictive chloride strategies and use of balanced crystalloids. Crystalloid solutions are equally as effective and much less expensive than colloid. Commonly used colloid solutions include those containing albumin or hydroxyethyl starch.

4.5.2   Septic shock

The management of sepsis and septic shock should be undertaken as a medical emergency. Screening patients for signs and symptoms of sepsis and septic shock facilitates earlier identification and intervention. Effective treatment should focus on timely intervention, including aetiology control. Aggressive assessment for an unrecognized aetiology or undrained abscess through appropriate laboratory testing and diagnostic imaging is a critical aspect of the initial management of sepsis. In addition, early initiation of appropriate antimicrobial therapy (ideally within one hour after recognition of septic shock), restoration of tissue perfusion via fluid resuscitation, and advanced interventions guided by assessment of the adequacy of resuscitation and resolution of organ dysfunction should be part of initial sepsis management. Prompt intravenous access should be obtained, blood and other appropriate cultures should be taken, and assessment for organ dysfunction and tissue hypoperfusion should be done.

4.5.3   Obstructive shock

The treatment of cardiac tamponade is the removal of pericardial fluid to help relieve the pressure surrounding the heart. This can be done by performing a needle pericardiocentesis at the bedside, performed either using traditional landmark technique in a sub-xiphoid window or using a point-of-care echo to guide needle placement in real-time. Often the removal of the first small amounts of fluid can make a large improvement in hemodynamics, but leaving a catheter within the pericardium can allow for further drainage. Surgical options include creating a pericardial window or removing the pericardium. Emergency department resuscitative thoracotomy and the opening of the pericardial sac is the therapy that can be used in traumatic arrests with suspected or confirmed cardiac tamponade.

For patients who have associated symptoms and are showing signs of instability in pneumothorax, needle decompression is the treatment of pneumothorax. This usually is performed with a 14- to 16- guage, and 4.5 cm in length angiocatheter just superior to the rib in the second intercostal space in the midclavicular line.

4.5.4   Cardiogenic shock

CS is an emergency requiring immediate resuscitative therapy before the irreversible damage of vital organs. Rapid diagnosis with prompt initiation of pharmacological therapy to maintain blood pressure and to maintain respiratory support along with reversal of underlying cause plays a vital role in the prognosis of patients with cardiogenic shock. Early restoration of coronary blood is the most important intervention and is the standard therapy for patients with CS due to myocardial infarction. The goal is to restore cardiac output and prevent irreversible end-organ damage rapidly.

Zhang Mao

Chapter 5

Multiple Organ Dysfunction Syndrome

5.1　Overview

The multiple organ dysfunction syndrome (MODS) is a term adopted at the consensus conference (1992) by the American College of Chest Physicians in collaboration with the Society of Critical Care Medicine to denote the evolving clinical syndrome associated with "development of otherwise unexplained abnormalities of organ function in critically ill patients". It is a leading cause of death in the ICU patients. There is no consensus among clinicians regarding whether MODS is a single pathological process with highly variable clinical expression or a limited phenotypical expression of numerous pathological processes (Figure 5-1).

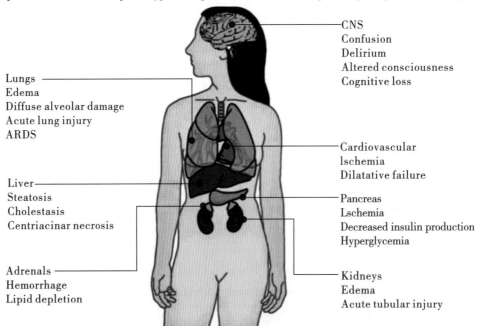

CNS
Confusion
Delirium
Altered consciousness
Cognitive loss

Lungs
Edema
Diffuse alveolar damage
Acute lung injury
ARDS

Cardiovascular
lschemia
Dilatative failure

Liver
Steatosis
Cholestasis
Centriacinar necrosis

Pancreas
Lschemia
Decreased insulin production
Hyperglycemia

Adrenals
Hemorrhage
Lipid depletion

Kidneys
Edema
Acute tubular injury

Figure 5-1　MODS

5.2   Epidemiology

General rate of incidence, morbidity, and mortality related to MODS has been on a steady decline within the past couple of decades, which is attributable to advancements in prehospital care and resuscitation. These change has led to better health outcomes and higher survival rates among patients with severe traumas. However, the elevated risk of late MODS risk (developing 4–10 days after the injury) still persists in patients who may develop sepsis. Such instances lead to prolonged ICU stay and high mortality. At present, the reported MODS incidence after injuries ranges from 7% –66% , with MODS–associated mortality rates constituting 31% –80% of cases among severe trauma patients.

5.3   Etiology

MODS etiology is still poorly understood, but a certain progress is evident in relating it to other condition of patients. For instance, at the 2005 International Pediatric Consensus Conference, the definitions of systemic inflammatory response syndrome (SIRS) , sepsis, septic shock, and MODS as a continuum were delineated. This recognition of the MODS continuum improved the overall etiological classification of the condition. With SIRS representing an inflammatory response mediated by cytokines to infections, trauma, burns, etc. , and sepsis being similar to SIRS but relating specifically to infections of bacterial, mycotic, and viral toxic nature, MODS can be the final and possibly the severest stage of the uncontrolled SIRS or sepsis.

5.4   Signs and symptoms

MODS is a syndrome characterized by a group of symptoms and signs occurring together, possessing a common mechanism, and having predictable outcomes. Its major signs include the simultaneous or subsequent failure or dysfunction of organs or organ systems including the respiratory, cardiovascular, neurological renal, hematological, and hepatic ones. The signs and symptoms of MODS depend on the affected organ system.

5.5   Pathophysiology

The earliest registered MODS cases were associated with occult or poorly controlled infection; in most cases, MODS resulted from peritonitis or pneumonia. The overall pathophysiology of MODS is complex and involves a range of inflammatory cells and mediators. There is still no precise data on the pathophysiology and underlying mechanisms of MODS; some researchers state that uncontrolled, occult sepsis is the primary trigger of MODS, while others believe that SIRS caused by host immune response to tissue injury is the primary cause of MODS.

The pro–inflammatory cytokines attack endothelial cells that possess an ability to produce vasoactive mediators (e. g. , arachidonic acid metabolites, nitric oxide, endothelin) with a range of local and systemic effects. Anti-inflammatory cytokines are usually produced by the human organism in a response to the release of pro-inflammatory agents and limit inflammation to prevent organ dysfunction and septic shock. Thus, overall, in the human organism affected by an inflammation, the inflammatory process is controlled by the balance of pro-and anti-inflammatory cytokines; If there is an excess of inflammatory mediators, the patient may suffer organ dysfunction. However, the excess of anti-inflammatory agents is also not beneficial, since the disproportionate presence of these mediators in the human body may cause anergy and death.

The researchers suggested three core pathophysiologic events depending on the time and extent of tissue injury to cause MODS. The first one is ischemia, a primary pathophysiologic event resulting from persistent and progressive splanchnic vasoconstriction and hypoperfusion. The second hypothesized cause of MODS is the gut-derived systemic inflammatory response caused by the ischemic gut; according to this mechanism, the injury erodes the gut barrier and causes translocation of gut microorganisms to distant organs, triggering SIRS and further transforming into MODS. The third one is the development of ionic disequilibrium leading to fluid shifts at the cellular and capillary level after injury.

5.6 Diagnostic method and process

Diagnostics of MODS is very challenging, since the syndrome's causation is multifactorial and underlying mechanisms are still poorly understood, while its course and outcomes are often unpredictable. Diagnosis of MODS may be established if two or more organ systems of the patient fail according to the following set of criteria (Table 5-1).

Table 5-1   Diagnostic definitions for organ system failure in MODS

Neurologic	Glasgow Coma Score <6 (in absence of sedation)
Cardiovascular	Heart rate <54 beats per minute Mean arterial blood pressure <49 mmHg (systolic blood pressure <60 mmHg) Ventricular tachycardia, ventricular fibrillation, or both Serum pH <7.24 with a $PaCO_2$ of <49 mmHg
Pulmonary	$PaCO_2$ >50 mmHg (acutely) $(A-a)DO_2$ >350 mmHg $(A-a)DO_2 = [713 \times FiO_2 - (PaCO_2/RQ)] - PaO_2$ Ventilator or continuous positive airway pressure dependence on the second day of organ dysfunction
Hepatic	Jaundice (bilirubin >6 mg/100 dL) $(A-a)DO_2 = [713 \times FiO_2 - (PaCO_2/RQ)] - PaO_2]$ Coagulopathy (prothrombin time, 4 sec greater tan control, in the absence of anticoagulation)
Renal	Urine output <479 mL/24 h or <159 mL/8 h Serum BUN >100 mg/100 dL
Hematologic	White blood count <1,000 cells/mm^3 Platelets <20,000 platelets/mm^3 Hematocrit <20%

Source: from Knaus and Wagner (1989).

In children, the new set of diagnostic criteria for MODS was developed at the 2005 consensus conference. These criteria define MODS as a concurrent dysfunction of two or more organ systems, with each of the system's failure established once meeting the following criteria(Table 5-2).

Table 5-2   Diagnostic criteria for MODS in children

Neurologic	Glasgow Coma Score ≤ 11 OR acute change in mental status with a change in Glasgow Coma Score ≥ 3 points from abnormal baseline
Cardiovascular	Despite administration of intravenous fluid bolus ≥ 40 mL/kg in 1 hour: · Decrease in BP (hypotension) <5th percentile for age or systolic BP <2 SD below normal for age (see Table) · OR need for vasoactive drug to maintain BP in normal range (dopamine >5 μg/(kg · min) or dobutamine, epinephrine, or norepinephrine at any dose) · OR two of the following: · Unexplained metabolic acidosis:base deficit >5.0 mEq/L · Increased lactate >2 times upper limit of normal · Oliguria:urine output <0.5 mL/(kg · h) · Prolonged capillary refill:>5 seconds · Core to peripheral temperature gap >3 ℃
Respiratory	· PaO_2/FiO_2 <300 torr in absence of cyanotic heart disease or preexisting lung disease · OR $PaCO_2$ >65 torr or 20 mmHg over baseline $PaCO_2$ · OR proven need for >50% FiO_2 to maintain saturation ≥ 92% · OR need for non-elective invasive or non-invasive ventilation
Hepatic	· Total bilirubin ≥ 4 mg/dL (not applicable for newborn) · OR ALT 2 times upper limit of normal for age
Renal	· Serum creatinine ≥ 2 times upper limit of normal level for age or 2 fold increase in baseline creatinine
Hematologic	· Platelet count <80,000/mm³ (<80 × 10⁹/L) or a decline of 50% in platelet count from highest value recorded over the past 3 days (for chronic hematology/oncology patients) · OR INR (International Normalized Ratio) >2

Source:from Goldstein et al. (2005).

5.7   Management of the disease

There are a number of interventions used to address MODS in the ICU;the major emphasis is on organ support and minimization of iatrogenic trauma and complications (e. g., nosocomial infection) because of the absence of a uniform standard for MODS management. Supportive ICU care includes adequate and early nutrition (replenishment of vitamins),skin care,physiotherapy,and infection control. Moreover,specific interventions are directed towards support of each organ system. For instance,cardiovascular care involves intravascular fluid loading for the sake of maintenance of adequate circulation. Respiratory support involves mechanical ventilation with lower tidal volumes,while renal support is usually directed towards hypoperfusion avoidance.

Zhang Mao

Section 3

Cardiac Emergencies

Chapter 6

Chest Pain

6.1 Introduction

Chest pain is the second most common emergency symptoms of patients searching help in emergency medicine. The causes of chest pain are quite varied, mainly including chest wall disease, mediastinal disease, respiratory system diseases, diseases of the cardiovascular system, etc. Symptoms (pain location, duration of pain, pain property, relief way and severity) in patients who have different causes of chest pain may be varied very much. Acute chest pain include a set of fatal diseases, known as "high-risk" chest pain, such as acute myocardial infarction, aortic dissection, pulmonary embolism, pneumothorax, etc. To avoid the grave error of discharging a patient from the emergency department with a potentially life-threatening illness, the physician must arrive at a reasonable diagnosis for every patient with chest pain.

According to different causes of chest pain, it can be divided into the following

(1) Chest wall lesions
- Costochondritis.
- Herpes zoster.
- Chest wall trauma.
- Cellulitis of the skin.
- Local skin, muscles, bones and neuropathy caused by tumour.

(2) Lung and pleural lesions
- Pleuritis.
- Pulmonary embolism and infarction.
- Spontaneous pneumothorax.
- Spontaneous tension pneumothorax.

(3) Diseases of the cardiovascular system
- Angina pectoris.
- Myocardial infarction.
- Pericarditis.

(4) Mediastinal and esophageal lesions

- Dissecting thoracic aortic aneurysm.

- Esophagitis.

- Diffuse esophageal spasm.

- Peptic ulcer disease.

(5) Others

- Cholecystitis.

- Hepatitis.

- Rhabdomyolysis.

The presence of risk factors for a particular disease is primarily of value as an epidemiologic marker for large population studies. Listed below are risk factors associated with potentially catastrophic causes of chest pain (Table 6-1).

Table 6-1   Risk factors associated with potentially catastrophic causes of chest pain

Acute coronary syndromes

    Past or family history of coronary artery disease

    Age

        Men older than 33 years

        Women older than 40 years

    Diabetes mellitus

    Hypertension

    Smoking or second hand smoking

    Elevated cholesterol [low-density lipoprotein(LDL)] or triglycerides

    Sedentary lifestyle

    Obesity

    Postmenopausal

    Left ventricular hypertrophy

    Cocaine abuse

Pulmonary embolism

    Prolonged immobilization

    Surgery longer than 30 minutes in last 3 months

    Prior deep vein thrombosis or pulmonary embolus

    Pregnancy or recent pregnancy

    Pelvic or lower extremity trauma

    Oral contraceptives with cigarette smoking

    Congestive heart failure

    Chronic obstructive pulmonary disease

    Obesity

Continue to Table 6-1

  Past medical or family history of hypercoagulability

Aortic dissection

  Hypertension

  Congenital disease of the aorta or aortic valve

  Inflammatory aortic disease

  Connective tissue disease

  Pregnancy

  Arteriosclerosis

  Cigarette use

Pericarditis or myocarditis

  Infection

  Autoimmune disease (e. g. ,systemic lupus erythematosus)

  Acute rheumatic fever

  Recent myocardial infarction or cardiac surgery

  Malignancy

  Radiation therapy to mediastinum

  Uremia

  Drugs

  Prior pericarditis

Pneumothorax

  Prior pneumothorax

  Valsalva's maneuver

  Chronic lung disease

  Cigarette use

6.2　History

  A history of prior pain and the diagnosis of that episode can facilitate the diagnostic process,but the physician should be wary of prior presumptive diagnoses that may be misleading. A prior history of cardiac testing, such as stress testing,echocardiography,or angiography,may be useful in determining if the current episode is suggestive of cardiac disease. Similarly,patients with previous spontaneous pneumothorax are at increased risk of recurrence (Table 6-1).

6.3　Symptoms

6.3.1　Pain

  If the patient can localize the pain to a very well-defined,discrete area,it is more likely resulting from processes that focally irritate or inflame the chest wall or pleura. The pain of pleuritis (used here to include all processes producing pleural irritation), pneumothorax, and costochondritis is often described as sharp and varying with respiration. Pain that aggravates or changes with deep inspiration suggests disorders that produce pleural, pericardial, or chest wall irritation.

6.3.2 Accompanying symptoms

Upper respiratory tract symptoms often precede vital pleuropericarditis and costochondritis. Fever, chills, dyspnea, and purulent sputum suggest pulmonary infection that may produce pleuritic discomfort, when involving lung segments adjacent to the pleura. Chest pain in young adults that lasts for only a few seconds, is well localized, and is described as sharp is probably caused by the rupture of small blebs in pulmonary lobules. Nausea, vomiting, diaphoresis, fatigue, light-headedness, palpitations, and dyspnea often accompany the angina of myocardial ischemia or infarction. Chest pain that is of sudden onset and is associated with varying degrees of dyspnea suggests pulmonary embolism or pneumothorax; the former diagnosis is more likely when the patient is female or she used to take birth control pill, pregnancy, or recent immobilization is obtained.

6.3.3 Exacerbation and alleviation

Patients with pericarditis often note that pain worsens with recumbency and improves with sitting up; patients with acid-induced esophagitis or gastritis frequently report improved chest pain with meals. Women are more likely to present with the complaint of chest pain than men.

6.3.4 Other associated symptoms

Diaphoresis should lead to an increased clinical suspicion for a serious or visceral cause. Hemoptysis, a classic PE sign, is rarely seen. Syncope lead to higher likelihood of a cardiovascular cause or PE. Dyspnea is seen in cardiovascular and pulmonary disease. Nausea and vomiting may be seen in cardiovascular and gastrointestinal complaints (Table 6-2).

Table 6-2　Significant symptoms of chest pain

Symptom	Finding	Diagnosis
Pain	Severe, crushing, pressure, substernal, exertional, radiation to jaw, neck, shoulder, Arm	Acute MI Coronary ischemia Unstable angina Coronary spasm
	Tearing, severe, radiating to or located in back, maximum at onset, may migrate to upper back or neck	Aortic dissection
	Pleuritic	Esophageal rupture Pneumothorax Cholecystitis Pericarditis Myocarditiss

Continue to Table 6-2

Symptom	Finding	Diagnosis
	Indigestion or burning	Acute MI
		Coronary ischemia
		Esophageal rupture
		Unstable angina
		Coronary spasm
		Esophageal tear
		Cholecystitis
Associated syncope or near –syncope		Aortic dissection
		PE
		Acute MI
		Pericarditis
		Myocarditis
Associated dyspnea (SOB,DOE,PND,orthopnea)		Acute MI
		Coronary ischemia
		PE
		Tension pneumothorax
		Pneumothorax
		Unstable angina
		Pericarditi
Associated hemoptysis		PE
Associated nausea,vomiting		Esophageal rupture
		Acute MI
		Coronary ischemia
		Unstable angina
		Coronary spasm
		Esophageal tear
		Cholecystitis

DOE:dyspnea on exertion;MI:myocardial infarction;PE:Pulmonary embolism;PND:paroxysmal nocturnal dyspnea;SOB:shortness of breath.

6.3.5 Physical examination

The physical examination,can be useful to identify higher-risk patients. The examination should also target potential noncardiac causes for the patient's symptoms,such as unequal extremity pulses (aortic dissection), prominent murmurs (endocarditis),friction rub (pericarditis),fever and abnormal lung sounds (pneumonia),or reproduction of chest pain with palpation of the chest wall (musculoskeletal disorders).

Typical,clustered,small vesicles on an erythematous base are noted in patients with herpes zoster (shingles);lesions classically occur in a radicular distribution,although in some patients presenting early,a single area of involvement may be noted. An occasional patient with severe discomfort will not manifest any rash when initially evaluated;in others presenting some what later,patches of simple erythema or an occasional vesicle will be noted. Localized chest wall tenderness at the costochondral junction suggests acute costochondritis;many patients report a subtle,subjective difference between the unaffected and affected sides with the application of pressure.

Fever,tachycardia,localized rales,dullness to percussion,decreased breath sounds,and egophony suggest pneumonia or other causes of pulmonary parenchymal consolidation. The presence of a pericardial friction rub, which may be transient, suggests pericarditis. Evidence of thrombophlebitis and confirmation that discomfort is pleuritic should be sought in patients with suspected pulmonary embolism. Pleural friction rubs may also be heard in patients with pleurodynia, a pleuralbased pneumonia, or pulmonary embolism.

6.4　Auxiliary examination

6.4.1　Electrocardiogram

The electrocardiogram(ECG) is the most informative tool for early risk stratification, and is probably the single most useful diagnostic test performed in the evaluation of chest pain. It should be obtained within 10 minutes of ED presentation. The ECG provides valuable diagnostic and prognostic information and will play a decisive role in the triage process. In patients presenting with a nonischemic ECG and no prior evidence of CAD, the frequency of MI was 2%, and in those with a history of CAD, it was 4%. However it should be reminded again and again that when initially evaluated in the emergency department, more than 50% of patients who are eventually ruled in for a myocardial infarction have nondiagnostic ECGs and some have completely normal ECGs. If the initial ECG is negative, repeat ECGs (e. g. ,5-10 minutes intervals) are recommended, because serial changes of ischemia or injury may evolve.

6.4.2　Chest roentgenogram

The chest roentgenogram is abnormal in 85%-90% of patients with aortic dissection and may reveal mediastinal widening, enlarged cardiac silhouette due to pericardial effusion, left pleural effusion, or calcification sign (≥1.0 cm displacement of intimal calcium from the soft tissue border of the aorta). It is helpful in diagnosing pneumothorax (an upright, posterior-anterior, expiratory film should specifically be requested) and pneumonia. In patients with PE, the chest roentgenogram may show focal lung oligemia, a peripheral wedge-shaped density above the diaphragm, or an enlarged descending right pulmonary artery, but more often than not, it is normal. Most patients with uncomplicated ACS have a normal chest roentgenogram. Other relevant entities evident on the chest roentgenogram include pneumonia, pneumothorax, and pneumomediastinum.

6.4.3　Cardiac biomarkers

Current guidelines recommend measurement of a cardiac injury marker (which should include a highly sensitive and specific cardiac troponin assay) in all patients with suspected myocardial ischemia. Serum markers for acute myocardial infarction are now rapidly available in the emergency department and include creatine kinase M and B subunits (CK-MB) and troponin T and I. Contemporary troponin assays have improved sensitivity, specificity, and precision at lower levels. When used serially to detect changes over short intervals, their sensitivity is higher than that of more traditional injury markers, which obviates the need for CK-MB or myoglobin measurement, even in patients with onset of symptoms shortly before presentation. It is important to remember that if sampling is performed immediately on arrival to the emergency department, sensitivity in detecting myocardial injury decreases to 50%. In patients who present early (within 6 hours of symptom onset), measurement should be repeated 6-8 hours after occurrence of symptoms in those with initially negative results. To achieve 100% sensitivity to be achieved in diagnosing myocardial infarction, an interval of up to 12 hours after the onset of pain is needed. Serum markers are discussed in more detail in section chapter 11.

Although an elevated cardiac troponin level is indicative of myocardial necrosis, it does not specify the mechanism of injury. An abnormal value alone may not indicate MI, because there are numerous nonischemic causes of elevated cardiac troponin. Confirmation of MI is based on evidence of myocardial necrosis afforded by the clinical setting and pattern of troponin values. Criteria include a rise or fall of cardiac troponin with at least 1 value above the 99th percentile of the upper reference limit and at least one of the following:

- Symptoms of cardiac ischemia.
- Characteristic ECG alterations.
- Imaging evidence of a new regional wall-motion abnormality (RWMA).

6.4.4　Echocardiography

Echocardiography can rapidly be obtained at the patient's bedside; regional wall motion abnormalities (RWMA) are often noted in patients with acute injury or ischemia. A major limitation of this technique includes a relatively low specificity for acute infarction in that ischemia, previous infarction, and acute infarction may have similar echocardiographic appearances. A pericardial effusion, if present in patients with acute pericarditis, is usually seen with this modality.

Acute PE may lead to RV pressure overload and dysfunction, which can be detected by echocardiography.

6.4.5　Arterial blood gases

In the past, arterial blood gases were used to make less probable the diagnosis of pulmonary embolus; because of the nonspecific nature of this particular test and the lack of sensitivity at virtually any level of PO_2, blood gases now are felt to have limited usefulness.

6.4.6　D-dimer testing

The levels of plasma D-dimer are elevated in the presence of acute thrombosis, because of simultaneous activation of coagulation and fibrinolysis, The negative predictive value of D-dimer testing is high and a normal D-dimer level renders acute PE unlikely. On the other hand, fibrin is also produced in a wide variety of conditions such as cancer, inflammation, bleeding, trauma, surgery and necrosis. Accordingly, the positive predictive value of elevated D-dimer levels is low and D-dimer testing is not useful for confirmation of PE.

6.4.7　Coronary angiography(CAG)

The diagnostic rate of CAG was only 65% in low-to intermediate-risk ED patients with acute chest pain. Performing of noninvasive test(NIV) provided only modest improvement in diagnostic rate of CAG. The unexpectedly low diagnostic rate might be attributable to the underuse of NIV and misinterpretation of physicians. The use of NIV are required as a gatekeeper to discriminate patients who require CAG and/or revascularization. If the patients with non-ST elevation acute coronary syndrome (NSTEACS) remain in pain despite receiving adequate treatment, they should be considered for urgent coronary angiography with a view to revascularization. If the pain is continuous and severe, alternative diagnoses should be re-explored, in particular aortic dissection.

6.4.8　Computed tomographic pulmonary angiography(CTPA)

CTPA is a useful method for imaging the pulmonary vasculature in patients with suspected PE. It allows adequate visualization of the pulmonary arteries down to at least the segmental level.

6.4.9　The process of initial assessment for critical diagnoses

See Figure 6-1.

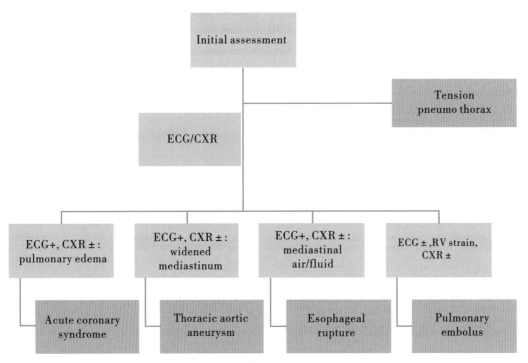

Figure 6-1 Initial Assessment for Critical Diagnoses

CXR:chest X-ray;ECG:electrocardiogram;RV:right ventricular.

6.5 Specific disorders

6.5.1 Cardiac chest pain

6.5.1.1 Acute coronary syndrome (ACS)

Chest pain is a common reason for patients to attend hospital among ACS patients,accounting for up to 5% of visits to the emergency department and 40% of hospital admissions. Around 50% of patients presenting with chest pain might have an underlying ACS,requiring hospitalization and intensive medical therapy. The remainders have other cardiac and non-cardiac causes for their symptoms,and require a different management approach. The diagnosis of ACS is usually made using a combination of clinical and ECG features. Cardiac troponin and cardiac functional tests can then be used to further risk-stratify the patient.

The medical history,physical examination,auxiliary examination,diagnosis and treatment of ACS will be discussed in detail in chapter 11.

6.5.1.2 Pericarditis

The causes of pericarditis (inflammation of the pericardium) include infections (viral,tubercular,and rarely,bacterial),autoimmune disorders (systemic lupus erythematosus,rheumatoid arthritis),renal failure,and neoplastic disorders (especially adenocarcinoma of the breast and squamous cell carcinoma of the lung).

(1)Medical history

Pericardial pain is retrosternal,severe,sharp,may worsen with inspiration,recumbency,coughing,and movement,and often eased by sitting forward. It is commonly seen following MI,or in a young adult with acute post-viral pericarditis.

(2)Physical examination

A pericardial rub is common, although it may be intermittent in these patients. Physical check may reveal a one-, two-, or three-componets of friction rub, frequently evanescent and often postural; it is usually heard clearly with the patient sitting forward at end expiration. If a hemodynamically significant pericardial effusion accompanies the inflammatory process, signs of cardiac tamponade may be noted, including hypotension, tachycardia, a narrow pulse pressure, distended neck veins that do not collapse on inspiration, and faint heart sounds.

(3)Diagnostic tests

The earliest change on the ECG is PR segment depression, after which J point and ST-segment elevation evolve, often globally. If a significant pericardial effusion is present, the ECG may reveal R waves of low voltage or electrical alternans. Chest roentgenograms may be normal or, if a large pericardial effusion is present, may demonstrate an enlarged cardiac silhouette with a "conical flask like" configuration. M-mode and two-dimensional echocardiography are the diagnostic procedures of choice if a pericardial effusion is suspected; however, aside from demonstrating mild pericardial thickening and a small infusion, echocardiography in many patients with simple pericarditis is unrevealing.

(4)Treatment

Treatment is directed at the underlying cause of the pericarditis, including antibiotics for bacterial and tuberculous infections, irradiation for carcinomatous etiologies, and hemodialysis in renal failure. When a viral infection is believed to be the cause (coxsackievirus A and B, adenovirus, echovirus), aspirin or a nonsteroidal antiinflammatory agent may be given (indomethacin, 50 mg four times daily, or ibuprofen, 400 mg four times daily, with food). It is important to note that if any suspicion exists that the effusion may be hemorrhagic, the use of these agents should be avoided. If hemodynamically significant tamponade exists, emergency pericardiocentesis may be lifesaving.

6.5.2 Non-cardiac chest pain

6.5.2.1 Acute dissecting thoracic aortic aneurysm and the aorta in acute dissection

Acute dissection of the aorta occurs when blood suddenly enters the aortic wall through a spontaneous intimal tear and dissects along its course. Patients (predominantly men in the fifth to seventh decades of life) give a history of the sudden onset of severe chest pain often radiating to the back; pain is frequently described feeling of "ripping" or "tearing". The intensity of discomfort associated with aortic dissection is typically maximal at its onset. Most patients are currently hypertensive (unless already compromised by complications) and/or have a history of hypertension or Marfan syndrome. Carotid pulses are normal and symmetric because retrograde extension from the site of origin of the dissection is rare. New aortic regurgitant murmurs are not noted. The pain of aortic dissection is severe and of sudden onset; it is tearing in nature, often radiates to the back, and may be associated with hypertension, aortic regurgitation, and neurological signs and pulse deficits.

6.5.2.2 Pulmonary embolism (PE)

The majority of patients with pulmonary embolus have no ECG changes apart from a tachycardia or atrial fibrillation (AF). The 'classic' ECG changes of $S_IQ_{III}T_{III}$ or right heart strain are associated with large PE and are often transient and easily missed.

6.5.2.3 Spontaneous pneumothorax and spontaneous tension pneumothorax

In spontaneous pneumothorax, there may be central chest pain with few auscultatory signs. Spontaneous pneumothorax is a strong possibility in patients with chronic obstructive pulmonary disease (COPD) who present with chest pain and dyspnoea in the absence of ECG evidence of acute myocardial ischaemia. A chest X-ray is critical to rule out the presence of air in the pleural space. Pain arising from the pleura is unilateral, sharp and stabbing, and worse on inspiration. A tension pneumothorax will develop from a relatively small fraction of spontaneous pneumothorax. Tension pneumothorax occurs when air continues to enter the pleural space through a ball-valve or "one-way" rent in the visceral pleura; progressively increasing pleural pressures eventually compromise venous return, resulting in rapidly evolving circulatory collapse. Spontaneous pneumothorax disorder most often occurs in young, healthy adults who present with a history of the sudden onset of unilateral, chest or back pain and varying degrees of associated dyspnea.

6.5.2.4　Pleuritis

Pleuritis is an inflammatory process involving the pleura that has many causes, including viral pleurodynia, pleural-based pneumonia, pulmonary infarction caused by pulmonary embolism, and neoplastic involvement of the pleura; pneumothorax, acute costochondritis, and intercostal muscle strain may also present with pleuritic discomfort and should also be considered. Regardless of the cause, patients typically report a history of sharp, often "knife-like" pain, usually well localized to a particular region of the chest or back that is typically increased with inspiration, cough, or sneeze.

6.5.2.5　Costochondritis

Costochondritis is an acute and self-limited inflammatory process involving the costosternal articulations. Patients report unilateral, pleuritic peristernal pain, the onset of which may be perceived as gradual or sudden, is typically increased by maneuvers that produce motion of the costochondral joints and frequently radiates along the course of the involved rib toward the side or back. A subjective sensation of breathlessness often accompanies the discomfort, and a history of a preceding upper respiratory tract infection is occasionally obtained.

6.5.2.6　Esophagitis

Esophagitis occurs as a result of the reflux of gastric acid from the stomach into the distal esophagus. Dyspeptic pain arising from the upper GI tract is usually burning in nature, may have a clear relationship to posture or food, and is often relieved by antacids. Oesophageal pain may, however, be very similar to the pain of cardiac ischaemia.

Treatment involves the use of antacids, the avoidance of large meals, particularly before bedtime, and elevation of the head of the bed; these latter measures simply decrease the probability of reflux. Some patients with particularly severe symptoms will respond to the addition of an H_2-receptor blocker at bedtime, or bethanechol at bedtime.

Li Nan

Chapter 7

Acute Coronary Syndromes

7.1 Epidemiology, definition and pathophysiology

7.1.1 Epidemiology

Coronary heart disease is the most common cause of death in the world. It is estimated that the incidence of acute coronary syndrome (ACS) is over 250,000 per year in the United Kingdom. Sudden death remains a frequent complication of ACS: approximately 50% of patients with ST elevation myocardial infarction (STEMI) do not survive, with around two-thirds of the deaths occurring shortly after the onset of symptoms and before admission to hospital.

7.1.2 Definition

The term 'acute coronary syndrome' (ACS) has been developed to describe the collection of ischaemic conditions that include a spectrum of diagnoses from unstable angina (UA) to non-ST elevation MI (NSTEMI) and STEMI. Patients presenting with ACS can be classified into two groups according to their electrocardiogram (ECG) (Figure 7-1): those with persistent STEMI and those without (non-ST elevation ACS or NSTEACS). The treatment of STEMI requires emergency restoration of blood flow within an occluded culprit coronary artery. Patients presenting with NSTEACS often have ECG changes including T-wave inversion, ST depression or transient ST elevation, although occasionally the ECG may be entirely normal.

Myocardial infarction can also be classified with regards to underlying etiology as defined by the European Society of Cardiology:

Type 1　Spontaneous myocardial infarction related to ischaemia due to a primary coronary event such as plaque erosion and/or rupture, fissuring or dissection.

Type 2　Myocardial infarction secondary to ischaemia due to either increased oxygen demand or decreased supply, e. g. , coronary artery spasm, coronary embolism, anaemia, arrhythmias, hypertension or hypotension.

Type 3　Sudden unexpected cardiac death, including cardiac arrest, often with symptoms suggestive of myocardial ischaemia, accompanied by presumably new ST elevation, or new LBBB, or evidence of fresh thrombus in

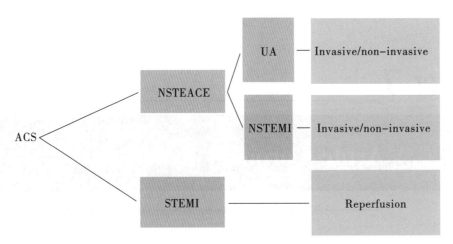

Figure 7-1   Definition, diagnosis and management of ACS

a coronary artery by angiography and/or at autopsy, but death occurring before blood samples could be obtained, or at a time before the appearance of cardiac biomarkers in the blood.

Type 4a   Myocardial infarction associated with PCI (percutaneous coronary intrervention).

Type 4b   Myocardial infarction associated with stent thrombosis as documented by angiography or at autopsy.

Type 5   Myocardial infarction associated with CABG (coronary artery bypass graft).

7.1.3   Pathophysiology

ACSs are caused by an imbalance between myocardial oxygen demand and supply that results in cell death and myocardial necrosis. Primarily, this occurs due to factors affecting the coronary arteries, but may also occur as a result of secondary processes such as hypoxaemia or hypotension and factors that increase myocardial oxygen demand. The commonest cause is rupture or erosion of an atherosclerotic plaque that leads to complete occlusion of the artery or partial occlusion with distal embolization of thrombotic material (Figure 7-2).

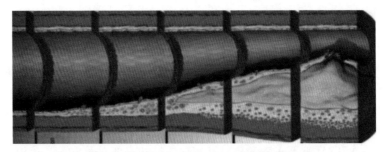

Figure 7-2   The process of plaque formation and rupture

Atherosclerosis is a disease of large and medium-sized arteries, affecting predominantly the arterial intima. The precise mechanism responsible for the generation of atherosclerotic arterial disease remains open to debate, but it is likely that arterial endothelial injury is an initiating factor. It is clear that the extent and stability of atherosclerotic lesions is influenced by the common risk factors of smoking, hypertension, hyperlipidaemia and diabetes. There are a large number of other modifiable risk factors, such as homocysteine, oxidative stress, fibrinogen and psychosocial factors, which may play an important role in atherogenesis in some individuals.

7.2   Clinical features

Accelerated or recent onset angina is present in 20% of patients with NSTEACS, where the pain is intermittent and related to stress or exertion. Typically, the discomfort is retrosternal, crushing and severe, radiating to the neck, arms or back. There is often associated nausea, sweating and vomiting related to the release of toxins from injured myocardial cells and autonomic activation. It is not usually affected by changes in posture, movement or respiration. The pain can be atypical (sited in the epigastrium, neck, arms or back or unusual in character). Particularly with inferior infarction, the pain can be difficult to distinguish from dyspepsia. Atypical symptoms are more likely to be presented in the young (aged 25-40 years old), elderly patients (aged>75), females, those with diabetes, chronic renal failure and those with dementia. In some patients, the pain is minimal or absent, with the dominant symptoms consisting of nausea, vomiting, dyspnoea, weakness, dizziness or syncope (or a combination of these). Occasionally ACS is recognized coincidentally (and often retrospectively) by the presence of ECG abnormalities in addition to raised plasma biochemical markers. It is also important to differentiate those with non-cardiac chest pain from those with anginal symptoms. Typical angina is defined by the presence of all three of the features listed below:

- A constricting discomfort across the chest and/or neck, shoulders, jaw or arms.
- Being precipitated by physical exertion or psychological stress.
- Re lieved by rest or by nitroglycerin within about 5 minutes.

7.3   Electrocardiographic changes

The majority of patients with an ACS will have an abnormal ECG at some stages. An initial normal ECG could not rule out the diagnosis, as ECG changes can develop, evolve and resolve rapidly. Patients with a suggestive history and a normal ECG should be admitted and the ECG monitored at regular intervals; if ECG changes then develops, appropriate treatment should be initiated.

7.3.1   Electrocardiographic changes in STEMI

STEMI is diagnosed for more than 30 minutes of chest pain and ST-segment elevation of $\geqslant$ 2 mV (2 mm) in two or more contiguous precordial leads or $\geqslant$ 1 mV (1 mm) in two or more adjacent limb leads or new left bundle branch block. In patients with this type of evolving MI:

- ST elevation develops rapidly (30-60 seconds) after coronary occlusion, and is usually associated with prolonged total occlusion of a coronary artery.
- The ST elevation resolves over several hours in response to spontaneous or therapeutic coronary reperfusion. Persistent ST elevation is a sign of failure to reperfuse, and is associated with a large infarct and an adverse prognosis. T-wave inversion, pathological Q waves and loss of R waves often develop in the infarct zone when reperfusion has been late or incomplete, indicating the presence of extensive myocardial necrosis. When successful reperfusion occurs early in the course of an evolving ST elevation MI, there may be less myocardial necrosis, preservation of the R waves and no Q-wave formation. Occasionally, reperfusion therapy may be administered so rapidly that any infarction is aborted.

In a small proportion of patients with chest pain and evolving MI (around 5%), the presenting ECG demonstrates bundle branch block (usually left). This is commonly associated with extensive anterior infarction and a poor prognosis. The distribution of ECG changes provides some information on the area of myocardium involved:

• Changes in V_2-V_6 indicate anterior ischaemia or necrosis in the territory of the left anterior descending (LAD) artery. Extensive infarction in this territory is associated with a high risk of heart failure, arrhythmias, mechanical complications and early death (Figure 7-3).

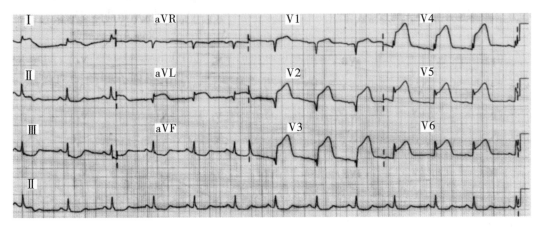

Figure 7-3   Note ST elevation in leads V_2-V_6, I and aVL

• Changes in I, aVL, V_5 and V_6 indicate lateral ischaemia or necrosis in the territory of the circumflex artery or diagonal branches of the LAD. Infarction in this territory has a better prognosis than extensive anterior infarction.

• Changes in II, III and a VF indicate inferior ischaemia or necrosis in the territory of the right coronary artery (Figure 7-4). Compared with patients with extensive anterior infarction, these patients have a lower incidence of heart failure, an increased incidence of bradyarrhythmias (since atrioventricular (AV) nodal ischaemia or vagal activation often accompanies occlusion of the right coronary artery) and a relatively good prognosis.

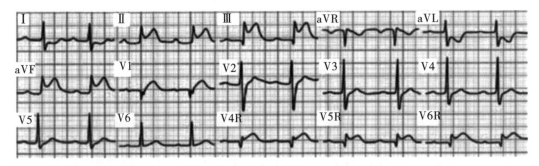

Figure 7-4   Note ST elevation in leads II, III, aVF

• Tall R waves in V_1-V_3 associated with ST depression indicate ischaemia or necrosis in the posterior wall, often associated with circumflex or right coronary artery occlusion.

7.3.2   Electrocardiographic changes in NSTEACS

NSTEACS are associated with transient ST segment changes (≥ 0.5 mm) that develop with symptoms at rest and which may resolve with the resolution of symptoms (Figure 7-5 and Figure 7-6). The degree of ST change correlates with the risk of further events and death. Transient ST elevation is also associated with a poorer outcome. T—wave inversion and ST changes of <0.5 mm are less specific at indicating and predicting events, though deep T—wave inversion in leads V_2–V_6 is associated with disease in the proximal LAD. Elderly patients with widespread severe ST depression often have multivessel disease and a poor prognosis.

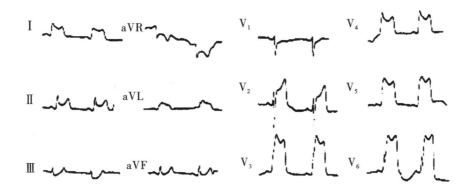

Figure 7—5   Electrocardiogram when chest pain occurs

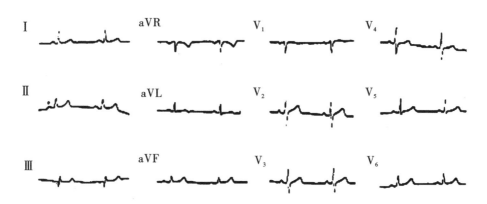

Figure 7—6   Electrocardiogram when chest pain relief for half an hour

7.4   Laboratory test

Cardiac enzyme tests are employed to substantiate or refute a provisional diagnosis of NSTEMI or UA and guide further therapy. Myocardial necrosis results in the release of intracellular proteins, which can be detected in blood samples. Measurement of total creatine kinase (CK) level has been employed as a common biochemical test in patients with suspected MI, with a temporally related increase to more than twice the upper limit of normal level and regarded as diagnostic. CK is widely distributed in non—cardiac tissues, and therefore has a significant rate of false—positive results. The isoenzyme, CK—MB, is predominantly located in the myocardium, and for this reason it was previously the gold standard marker for myocardial necrosis. A low—molecular—weight protein, myoglobin, is released as a result of damage to any muscle. Myoglobin release occurs relatively soon after MI, and the plasma levels can be detectable within 2 hours, which makes it as a useful early biomarker in the triage of patients with chest pain in the emergency department.

Any patient who demonstrates a typical rise and gradual fall of troponin in association with ischaemic symptoms or ECG changes should be diagnosed as definite MI. The troponin complex is an integral part of the cardiac myofibril and is released following damage of myocardium. Two regulatory components, troponin I and T, released by myocardial micro-infarction, can be detected peripherally, indicating that myocardial necrosis has occurred. As well as their specificity, cardiac troponins are highly sensitive, with detectable elevations occurring after necrosis of less than 1 g of myocardial tissue. Troponins are detectable 3−4 hours after the onset of infarction, peak at 12 hours, and can remain elevated for up to 2 weeks.

7.5   Diagnosis

The diagnosis of ACS is usually made using a combination of clinical and ECG features. Cardiac troponin studies and functional tests can then be used to further risk-stratifying the patient. As a general principle, all patients with symptoms that may be due to an ACS should be admitted to hospital. These patients should preferably be admitted to a chest pain assessment unit or heart attack centre, as those at high risk of early adverse events need to be carefully monitored and selected for early invasive therapy

STEMI is diagnosed by the presence of characteristic chest pain for more than 30 minutes and ST-segment elevation of $\geqslant$ 2 mV (2 mm) in two or more contiguous precordial leads or $\geqslant$ 1 mV (1 mm) in two or more adjacent limb leads or new left bundle branch block. In patients with this type of evolving MI.

NSTEACS are associated with transient ST segment changes ($\geqslant$ 0.5 mm) that develop with symptoms at rest and which may resolve with the resolution of symptoms.

7.6   Differential diagnosis

Since acute chest pain can have many possible causes, a careful history and comprehensive physical examination along with inspection of the ECG and chest X-ray are mandatory in all cases where diagnostic uncertainty exists.

Sometimes physicians need to identify the false-positive results of troponins which can be due to:
- Renal failure.
- Pulmonary embolism.
- Septicaemia.
- Rhabdomyolysis.
- Acute neurological disease (stroke or subarachnoid haemorrhage).
- Significant valvular disease (aortic stenosis).
- Acute and chronic heart failure.
- Cardiomyopathy (hypertrophic, apical ballooning).
- Infiltrative disease (amyloidosis, sarcoid, haemochromatosis, scleroderma).
- Inflammatory disease (myocarditis or myocardial extension of pericarditis and endocarditis).
- Cardiotoxic drugs (anthracyclines, herceptin and 5-fluorouracil).
- Cardiac contusion.
- Tachycardia or bradycardia.

7.7   Treatment

7.7.1   Initial treatment

If a patient with suspected ACS arrives in hospital, rapid processing is necessary to establish an early diagnosis and allow effective emergency care to be instituted. The initial assessment should be rapid, and aimed at establishing the diagnosis, assessing the haemodynamic state and determining suitability for reperfusion therapy. Patients with clear-cut clinical features of STEMI with an ECG that demonstrates ST elevation or bundle branch block should enter a 'fast track' system, designed to ensure that they receive appropriate emergency care; any reperfusion therapy required should be instituted within 90 minutes of the initial call for medical assistance. The main aims for treatment of ACS are to prevent continued ischaemia, limit myocardial damage, reduce the incidence of left ventricular dysfunction, heart failure and death. This is achieved with early identification of patients who require revascularization and treatment of complications of ischaemia including arrhythmia (VF/VT and bradycardia), heart failure and shock. Initially, in all patients with ACS, emergency care consists of symptom relief, administration of antithrombotic agents, and instigating reperfusion therapy as early as possible for STEMI. The priorities are to:

- Establish venous access with a large-bore cannula in an arm vein providing ready access for drug administration, and institute rhythm monitoring to aid in the rapid detection and treatment of arrhythmias.

- Provide adequate analgesia, which is vital. Uncontrolled pain and anxiety are associated with sympathetic activation, with resultant detrimental effects on cardiac performance, oxygen consumption and the arrhythmia threshold.

- Treat pulmonary oedema with frusemide 40-80 mg via IV path.

- Consider supplemental oxygen.

- Commence treatment with oral antiplatelets. Aspirin (loading dose of 300 mg) and a thienopyridine (currently usually clopidogrel 600 mg, though recently published trials indicate that prasugrel 60 mg and ticagrelor may offer significant benefits).

- STEMI patients should be considered for immediate reperfusion therapy. This ideally should be primary PCI, but where this is not available, thrombolysis with fibrin-specific agents should be used.

- NSTEACS patients should be treated with low-molecular-weight heparin (LMWH) and antianginals such as beta-blockers, calcium channel antagonists and nitrates. They should have continuous rhythm monitoring and repeated 12-lead ECGs whilst in pain. If they develop ST elevation, they should then be treated as a STEMI. If they remain in pain despite adequate treatment, they should be considered for urgent coronary angiography with a view to revascularization. If the pain is continuous and severe, alternative diagnoses should be re-explored, in particular aortic dissection.

7.7.2   Treatment of STEMI

Prior to the advent of thrombolysis or primary PCI, the only means of achieving therapeutic reperfusion in patients with evolving MI was emergency CABG. With the advent of thrombolysis and primary PCI, emergency CABG is now rarely performed in patients with evolving MI, unless there is an associated early mechanical complication such as a ventricular septal rupture or acute severe mitral regurgitation. Achieving reperfusion as soon as possible is fundamental to improving outcomes.

7.7.2.1 Primary PCI

Primary PCI involves arterial access, either via the femoral or radial artery and passage of a catheter to selectively engage the coronary ostia under X-ray visualization. Once the culprit vessel has been identified, a small guide wire is passed along the vessel and past the occlusion. Balloons, stents and other devices can then be delivered to the point required in order to successfully treat the artery. This requires the patient to be anticoagulated, usually with unfractionated heparin, to reduce the incidence of thrombus formation on the equipment in situ.

7.7.2.2 Thrombolysis

The benefit with thrombolysis is even more time dependent than that of primary PCI. Therefore minimizing the symptom-to-needle time is key to producing good outcomes where thrombolysis is used. If thrombolysis is the default reperfusion strategy pre-hospital thrombolysis is recommended. A high proportion (85.4%) of the thrombolysis group also underwent coronary early angiography, which supports the use of early adjuvant PCI in patients who have had successful thrombolysis.

(1) Selection of thrombolytic agents

Most of the beneficial effect on reducing mortality was obtained in patients with anterior infarction treated within 6 hours of symptom onset. Newer plasminogen activators, produced by bioengineering techniques applied to rt-PA, have been developed to overcome the disadvantages of earlier thrombolytic agents. Fibrin-specific compounds, reteplase (r-PA) and tenecteplase (TNK), have longer half lives than the original compound, allowing for single or double bolus administration. These simplified regimens have been shown to shorten door-to-needle times. Accelerated rt-PA or TNK with concomitant heparin are the regimens with the best record for mortality reduction. The modified plasminogen activators have the simplest dosing regimens, to reduce door-to-needle time.

(2) Inclusion criteria

Where primary PCI is not available or where an additional time delay to primary PCI of 90 minutes or more is expected, thrombolysis should be given if presentation within 12 hours of onset of ischaemic cardiac pain in a patient with:

- ST-segment elevation of at least 2 mm in two adjacent chest leads.
- ST-segment elevation of 1 mm in two adjacent limb leads.
- True posterior infarction or new bundle branch block.

If the presentation is >12 hours after onset of pain with ongoing symptoms and ECG evidence of evolving infarction, primary PCI should be considered first. Additionally, patients presenting with shock should be treated with primary PCI, rather than thrombolysis. The SHOCK trial showed a 20% reduction in mortality at 6 months in those treated with PCI (see Cardiogenic shock).

(3) Exclusion criteria

These continue to evolve, and are in general decreasing as our experience with thrombolytic agents increases. At present, there are few absolute contraindications. Many are now regarded as relative, to be interpreted within the clinical context. Criteria include:

- Known coagulation disorder, including uncontrolled anticoagulation therapy.
- Active peptic ulceration, varices or recent GI haemorrhage (dyspepsia alone is not a contraindication).
- Severe hypertension (systolic >180 mmHg and/or diastolic >110 mmHg).
- Traumatic cardiopulmonary resuscitation (CPR) (CPR performed by trained staff is not regarded as a contraindication).

- Recent internal bleeding from any site (menstruation is not an absolute contraindication).

- Previous haemorrhagic stroke at any time.

- Ischaemic stroke within the last year.

- Transient ischaemic attack (TIA) in last 3 months.

- Surgery, major trauma or head injury within the last month.

- Pregnancy.

- Diabetic retinopathy (now only a relative contraindication, as the risk of intraocular bleeding is very small and the potential benefit of thrombolysis in diabetics far outweighs this risk).

(4) Complications

1) Allergy

Allergic reactions to streptokinase are due to the effect of pre-existing an tistreptococcal antibodies. Mild urticarial reactions are the most common allergic response, and should be treated with 200 mg Ⅳ hydrocortisone and 10 mg Ⅳ chlorpheniramine. If a more severe reaction with bronchospasm occurs, 250-500 mg of intramuscular adrenaline should be administered along with nebulized bronchodilators. Major anaphylaxis is very rare (0.1%). If this occurs, with associated cardiovascular collapse, 5 mL of 1 ∶ 10,000 adrenaline Ⅳ is the first-line therapy, followed by rapid volume loading with Ⅳ plasma expanders, steroids and antihistamines.

2) Haemorrhage

Minor bleeding at venepuncture sites is relatively common, but rarely requires any specific therapy other than direct compression at the site. Major haemorrhagic episodes requiring transfusion are rare. If a major bleeding occurs, the following action should betaken.

- Stop thrombolytic infusion (or heparin).

- Reverse heparin with protamine sulphate (10 mg per 1,000 u heparin).

- Give two units of plasma immediately.

- Consider the administration of tranexamic acid 10 mg/kg by slow Ⅳ injection.

3) Cerebrovascular events

The overall incidence of stroke is only minimally increased, since thrombolytic therapy causes a slight increase in cerebral haemorrhages, which is offset by a reduction in cerebral infarcts. Plasminogen activators are associated with a greater risk of haemorrhagic stroke than streptokinase. Stroke is more common in elderly patients. If a stroke occurs, thrombolytic or anticoagulant therapy should be discontinued. A CT scan and neurological opinion will help to determine the mechanism of the stroke and guide therapy.

7.7.2.3 Failed reperfusion

(1) Detection and implications of failed reperfusion

Patients treated with thrombolysis who achieve effective reperfusion have a good prognosis, with hospital mortality rates of less than 5%. In a substantial proportion of patients, however, reperfusion fails. In some of these patients the IRA is persistently occluded by an extensively disrupted plaque or residual thrombus. In other patients (particularly those treated late), platelet microthrombi or capillary disruption prevents reperfusion of myocardium at the tissue level despite restoration of blood flow in the epicardial IRA. Failure of reperfusion is associated with continuing chest pain, extensive infarction, electrical and haemodynamic instability, mechanical complications and a poor prognosis. Detecting failed reperfusion in current clinical practice is based on serial evaluation of ST-segments. Persistent ST elevation occurs in about one-third of patients, and is associated with failure of reperfusion, and portends an adverse prognosis.

(2) Rescue angioplasty

The REACT trial as well as meta-analysis of angioplasty strategies after thrombolysis support the role of rescue angioplasty for STEMI patients who fail to reperfuse after thrombolysis. Accordingly, all patients should have an ECG recorded 90 minutes after commencing thrombolysis. Patients who have less than 50% ST-segment resolution in the infarct zone should be considered for rescue angioplasty.

7.7.2.4 Recurrent ischaemia and early PCI after thrombolysis

Following successful thrombolytic therapy, patients are often left with a residual high grade stenosis or an 'inflamed' ruptured plaque. Recurrent ischaemia occurs in up to one-third of thrombolyzed patients, and is associated with increased hospital mortality.

7.7.3 Treatment of NSTEACS

The management of NSTEACS is different from that of acute STEMI. Treatment is aimed at reducing persistent ischaemia and the risk of reinfarction as opposed to opening an occluded artery to abort an infarction. Medical therapy has limited impact on mortality but does lead to a reduction in subsequent infarction and persistent ischaemia by stabilizing coronary plaques. The addition of coronary angiography provides anatomical information on the culprit lesion, the extent of disease, global and regional left ventricular function and provides a starting point for subsequent revascularization.

7.7.3.1 The characteristics in NATEACS

The characteristics that increase the likelihood of failure of medical therapy are:

- Reversible ST-segment change.
- Previous angina.
- Prior aspirin use.
- Family history of premature coronary disease.
- Increased age.

If all these characteristics are present, medical failure occurs in 90% of cases. If none is present, the majority of patients settle with medical therapy.

7.7.3.2 Clinical features and the 12-lead ECG

The medical history and physical examination provide some help for risk stratification. Patients with multiple risk factors for vascular disease are at increased risk of adverse events. Older age and previous aspirin use are also indicators of adverse risk. A highly unstable pattern of symptoms with recent rest pain is also an risk factor. Evidence of haemodynamic instability or compromise indicates a poor prognosis.

The primary ECG abnormality necessitating admission is ST-segment depression or elevation greater than 1 mm. In the presence of lesser changes such as.

- ST elevation 0.5-1 mm.
- ST depression 0.25-1 mm.
- T-wave inversion in >2 leads.
- Q waves.
- Left ventricular hypertrophy.
- Abnormal rhythm.

7.7.3.3 Risk scores in NATEACS

Fundamental to the development of modern risk scores in NSTEACS is the quantification of serum troponin. As described earlier, troponin measurement is now the gold standard test for detection of myocardial injury. In ACS, troponin levels rise about 4 hours after the onset of chest pain in 30% –50% of patients, of which, 100% of MI patients have positive result at 12 hours of onset of the disease. The elevation of cardiac troponin indicates the presence of minor myocyte damage, which is associated with a high risk of subsequent progression to MI and death in patients with unstable angina.

(1) Risk assessment in NATEACS

Risk assessment can be further refined using clinical scoring systems which have been developed from the analysis of large cohorts of patients with NSTEACS. They use features from the history, clinical examination, ECG changes and biomarkers to predict the risk of further events. It assigns one point to each of the following risk factors.

- Age ⩾ 65.
- Three or more risk factors for coronary artery disease (family history/diabetes/current smoker/hyperlipidaemia/hypertension).
- Known coronary stenosis ⩾50%.
- Aspirin use in the preceding 7 days.
- Two or more episodes of severe angina during the previous 24 hours.
- ST segment deviation on ECG of ⩾0.5 mm.
- Elevated serum cardiac biomakers.

(2) High-risk patients in NATEACS

The American Heart Association/American College of Cardiology (AHA/ACC) guidelines recommend an invasive strategy in NSTEACS in the following situations.

- Recurrent angina/ischemia at rest or low-level exercise despite intensive medical therapy.
- Signs or symptoms of heart failure or new or worsening mitral regurgitation.
- High-risk findings on non-invasive stress testing.
- Reduced left ventricular function (EF<40%).
- Haemodynamic instability.
- Sustained ventricular tachycardia (VT).
- PCI within the previous 6 months.
- Prior CABG.
- High-risk score (e. g. , TIMI or GRACE).
- New or presumably new ST-segment depression.
- Elevated cardiac biomarkers (troponin I and T).

(3) Low-risk patients in NATEACS

Non-invasive stress testing with a low-level treadmill exercise test (two stages of the Bruce protocol) should be performed in patients free of ischaemia at rest or on minimal exertion for 12–24 hours. Where the baseline ECG has resting ST-segment depression (>0.1 mV), bundle branch block, left ventricular hypertrophy, an intraventricular conduction defect, a paced rhythm, or the patient is on digoxin therapy, stress perfusion imaging or stress echocardiography may be done to identify a substrate for ischaemia. Those that subsequently have a positive stress test should undergo coronary angiography with a view to revascularization.

7.7.4　Bleeding risk in ACS

Bleeding is the most common non-cardiac complication associated with coronary intervention. The use of antithrombotic agents increases the risk of both access site-related bleeding, and non-access site-related bleeding such as gastrointestinal, cerebral and retroperitoneal haemorrhage. Bleeding is also commoner among older, more frail subjects with significant co-morbidities, who are also at higher risk of ischaemic events. Therefore the benefit gained from treatment has to be balanced against the risks of bleeding and treatment needs to be tailored to individual patients. Several risk scores have been developed to predict the risks of bleeding in an effort to assist with the decision-making. More recently, a system from over 302,000 patients who underwent PCI has been developed, which assigns points to the following nine variables(Table 7-1).

Table 7-1   Bleeding risk factor in ACS

Risk factor	Score
ACS type	STEMI 10 points/NSTEACS 3 points
Cardiogenic shock	8 points
Female gender	6 points
Previous congestive heart failure	5 points
No previous PCI	4 points
NHYA class IV heart failure	4 points
Peripheral vascular disease	2 points
Age(years)	66-752 points 76-855 points ≥858 points
Renal function	1 point for every 10 unit decrease in eGFR if <90

7.7.5   Adjunctive medical therapy

7.7.5.1   Antiplatelets

(1)Aspirin

Unless there is a contradidication, aspirin should be administered to all patients with NSTEACS and STEMI at presentation. It should be continued indefinitely in all patients with suspected or proven coronary disease. Aspirin inhibits the cyclooxygenase enzyme in platelets which leads to the formation of thromboxane A_2, a potent stimulus to platelet activation. Aspirin reduces platelet aggregation, enhancing recanalization in STEMI, and reducing the risk of further vascular events in patients with previous MI. A loading dose of 150 mg produces rapid and complete inhibition of thromboxane-mediated platelet inhibition. For long-term treatment, higher doses are more gastrotoxic. A dose of 75 mg/d maintains virtually complete long-term cyclooxygenase inhibition, and is suitable for chronic therapy.

There are few contraindications to the use of aspirin, it should not be given to patients with:

- Known hypersensitivity to aspirin.
- Bleeding peptic ulcer.
- Coagulation disorder.
- Severe hepatic disease.

(2)Clopidogrel

Clopidogrel is a thienopyridine which blocks ADP-mediated platelet aggregation and the activation of the GpIIb/IIIa receptor, which cross-links platelets through fibrinogen. A loading dose of at least 300 mg should be given to all patients presening with ACS, with 600 mg being preferable in those likely to require urgent PCI.

(3) Other thienopyridines

Prasugrel, a third generation thienopyridine, has been shown in vivo to have a faster onset and be more potent than clopidogrel. Ticagralor was studied in the PLATO trial, where it was given as a loading dose of 180 mg followed by maintenance of 90 mg twice a day.

(4) Duration of antiplatelets

Following NSTEACS, it is recommended that DAPT, with aspirin and clopidogrel, should be continued for at least 1 year whether treated by PCI or medically (CURE study). For STEMI, there is strong evidence for benefit for DAPT up to one month (COMMIT and CLARITY studies) and considering the effect on NSTEACS it is reasonable to continue DAPT for one year for all ACS, including STEMI. In addition, most patients will be treated with PCI and therefore the duration will depend on the type of stent used as well as the risk of reinfarction (which will be dependent on other factors such as diabetes and impaired left ventricular function) that should be weighed up against the risk of bleeding. Patients who receive a DES need to continue DAPT for at least one year, as premature cessation is strongly associated with a risk of stent thrombosis, which induces high mortality. In any patients who are going to require non–cardiac surgery or who have a bleeding, the cessation of antiplatelets should be discussed with a cardiologist first.

7.7.5.2 Anticoagulants

Heparin is required for 48 hours after thrombolysis with plasminogen activators. The use of UFH is recommended during PCI procedures as it is rapidly effective with a measurable change in the ACT and it can be promptly reversed with protamine if necessary. Bivalirudin, a direct thrombin inhibitor, is also effective in STEMI and NSTEACS patients and can be continued during PCI. Overall, anticoagulants are recommended in all patients with ACS, but the doses and agents used need to be carefully considered in relation to the risk of bleeding in patients.

7.7.5.3 Glycoprotein IIB/IIIA inhibitors

Because activation of the GpIIb/IIIa receptor is the final common pathway of platelet aggregation through its ability to cross–link with other GpIIb/IIIa receptors via fibrinogen or von Willebrand factor, different agents have been developed specifically to inhibit this process. These are the chimeric (murine–human) antibody fragment to the GpIIb/IIIa receptor, abciximab (Reopro^{TM}), synthetic peptides such as eptifibatide (Integrelin^{TM}) and synthetic non–peptides such as tirofiban (Aggrastat^{TM}). Abciximab is a Fab antibody fragment of a human–murine (chimeric) monoclonal antibody (c7E3) with a short plasma half–life but strong receptor affinity, persisting for weeks (although platelet aggregation returns to normal within 48 hours). Abciximab is relatively non–specific and also inhibits the vitronectin ($\alpha v \beta 3$) receptor which is on endothelial cells and the MAC–1 receptor on leucocytes. By contrast, the synthetic (small molecule) GpIIb/IIIa inhibitors have half–lives of 2–3 hours and are more specific to the receptor. There is an increased risk of bleeding with these agents, which is typically mucocutaneous or at access sites, particularly at the site of a femoral artery sheath.

7.7.5.4 Beta–blockers

Beta–blockers have antiarrhythmic, anti–ischaemic and antihypertensive properties. Some studies indicated that these beneficial effects reduce chest pain, myocardial wall stress and infarct size in patients with STEMI. However, routine use of intravenous beta–blockers should not be recommended for all patients with STEMI. As maximum benefit in reducing mortality from beta–blocker therapy is obtained in higher–risk patients, whose infarctions are complicated by arrhythmias or heart failure; treatment should be directed to specific problems such as ongoing chest pain, poorly controlled hypertension and tachy-arrhythmia. However, patients should be carefully selected to avoid those at risk of developing shock.

All patients should be considered for longterm oral beta-blocker after STEMI. Contraindications to beta-blocker therapy present in around 15% of patients, and consist of:

- Resting heart rate <55 bpm.
- Second or third degree atrioventricular heart block.
- A history of asthma.

7.7.5.5   Calcium channel blockers

Calcium channel blocking drugs have anti-ischaemic, vasodilating and antihypertensive properties that may be beneficial in patients with acute MI. There are some evidences that the type of calcium antagonist used may be important. Dihydropyridine calcium antagonists are powerful vasodilators and may induce tachycardia. Since they have no effect on the cardiac conduction system and showed a trend towards increased mortality, they should be avoided in MI patients. Both diltiazem and verapamil have effects on the cardiac conduction system, slowing heart rate, potentially improving their efficacy in MI patients. However, for their rate-slowing function, they should not be given to patients with significant left ventricular dysfunction. For patients in whom a beta-blocker is contraindicated or poorly tolerated, and left ventricular function is well preserved, a rate-slowing calcium antagonist can be safely used for symptom control if required.

7.7.5.6   ACE inhibitors

Activation of the renin-angiotensin system is an early compensatory response to an evolving MI. Activation of the renin-angiotensin system leads to vasoconstriction, increased heart rate and sympathetic activation. In the early phases of evolving MI these deleterious changes will increase ventricular wall stress, increase oxygen consumption and reduce electrical stability. In the longer term, persistent activation of the renin-angiotensin system potentiates adverse remodelling, leading to ventricular dilatation and heart failure. The adverse consequences of renin-angiotensin activation can be blocked by the use of ACE inhibitors with potentially beneficial effects on lowering mortality. ACE inhibitors should be prescribed early after ACS in patients who are clinically stable with an adequate blood pressure. If possible, treatment should be initiated within 24 hours of admission, intravenous drip up to target doses. Current ACE inhibitors licensed post-MI are ramipril (target dose 5 mg bd or 10 mg od) and perindopril (target dose 8 mg od). Renal function and electrolytes should be monitored to ensure there is no significant ACE inhibitor-induced deterioration in renal function (a 20% reduction in eGFR on and ACE inhibitor is acceptable). In patients who are intolerant to ACE inhibitors, angiotensin-2 receptor blocker may be used instead.

7.7.5.7   Statins

The benefit of statin therapy in the primary prevention of coronary heart disease and in the secondary prevention of further events in patients with angina, and previous unstable angina or infarction is well-established. There is also evidence to support their role as adjunctive therapy in ACS. On the basis of these trial data, all patients with ACS should be commenced on a high dose of statin early in their hospital admission.

7.7.5.8   Nitrate therapy

Nitrates have a number of potentially beneficial effects (systemic vasodilatation and coronary artery dilatation), and early studies suggested that their routine administration to patients with acute infarction may reduce mortality. Although nitrates are safe and effective in the treatment of post-infarction ischaemia or heart failure, they should not routinely be administered to uncomplicated patients.

7.7.5.9　Prophylactic antiarrhythmic therapy

Ventricular tachyarrhythmias are an important cause of death early after the onset of MI. Class I antiarrhythmic drugs can suppress these arrhythmias, but this beneficial effect may be offset by adverse effects such as the induction of bradyarrhythmias, induction of tachyarrhythmias and depression of ventricular function. Routine prophylactic therapy with class I antiarrhythmic drugs early in the course of evolving MI is not recommended.

7.7.5.10　Pre–existing drug therapy

Patients admitted with evolving acute MI are often already on treatment with oral beta–blockers for pre–existing angina or hypertension. Given the beneficial effects of beta–blockers following infarction and the potential adverse effects associated with abrupt beta–blocker withdrawal, administration of these agents should continue uninterrupted unless severe heart failure or a symptomatic bradyarrhythmia develops. Combined oral contraceptives and HRT are associated with an increased risk of thromboembolism and reinfarction, and should be withdrawn. Non–steroidal anti–inflammatories not only increase the risk of bleeding from the GI tract, but also reduce the effectiveness of aspirin and are associated with higher rate of myocardial infarction and death. Similarly, COX–2 inhibitors should be avoided in the post–infarct period.

7.7.5.11　Symptomatic treatment

Hypokalaemia is common in patients with acute infarction, and is related to prior treatment with diuretics or catecholamine effects on electrolyte handling. Hypokalaemia is associated with myocardial electrical instability and should be corrected. If serum potassium is below 4.0 mmol/L in the absence of an important arrhythmia, then oral potassium supplements are given (e.g., slow K, three tablets three times daily, providing approximately 72 mmol potassium daily) and potassium needs to be rechecked after 12–18 hours.

A number of studies (including LIMIT–2) suggested that routine administration of magnesium may reduce mortality of acute infarction by beneficial effects on heart rate, contractility, electrical stability and platelet activity, but there is no good evidence to support the routine use of magnesium in patients with evolving acute MI. Magnesium is, however, still indicated for the treatment of arrhythmias.

Li Nan

Chapter 8

Heart Failure

Heart failure (HF) is a complex clinical syndrome resulting from structural and functional impairment of ventricular filling or ejection of blood. Although most patients have impairment of myocardial performance, heart failure can occur ranging from normal ventricular size and function to marked dilation and reduced function.

8.1　Etiology

Any condition that causes changes in the structure or function of the heart can cause heart failure. Coronary arteriosclerotic cardiopathy(CAD), hypertension, rheumatic heart disease, cardiomyopathy, valve disease, infect and so on can be the causes of heart failure. The common causes of acute heart failure include: ①acute exacerbation of chronic heart failure(About 80% of the causes); ②acute myocardial necrosis and/or injury: acute coronary syndrome, acute severe myocarditis, perinatal cardiomyopathy, myocardial injury or necrosis caused by drugs or poisons, etc. ; ③acute hemodynamic disorder: valvular injury (valve stenosis, regurgitation, rupture of chordae tendineae) and acute injury of artificial valve, hypertension crisis, aortic dissection, cardiac tamponade, fluid infusion too quickly with basic heart disease, etc.

8.2　Nosogenesis

8.2.1　Acute myocardial injury and necrosis

Reduction of contractile units in the myocardium.

8.2.2　Hemodynamic disorder

Decreased cardiac output, inadequate perfusion of peripheral tissues and organs, leading to organ dysfunction and peripheral circulatory disorder, cardiogenic shock. Increased left ventricular end-diastolic pressure and pulmonary capillary wedge pressure can lead to hypoxemia. Increased right ventricular filling pressure, resulting in water and sodium retention and edema.

8.2.3　Neuroendocrine activation

Long-term hyperstimulation of sympathetic nervous system and renin-angiotensin-aldosterone system (RAAS) may lead to increased myocardial injury, decreased cardiac function and hemodynamic disorders.

8.2.4　Cardiorenal syndrome

Heart failure and renal failure often coexist and reciprocal causation, which is called cardiorenal syndrome.

8.3　Clinical manifestations

8.3.1　Acute pulmonary edema

Cough, wheezing, dyspnea (exertional, paroxysmal nocturnal dyspnea, orthopnea), Breathing frequency up to 30-50 times/min, frothy pink or white sputum, moist and/or wheezes pulmonary rales, tachycardic, hypertensive, arrhythmia(such as atrial fibrillation or premature ventricular contractions), and a third heart sound (S3) or fourth heart sound (S4).

8.3.2　Tissue hypoperfusion

①Skin wet and cold, pale and cyanotic. ②Tachycardic(>110 beats/min), pulse pressure (low), pulsus alternans. ③Significant reduction in urine discharge or even anuria. ④Disturbance of consciousness, often restlessness, agitation, anxiety, fear, and feeling of impending death. ⑤Hypoxemia and metabolic acidosis.

8.3.3　Other signs and symptoms

Depression, sleep disturbances, palpitations, orthostatic hypotension, peripheral edema (legs, sacral), ascites, hepatomegaly, jugular venous distention, hepatojugular reflex, sympathetic nervous excite, etc.

8.4　Ancillary inspction

8.4.1　Chest radiography

Chest radiography could show the degree of pulmonary congestion and pulmonary edema, and evaluate basic or accompanying heart and lung diseases based on enlargement of the cardiac image and its morphological changes.

8.4.2　Electrocardiogram(ECG)

Electrocardiogram provides information on heart frequency, rhythm, conduction, etc. ECG abnormalities are extremely common in patients with AHF. It could show myocardial ischemia, ST-segment elevation or non-ST-segment elevation myocardial infarction, etc. Careful attention for ECG changes suggestive of ischemia is of importance, because troponin elevation is common in AHF regardless of cause and thus may not be a reliable marker of acute coronary syndromes.

8.4.3 Echocardiogram

Echocardiogram is perhaps the single most useful test in investigation of the cause of AHF, echocardiography can assess global systolic and diastolic function, regional wall motion abnormalities, valvular function, hemodynamics including estimation of filling pressures and cardiac output, and pericardial disease.

8.4.4 Heart failure markers

The increased concentration of brain natriuretic peptide (BNP) and N-terminal pro-brain natriuretic peptide (NT-proBNP) has been recognized as an objective indicator for diagnosis of heart failure. If BNP< 100 ng/L or NT-proBNP<400 ng/L, the likelihood of heart failure is very low, with a negative predictive value of 90%. If BNP>400 ng/L or NT-proBNP>1,500 ng/L, the likelihood of heart failure is high, with a positive predictive value of 90%. If BNP is normal or low, the possibility of acute heart failure almost could be excluded.

8.4.5 Myocardial injury marker

The purpose of testing the biological makers to evaluate the presence and severity of myocardial injury or necrosis. The specificity and sensitivity of cardiac troponin T or I(cTnT or cTnI) monitoring myocardial damage are higher. Chronic heart failure can also be elevated. Creatine phosphokinase isoenzyme(CK-MB) and myohemoglobin can also be used as auxiliary indexes.

8.4.6 Other Laboratory Tests

Blood routine, liver function, renal function, electrolyte, blood sugar, blood gas analysis, etc.

8.5 Severity classification

Killip classification is suitable for evaluating the severity of heart failure in acute myocardial infarction.

Grade I : No clinical symptoms and signs of heart failure.

Grade II : Have clinical symptoms and signs of heart failure, lung field moist rales less than 50%, cardiac third heart sound (S3), pulmonary venous hypertension, chest radiographs showing pulmonary congestion.

Grade III : Clinical symptoms and signs of severe heart failure, severe pulmonary edema, lung field moist rales above 50%.

Grade IV : Cardiogenic shock.

8.6 Diagnosis

According to the typical symptoms and signs, the diagnosis can be made. The main points of diagnosis are: ①used to be basic heart disease, or no basic heart disease. ②Burst with dyspnea, orthopnea, cough frothy pink sputum. ③Pallor, cyanosis of lips, sweat profusely, heart rate 130-140 beats/min. ④Chest Radiography show pulmonary interstitial edema.

8.7　Differential diagnosis

In the differential diagnosis, we should consider the common causes of acute respiratory distress: asthma, chronic obstructive pulmonary disease, pneumonia, pulmonary embolus, allergic reactions, and other causes of respiratory failure. Other causes of noncardiogenic pulmonary edema also should be considered in differential diagnosis, such as drug-related alveolar capillary damage or acute respiratory distress syndrome.

8.8　Treatment

Acute heart failure is life-threatening and should be saved quickly. The goals of emergency treatment include: relieving dyspnea, stabilizing hemodynamic state, correcting electrolyte disorders and acid-base imbalance, removing the cause and precipitating triggers for the episode of AHF, protecting of liver, kidney, lung and other important organs function.

8.8.1　General treatment

8.8.1.1　Body position

The patient maintains a sitting or semi-lying position, the drooping of the legs reduces the amount of blood returned to the heart to reduce the preload of the heart.

8.8.1.2　Oxygen therapy

High flow nasal catheter oxygen inhalation at 4-8 L/min, 20%-40% alcohol or silicone defoamer can be added to the humidifying bottle to improve alveolar ventilation. Twenty-eight percent of concentration oxygen is given to COPD patients by inhalation mask. If hypoxia persists despite oxygen therapy, or if the patient is showing signs of respiratory distress (tripod stature, accessory muscle use, inability to speak), continuous positive airway pressure (CPAP) or biphasic positive airway pressure (BiPAP) should be applied.

8.8.2　Medications treatment

8.8.2.1　Morphia

Morphia could relieve pain and anxiety, attenuate central sympathetic impulse, dilate peripheral veins and arterioles, reduce myocardial oxygen demand. The close of 2.5-5 mg could be given slowly via intravenous injection, also hypodermic or intramuscular injection and could be repeat after 15 minutes. But attention should be paid for the side effects of its respiratory suppression Taboo application in, especially for the patients who are smoker and under shock condition, or have disturbance of consciousness, chronic obstructive pulmonary disease, etc. Elderly patients should be carefully given at relatively low dose.

8.8.2.2　Diuretics

Diuretics are the primary drugs for treatment of volume overload in patients of AHF and generally produce rapid symptom relief in most patients. Diuretics have rapid diuretic effect, can reduce circulating blood volume and improve oxygen supply. Furosemide at dose of 20-40 mg could be given intravenously within 2 minutes and the dosage could be in creased or reused if it is necessary. Diuretic action usually starts within 5 minutes and lasts about 2 hours. Doctors should pay a great attention when using diuretic to the AMI patients with acute left ventricular failure to avoid inducing hypotension.

8.8.2.3 Vasodilators

Vasodilators can be used in combination with diuretics to treat patients without hypotension of AHF and improve congestive symptoms. Vasodilators can be classified as predominantly venous dilators, with consequent reduction in preload; arterial dilators, leading to a decrease in afterload; and balanced vasodilators, with combined action on both the venous and the arterial system. Currently available vasodilators include the organic nitrates (nitroglycerin and isosorbide dinitrate), sodium nitroprusside (SNP), and nesiritide. All these medications act by activating soluble guanylate cyclase in smooth muscle cells, leading to higher intracellular concentrations of cyclic guanosine monophosphate and consequent vessel relaxation. Caution should be taken in patients who are preload−or afterload−dependent(severe diastolic dysfunction, aortic stenosis, coronary artery disease), because they may cause severe hypotension.

(1)Nitrates

Organic nitrates are one of the oldest therapeutic agents for management of AHF. These drugs are potent venodilators that can rapidly reduce pulmonary and ventricular filling pressures, and improve pulmonary congestion, dyspnea, and myocardial oxygen demand at low doses. At slightly higher doses, nitrate is also a vasodilator for arterioles, reducing the afterload and increasing cardiac output in the presence of vasoconstrictive drugs. The starting dose of nitroglycerin usually is 20 μg/min with rapid uptitration occurring every 5−15 minutes in either 20−40 μg/min increments or doubling of the dose. The dose may initially be titrated to the goal of immediate symptom relief, but a blood pressure reduction of at least 10 mmHg in mean arterial pressure with a systolic blood pressure (SBP) greater than 100 mmHg may be preferable. The nitrate dose may need to be reduced if SBP is 90−100 mmHg and often will need to be discontinued when SBP below 90 mmHg.

(2)Sodium nitroprusside

Sodium nitroprusside, with a very short half−life, can reduce both the afterload and preload, particularly effective in the setting of markedly elevated afterload (hypertensive AHF). Titration of the Sodium nitroprusside dose could rapidly improve symptoms. The initial dose is 10−15 μg/min, and at the interval of every 5−10 minutes increases 5−10 μg/min until pulmonary edema is alleviated or the arterial systolic pressure drops to 100 mmHg.

(3)Nesiritide

Nesiritide induces potent vasodilation in the venous and arterial vasculatures, leading to significant reductions in venous and ventricular filling pressures and mild increases in cardiac output. Nesiritide may be used for treatment of patients with acutely decompensated congestive heart failure who have dyspnea with minimal activity or at rest, but it's no substitute for diuretics. It could enhance diuresis, protect renal function, and improve survival. An optional bolus of 2 μg/kg followed by a 0.01 μg/(kg · min) infusion is the recommended starting dose for nesiritide. However, its high cost and lack of clear clinical benefit over other less expensive and more readily titratable agents make its application limited.

8.8.2.4 Positive inotropic drugs

(1)Inodilators

Inodilators (inotropic drugs with vasodilatory properties) increase cardiac output and reduce PCWP. However, even the short term use (hours to a few days) of intravenous inotropes (except for digoxin) is associated with significant side effects such as hypotension, atrial or ventricular arrhythmias, an increased hospitalization and possibly high mortality for long term. The risk of adverse events may be higher in patients with coronary heart disease due to decreased coronary artery perfusion and increased myocardial oxygen demand along with possible myocardial ischemia and injury.

(2) Digitaloid drugs

The most commonly used digitalis drugs are digoxin and cedilanid. Cedilanid rapidly improves hemodynamics without increasing heart rate or decreasing blood pressure and may be considered to give the patients with a low blood pressure resulting from a low cardiac output. Cedilanid is generally used intravenously with an initial dose of 0. 2–0. 4 mg, it could be reused 0. 2 mg after 2–4 hours if it is necessary. Cedilanid is especially suitabled for the patients with rapid atrial fibrillation and heart failure ischemia. Hypokalemia and hypomagnesemia may increase the likelihood of developing digitalis poisoning, even at the therapeutic doses.

(3) Dobutamine

Dobutamine is the most commonly used positive inotrope in Europe and the United States, despite evidence that it increases mortality. Dobutamine at a dose of 1–2 μg/(kg · min) could improve renal perfusion in most patients. However, patients with more profound hypoperfusion may need a high dose of 5–10 μg/(kg · min). Tachyphylaxis may occur with infusions lasting for longer than 24–48 hours, owing in part to receptor desensitization. In general, dobutamine (or dopamine) is generally the first choice of inotropic drugs in patients with significant hypotension and in the setting of significant renal dysfunction, in keeping with the renal excretion of milrinone. The lowest effective dose of dobutamine should be used with continuous blood pressure and rhythm monitoring.

(4) Dopamine

As a precursor of norepinephrine, an agonist of both adrenergic and dopaminergic receptors, and an inhibitor of norepinephrine uptake, dopamine has complex effects that vary significantly with dose. The onset of dopamine therapy leads to the rapid release of norepinephrine, which can lead to tachycardia, atrial arrhythmias and ventricular arrhythmias. In addition, moderate to high doses can lead to severe vasoconstriction, precipitating heart failure and low perfusion. Dopamine is usually given at the dose of 250–500 μg/min through intravenous infusion, but the individual difference of drug effect is large, generally starting from low doses, gradually increasing the dose, and keeping short–term application. Dopamine dosing should be gradually decreased from these doses down to 3–5 μg/(kg · min) and then discontinued to avoid potential hypotensive effects of low–dose dopamine.

(5) Epinephrine

Epinephrine is a full beta receptor agonist and a potent inotropic agent with balanced vasodilator and vasoconstrictor effects. The direct effect of epinephrine on increasing inotropy independent of myocardial catecholamine stores makes it a useful agent in the treatment of transplant recipients with denervated hearts.

(6) Phosphodiesterase inhibitors

Cyclic AMP is a ubiquitous signaling molecule that increases inotropy, chronotropy, and lusitropy in cardiomyocytes and causes vasorelaxation in vascular smooth muscle. Phosphodiesterase IIIA is decomposed in the cardiac and vascular smooth muscle, and the signal activity of cAMP is terminated by degrading it into AMP. The commonly used drugs are milrinone and amrinone.

(7) Levosimendan

Levosimendan is a calcium sensitizer that increases myocardial contractility and produces peripheral vasodilation, it is suitable for a poor therapeutic effect from traditional therapy (diuretics, digitalis, vasodilators, etc.), and a short–term treatment of acute decompensated heart failure requiring increased myocardial contractility. It is used in patients with reduced LV systolic function and hypoperfusion in the absence of severe hypotension. It can significantly increase cardiac output, reduce PCWP and afterload, and decrease dyspnea. The first dose is 12–24 μg/kg intravenous injection, followed by 0.1 μg/(kg · min) intravenous drip, which can be halved or doubled as appropriate.

8.8.2.5   Bronchial antispasmodic

Aminophylline 0.125–0.25 g, diluted with glucose solution, slowly intravenous injection (10 minutes) or intravenous drip. Can be repeated once after 4–6 hours.

8.8.3   Non-medication therapy

For patients with poor or ineffective medication therapy, non-drug therapy may be considered, including intra-aortic balloon repulsive surgery, mechanical ventilation, blood purification therapy, and mechanically assisted circulation, etc.

Deng Ying

Chapter 9

Aortic Dissection

Acute aortic syndromes include aortic dissection, aortic intramural hematoma (IMH), and penetrating atherosclerotic ulcer (PAU). Aortic dissection refers to intimal disruption leading to a dissection plane in the aortic wall that may propagate anterogradely (or less commonly, retrogradely) throughout the length of the aorta, and form two layers separation of the aorta wall.

9.1 Etiology

Hypertension occurs in approximately 80% of all patients who suffer aortic dissection. Genetically triggered aortic syndromes, congenital heart diseases, atherosclerosis, inflammatory vascular diseases, cocaine use, and iatrogenic causes are also risk factors for aortic dissection.

9.2 Nosogenesis

Hypertension leads to changes in arterial wall structure, including intimal thickening, calcification, and adventitial fibrosis. These alterations may affect the elastic properties of the arterial wall and increase stiffness and thereby predispose to aneurysm or dissection. In the early stage of intimal tear, the blood from the true lumen flows into the middle or outer membrane of the aorta, forming a false lumen. The true and false lumina is separated by a layer of internal diaphragm. Dissection may extend to the proximal or distal end of the aorta, resulting in stenosis or blockage of branches of the aorta.

9.3 Clinical manifestations

9.3.1 Pain

The most common symptom of acute aortic dissection is pain. The pain is usually intense and unbearable, reaching a peak when the disease begins, taking the form of a knife cut and torn. The pain may be accompanied by a "sense of doom." The quality of the pain is most commonly described as "sharp" "severe" or "stabbing". The pain is not significant in a few slow onset patients. Some aortic dissections are characterized by chest burning, pressure, or pleuritic pain, even complications of aortic dissection, such as syncope, heart failure, or stroke.

9.3.2 Hypertension

Most of the patients are accompanied by hypertension. For the patients with primay hyertension, the aortic dedissection can make the blood pressure higher due to the sharp pain. Some patients may have differences in blood pressure and pulse in two upper limbs. Blood pressure drops if the outer membrane is ruptured and haemorrhaged.

9.3.3 Cardiovascular symptoms

Dissection involved aortic valve may lead to aortic valve insufficiency, diastolic blowing murmur could be heard in the valvular auscultation area, and increased pulse pressure might present. Aortic valve reflux can cause heart failure. The branches of the aorta were compressed compressed aortic branches could cassce weaken or disappenred pulse at the affected side. Dissection rupturing into pericardial cavity, and pleural cavity can cause cardiac tamponade and pleural effusion.

9.3.4 Nervous system symptoms

Impairment of nerve function with occours in about 15% -20% of aortic dissection patients. Dissection that extends to the branches of the aorta(such as arteria carotis) or intercostal artery can cause cerebral or spinal cord ischemia, which further causes hemiplegia, mental retardation, paraplegia, limb numbness, etc. Two to seven percents of the patients have syncope, but have no other neurological symptoms.

9.3.5 Other symptoms

Nausea, vomiting, abdominal distension, diarrhea, black stool and so on might be caused by abdominal and mesenteric artery compressioned by separation of aortic dissection; Horner syndrome is caused by compression of sympathetic nerve; hoarseness is caused by compression of recurrent laryngeal nerve; superior vena cava syndrome is caused by compression of superior vena cava; aortic dissection involved renal artery may cause hematuria, oliguria or anuria.

9.4 Accessory examination

9.4.1 Chest radiograph

The most common abnormality seen on the chest radiograph is an abnormal aortic contour or widening of the aortic silhouette. If calcification of the aortic knob occurs, one may detect the separation of the intimal calcification from the outer aortic soft tissue border by more than 0.5-1.0 cm the "calcium sign". Even though most patients with aortic dissection will have abnormal findings on the chest radiograph, but 12% -15% have chest radiographs with normal findings. Thus normal chest radiograph results can not exclude the presence of an aortic dissection.

9.4.2   Electrocardiogram

In patients with aortic dissection the electrocardiogram findings are nonspecific but may indicate acute complications such as myocardial ischemia or infarction related to coronary artery involvement or acute pericarditis and so on, But one third of the patients has normal electrocardiogram.

9.4.3   Laboratory examination

The increase of serum myosin heavy chain concentration in smooth muscle is the most important biochemical index for the diagnosis of aortic dissection. The leukocyte count is increased and the creative protein is increased, bilirubin and lactate dehydrogenase are increased. Gross hematuria or red blood cells appear in urine.

9.4.4   CT examination

The most commonly used method for the diagnosis of aortic dissection is CT examination. CT without contrast enhancement, aortic dissection may go undetected. Contrast-enhanced CT is the modality most commonly used for evaluating aortic dissection. CT can show dilatation of diseased aorta can find and calcification of the aorta intima. If the intima moves toward the center, the aortic dissection is indicated, and the outward displacement indicates the aneurysm. It can also show the intima film caused by aortic intimal tear. The accuracy of CT in the diagnosis of descending aortic dissection is higher than that in other sites, but it is difficult to judge the existence of aortic insufficiency. Contrast-enhanced CT is highly accurate in diagnosing aortic dissection, with a sensitivity and specificity of 98%–100%.

9.4.5   Magnetic resonance imaging

MRI is highly accurate in evaluating aortic dissection, its accuracy being similar to or higher than that of CT, and does not require intravenous iodinated contrast agent or ionizing radiation. MRI may detect pericardial effusion, aortic rupture, entry points, and exit points with a high level of accuracy and is considered to be " the gold standard " for the diagnosis of aortic dissection. But the examination takes a long time (30–60 minutes) and is not safe for patients with emergency and hemodynamic instability. It is contraindicated in patients with certain implantable devices (pacemaker, defibrillator) and other metallic implants.

9.4.6   Echocardiography

Echocardiography is valuable in the diagnosis of ascending aortic dissection and can identify complications of pericardial hemorrhage, aortic valve insufficiency and pleural hemorrhage, but the sensitivity of diagnosis of descending aortic dissection is low. In recent years, Transesophageal Echocardiography (TEE) is highly accurate in the evaluation and diagnosis of acute aortic dissection. It has high sensitivity and specificity in judging aortic valve insufficiency and pericardial effusion and has high sensitivity in judging intimal tear and pseudoluminal thrombus, can be used in patients with hemodynamic instability, but its accuracy is operator dependent.

9.4.7   Other inspections

Aortography and intravascular ultrasound are invasive examinations, which are dangerous and rarely used in clinical practice.

9.5 Classification

The classification of aortic dissection is shown in Table 9-1.

9.6 Diagnosis

Diagnosis can be made by combining clinical manifestation with related auxiliary examination (such as echocardiography, CT, magnetic resonance imaging).

Table 9-1　The classification of aortic dissection

DeBakey classification		Stanford classification	
I classification	The intimal tear is located in the ascending aorta, and expanded into the abdominal aorta	A classification	Intimal tear may be located in ascending aorta, aortic arch or proximal descending aorta
II classification	Intimal tear is located in ascending aorta, and expansion is limited in ascending aorta	B classification	The laceration of the intima is often located at the isthmus of the aorta and beyond
III classification	Intimal tear is located at the isthmus of the aorta and beyond		
IIIa classification	Expansion only invdves descending aorta		
IIIb classification	Expansion reaches to the abdominal aorta		

9.7 Differential diagnosis

Diseases that need to be distinguished from aortic dissection include: acute coronary syndrome, pulmonary embolism, pneumothorax, aortic aneurysm without dissection, aortic insufficiency without dissection, musculoskeletal pain, pericarditis, pleurisy, mediastinal tumor, cholecystitis, cerebral apoplexy and so on.

9.8 Treatment

Anyone diagnosed or suspected of this disease should be admitted to the intensive care unit immediately. The treatment is divided into two stages: emergency treatment and follow-up treatment.

9.8.1 Emergency treatment

9.8.1.1 General treatment

Keep calm, take a rest and avoid emotional agitation. The patients with severe pain could be given morphine to relieve pain. Doctors should pay close attention to the changes of nervous system, pulse, heart sounds, monitor life indicators, electrocardiogram, urine volume, etc. Avoid to provide too much fluid, intravenously and lest cause hypertension and pulmonary edema and other complications.

9.8.1.2 Controlling blood pressure and lowering heart rate

Both blood pressure and heart rate are involved in the shear force applied to the aorta, which is the main factor in the occurrence of aortic dissection. Beta receptor blockers and vasodilators could be to reduce vascular resistance, vessel wall tension and ventricular contractility, and reduce the rate of changes of left ventricular systolic pressure in aorta. The targets are systolic blood pressure at 100–120 mmHg and heart rate at 60–75 beats/min. Commonly used drugs include esmolol, labetolol and so on. Vasodilators, such as nitroprusside, should be used only after adequate inotropic blockade has been made with β–receptor or calcium channel blockers. When a patient being suspected with aortic dissection has significant hypotension, yapid and large volume liquid expansion should be given as the dropped blood pressure might be resulted from cardiac tamponade or aortic rcepture with hemorrhage into the medastinum plearoll space of abdomen. Pain relief and disappearance after blood pressure drop are the signs that aortic dissection stops expanding.

9.8.1.3 Surgical treatment

Definitive therapy for acute aortic dissection includes emergency surgery. In general, patients with dissection of the ascending aorta require prompt surgical intervention. Immediate surgical treatment improves survival in patients with acute type A aortic dissection compared with medical therapy. The operative care of dissection of only the descending aorta is controversial and should be evaluated on a case–by–case basis. Patients with aortic dissection require emergent vascular or thoracic surgical consultation that assesses the possibility, advantages and disadvantages, risks and so on of the operation.

9.8.1.4 Other treatments

Patients with severe hemodynamic instability should be given immediate endotracheal intubation, and supplementary blood volume. For the patients with dissection rupture and bleeding into the pericardium and thorax blood transfusion should be given. It is important to monitor the blood pressure of bilateral upper limbs in order to eliminate pseudohypotension caused by blockage of branches of aortic arch. As soon as cardiac tamponade is found, sternotomy should be performed immediately. Pericardial puncture and drainage before operation may be harmful and may cause rebleeding after lower pericardial pressure.

9.8.2 Follow–up treatment

After stabilization, oral antihypertensive drugs can be used to control blood pressure, and the CT, MRI and other examinations in time should be done to decide the next treatment plan (surgical or interventional treatment, etc.). β–receptor blockers and strict blood pressure control are the basis of treatment to the survival patients of aortic dissection. Regardless of the initial treatment plan, doctors should review MRI or CT at every 6 to 12 months interval to detect aortic diameter, tear and repair status.

Deng Ying

Chapter 10

Influenza

10.1 Introduction

The outbreak of influenza is urgent, although most of it is self limiting, but some complications such as pneumonia can be developed from severe influenza, a few severe cases are patients progressed rapidly, and can be died of acute respiratory distress syndrome (ARDS) or multiple organ failure. Severe influenza mainly occurs in the elderly, young children, pregnant women or those with chronic underlying diseases and so on, and can also occur in the general population.

10.2 Epidemiologye

Influenza viruses belong to the RNA virus. They have a lipid envelope from the surface of which the hemagglutinin(H) and neuraminidase(N) glycoproteins project. Influenza A and B viruses constitute one genus, and influenza C viruses make up the other. The designation of influenza viruses as type A, B, or C is based on antigenic characteristics of the nucleoprotein (NP) and matrix (M) protein antigens. The most extensive and severe outbreak are caused by influenza A viruses.

10.2.1 Source of infection

Influenza patients and recessively infected patients are the main sources of influenza. It is contagious from the end of incubation period to the acute stage. Infected animals can also become sources of infection. Close contact may cause human influenza infection by infecteds animals.

10.2.2 Route of transmission

Influenza mainly spreads through droplets such as sneezing and coughing, and can also be transmitted directly or indirectly through mucous membranes such as oral cavity, nasal cavity and eye. Exposure to substances contaminated by viruses can also cause infection. Human infection with avian influenza is mainly achieved through direct contact with infected animals or contaminated environment.

10.2.3　Susceptible population

The crowd is generally susceptible.

The following groups of people infected with influenza virus are more likely to develop into severe cases.

(1) Children below 5 years of age.

(2) People over 65 years of age.

(3) The patients with the following diseases or conditions: chronic respiratory disease, cardiovascular diseases, nephropathy, hepatopathy, hematological diseases, nervous system and neuromuscular diseases, metabolic and endocrine system diseases, immune function inhibition.

(4) Obese patients (BMI>30 kg/m^2).

(5) Pregnant women.

10.3　Pathophysiology

The initial event of influenza is infection of the respiratory epithelium with influenza virus acquired from respiratory secretions of acutely infected individuals. Viral infection involves the ciliated columnar epithelial cells, the viral genome is transcribed and replicated in the nucleus. The hemagglutinin is the site by which virus binds to cell receptors, whereas the neuraminidase degrades the receptor and probably plays a role in the release of virus from infected cells after replication has taken place. Influenza viruses enter cells by receptor-mediated endocytosis, forming a virus-containing endosome. The viral hemagglutinin mediates fusion of the endosome membrane with the virus envelope, and nucleocapsids are subsequently released into the cytoplasm. In infected cells, virus replicates within 4-6 hours, after which infectious virus is released to infect adjacent or nearby cells. In this way, infection spreads from a few foci to a large number of respiratory cells over several hours. Histopathologic study reveals degenerative changes, including granulation, vacuolization, swelling, and pyknotic nuclei, in infected ciliated cells. The cells eventually become necrotic and desquamated; in some areas, previously columnar epithelium is replaced by flattened and metaplastic epithelial cells.

10.4　Clinical manifestation

The incubation period is usually 1-7 days, The most are 2-4 days.

Influenza has frequently been described as an illness characterized by the abrupt onset of systemic symptoms, such as headache, feverishness, chills, myalgia, or malaise, and accompanying respiratory tract signs, particularly cough and sore throat. However, the spectrum of clinical presentations is wide, ranging from a mild, afebrile respiratory illness similar to the common cold to severe prostration with relatively few respiratory signs and symptoms. In most of the cases, the patient has a fever, with a temperature of 38-41 ℃. A rapid temperature increase within the first 24 hours of illness is generally followed by gradual defervescence over 2-3 days, although, on occasion, fever may last as long as one week. Headache, either generalized or frontal, is often particularly troublesome.

Respiratory symptoms often become more prominent as systemic symptoms subside. Many patients have a sore throat or persistent cough, which may last for ≥ one week or even longer which is often accompanied by substernal discomfort. Ocular signs and symptoms include pain on motion of the eyes, photophobia, and burning of the eyes.

In uncomplicated influenza, the acute illness generally resolves over 2−5 days, and most patients have largely recovered in one week, although cough may persist for 1−2 weeks or longer.

10.5　Complications

Pneumonia is the most common complication of influenza. Other complications include nervous system damage, heart damage, myositis, rhabdomyolysis and septic shock.

10.5.1　Pneumonia

The most significant complication of influenza is pneumonia："primary" influenza viral pneumonia, secondary bacterial pneumonia, or mixed viral and bacterial pneumonia.

The disease is aggravated within 2−4 days after the onset of influenza, or worsened after the recovery period of the influenza. High fever, severe cough, pyogenic sputum, dyspnea, and pulmonary moist rales will present. The total number of leukocytes and neutrophils are increased significantly in peripheral blood. The main pathogens were streptococcus pneumoniae, staphylococcus aureus and haemophilus influenzae.

10.5.2　Nervous system injury

Central nervous system diseases, including encephalitis, transverse myelitis, and Guillain−Barré syndrome, have been reported during in influenza cases. The etiologic relationship of influenza virus to such CNS illnesses remains uncertain.

10.5.3　Heart injury

Heart injury is not common in influenza, mainly include myocarditis and pericarditis, which may be accompanied with increatine kinase and ECG abnormalities, severe cases can have heart failure.

10.5.4　Myositis and rhabdomyolysis

The main symptoms are myalgia and myasthenia, serum levels of creatine phosphokinase and aldolase are markedly elevated, and occasionally patients develop renal failure from myoglobinuria.

10.5.5　Septic shock

The severe inf luenza might develop septic shock which is manifested as hyperthermia, shock and multiple organ dysfunction.

10.6　Laboratory findings and diagnosis

During acute influenza, virus may be detected in throat swabs, nasopharyngeal washes, or sputum. Most commonly, the laboratory diagnosis is established with rapid viral tests that detect viral nucleoprotein or neuraminidase by means of immunologic or enzymatic techniques that are highly sensitive and 60% –90% as specific as tissue culture. Viral nucleic acids can also be detected in clinical samples by reverse transcriptase polymerase chain reaction. The type of the infecting influenza virus may be determined by either immunofluorescence or HI techniques, and the hemagglutinin subtype of influenza A virus may be identified by HI with use of subtype–specific antisera.

10.7   Treatment

In uncomplicated cases of influenza, symptom–based therapy with acetaminophen for the relief of headache, myalgia, and fever may be considered, but the use of salicylates should be avoided in children below 18 years of age because of the possible association of salicylates with Reye's syndrome. Because cough is ordinarily self–limited, treatment with cough suppressants generally is not indicated, although codeine–containing compounds may be used if the cough is particularly troublesome.

Patients should be advised to rest and maintain hydration during acute illness and to return to full activity only gradually after illness has resolved, especially if it has been severe.

10.8   Prophylaxisp

10.8.1   Vaccinations

Influenza vaccination is the most effective way to prevent influenza, which can significantly reduce the risk of influenza and serious complications. The vast majority of currently used vaccines are inactivated preparations derived from influenza A and B viruses that spread during the previous influenza season. Vaccine should be administered early in the autumn before influenza outbreak occur and should then be given annually to maintain immunity against the most current influenza virus strains.

10.8.2   Drug prevention

Antiviral drugs may be used as chemoprophylaxis against influenza, but it is not a substitute for vaccination. It can only be used as an emergency temporary preventive measure for high–risk groups of severe influenza without vaccination or have not gained immunity after vaccination.

Zhang Guoxiu

Chapter 11

Dyspnea

11.1 Introduction

Dyspnea, or breathing discomfort, is a common symptom that afflicts millions of patients with pulmonary disease and may be the primary manifestation of lung disease, myocardial ischemia or dysfunction, anemia, neuromuscular disorders, obesity, or deconditioning. The term of dyspnea suggests that this symptom represents a number of qualitatively distinct sensations, and that the words utilized by patients to describe their breathing discomfort may provide insight into the underlying pathophysiology of the disease.

11.2 Deffintion of dyspena

Dyspnea may be acute when it develops over hours to days and chronic when it has been for more than four to eight weeks. Some patients present with acute worsening of chronic breathlessness that might be caused by a new problem or a worsening of the underlying disease.

11.3 Pathophysiology

Most patients with breathing discomfort can be categorized into one of two groups: respiratory system dyspnea or cardiovascular system dyspnea. Respiratory system dyspnea includes discomfort related to disorders of the central controller, the ventilatory pump, and the gas exchanger, while cardiovascular system dyspnea includes cardiac diseases, anemia, and deconditioning. More than one process may be active in a given patient, and the basic physiology of dyspnea does not always adhere to this structure; for example, stimulation of pulmonary receptors can result from interstitial inflammation (respiratory system) or interstitial edema (cardiovascular system).

11.3.1   Respiratory dyspnea

The respiratory system is designed to move air by bulk transport from the atmosphere to the alveoli, where oxygen uptake into the blood and elimination of carbon dioxide occurs by diffusion across the alveolar –capillary membrane. Carbon dioxide is then removed from the lungs by bulk transport to the atmosphere. Several components must be functioning smoothly for this process to occur; derangements in any of these elements can lead to dyspnea.

11.3.2   Cardiovascular dyspnea

The cardiovascular system is designed to move oxygenated blood from the lungs to metabolically active tissues, and then transport carbon dioxide from the tissues back to the lungs. For this system to work optimally and avert breathing discomfort, one must have a pump that functions without generating high pulmonary capillary pressures. There must also be sufficient hemoglobin to carry oxygen and appropriate enzymes to utilize oxygen in the tissues.

11.3.3   Heart failure

Heart failure is a clinical syndrome that can result from any structural or functional cardiac disorder that impairs the ability of the ventricle(s) to fill with or eject blood. Symptoms of heart failure fall into two major classes: those due to a reduction in cardiac output (fatigue, weakness) and those due to increased pulmonary or systemic venous pressure and fluid accumulation (dyspnea, edema, hepatic congestion, and ascites). When heart failure causes an increase in pulmonary venous pressure, it can lead to dyspnea either by producing hypoxemia or by stimulating pulmonary vascular and/or interstitial receptors (e. g. , unmyelinated J–receptors, also called C–fibers). Causes of heart failure include ventricular systolic dysfunction, ventricular diastolic dysfunction, and valvular disease.

11.4   Clinical assessment

While clinical history is often insufficient to make a affirmatory diagnosis, it provides guidance in narrowing the diagnostic scope and selecting diagnostic tests. In one study of 85 patients presenting to a pulmonary unit with a complaint of chronic dyspnea, the initial diagnosis of the etiology of dyspnea based upon the patient history alone was correct in only 66% of cases. Thus, a systematic diagnostic approach to these patients is necessary.

11.4.1   Exertional and nocturnal dyspnea

Chronic exertional dyspnea and paroxysmal nocturnal dyspnea (PND) are both associated with heart failure, although nocturnal dyspnea is more specific to heart failure. Asthma is also associated with exertional and nocturnal dyspnea, and does not usually improve with sitting or standing, which is not like PND.

Dyspnea that is not exacerbated by exertion is more often due to a functional or perceptual problem than to cardiopulmonary disease.

11.4.2   Intermittent dyspnea

Intermittent dyspnea associated with cold air or animal dander exposure suggests asthma; work–related dyspnea may suggest occupational asthma; and dyspnea following upper respiratory infections may be due to asthma or chronic obstructive pulmonary disease (COPD).

In addition to asthma, intermittent symptoms that resolve completely between episodes can be seen with recurrent aspiration; recurrent pulmonary emboli and heart failure can also wax be and wane, but generally are characterized by a baseline level of dysfunction. The presence of specific, reproducible inciting events such as exercise or cold air exposure is common with airways hyperreactivity.

The rapidity with which symptoms develop during exercise can also provide useful diagnostic information. For example, patients who develop shortness of breath and wheezing after walking 50-100 feet often have acute elevations in pulmonary capillary wedge pressure (usually due to cardiac diastolic dysfunction) or pulmonary hypertension. In contrast, symptoms of exercise-induced asthma usually are precipitated by more intense activity, beginning three minutes into after exercise, peaking within 10-15 minutes, and resolving by 60 minutes. Respiratory muscle weakness generally leads to gradually progressive dyspnea, sometimes with an acute worsening at a time of illness, particularly a respiratory infection.

11.4.3 Severity of dyspnea

For patients with chronic dyspnea, formal assessment of the severity of dyspnea can help create a baseline for future comparisons. A number of instruments are available to help assess the severity of dyspnea, such as the Baseline Dyspnea Index, the Modified Medical Research Council (mMRC) dyspnea scale, and the Borg scale. It is important to note that scales like the mMRC do not measure dyspnea directly; rather, they assess the intensity of exercise that provokes dyspnea and, indirectly, the degree of disability resulting from dyspnea.

Associated symptoms such as cough, sputum production, nasal congestion, chest pain, peripheral edema, Raynaud phenomenon, joint swelling, and muscle weakness can help identify areas for further investigation. As examples, asymmetric lower extremity edema might suggest venous thromboembolic disease; Raynaud phenomenon is seen in a number of rheumatic diseases that are associated with interstitial lung disease or pulmonary hypertension; and symmetric swelling of the metacarpophalangeal joints may be a clue to rheumatoid lung disease.

11.5 Evaluation of acute dyspnea

Breathing discomfort arising over the course of minutes to hours is generally due to a limited number of conditions and generally involves processes that require prompt evaluation and treatment. Clues to the need for an urgent evaluation include heart rate >120 beats/min, respiratory rate >30 breaths/minute, pulse oxygen saturation (SpO_2) <90%, use of accessory respiratory muscles, difficulty speaking in full sentences, stridor, asymmetric breath sounds or percussion, diffuse crackles, diaphoresis, and cyanosis.

11.6 Initial testing in chronic dyspnea

When evaluating chronic dyspnea, we follow a step-wise diagnostic approach of initial testing, follow-up testing, and advanced testing, starting with the tests that are the least invasive and most likely to yield a diagnosis.

The majority of patients with chronic dyspnea of unclear etiology has one of five diagnoses, although the spectrum of potential causes is broad and more than one etiology may be present. It is also important to remember that the presence of a known chronic cardiopulmonary disease does not guarantee that the patient's symptoms or the etiology of their exercise limitation are due to that condition, particularly in patients with coexisting conditions.

The five most common causes of chronic dyspnea are the following.

- Asthma.
- Chronic obstructive pulmonary disease (COPD).
- Interstitial lung disease.
- Myocardial dysfunction.
- Obesity/deconditioning.

11.6.1   Pace of testing

For patients with chronic dyspnea, the severity of dyspnea and rate of worsening are important determinants of the pace and location of diagnostic testing. The optimal sequence of diagnostic testing for chronic dyspnea has not been determined. We typically follow an algorithm that utilizes three tiers of testing: initial testing, follow-up testing based on results of initial tests, and advanced testing if the diagnosis remains uncertain. Within each tier, we select tests based on the patient's clinical features, results of prior tests, and likelihood of a diagnostic result. One study found that the most informative tests for adults (age 45-84) with dyspnea, but no known cardiopulmonary disease are the forced expiratory volume in one second (FEV_1) obtained by spirometry, the N-terminal pro-brain natriuretic peptide (NT-proBNP), and emphysema on chest computed tomography.

11.6.2   Specific tests

If the clinical evaluation could not narrow the scope of differential diagnosis we usually obtain the following "initial tests".

- Blood count (to exclude anemia): the degree of dyspnea associated with anemia may depend on the rapidity of blood loss and the degree of exertion that the patient undertakes.
- Blood glucose, blood urea nitrogen, creatinine, electrolytes.
- Thyroid stimulating hormone (TSH).
- Spirometry pre and post inhaled bronchodilator OR full pulmonary function tests (PFTs) if the clinical evaluation does not suggest asthma or COPD.
- Pulse oximetry during ambulation at a normal pace over approximately 200 meters and/or up two to three flights of stairs.
- Chest radiograph.
- Electrocardiogram.
- Plasma BNP or NT-proBNP.

Spirometry can identify the presence and severity of airflow obstruction, and when both FEV_1 and forced vital capacity (FVC) are reduced proportionately (i. e., the FEV_1/FVC ratio is normal or high), restrictive disease is suggested. When intrathoracic airflow limitation is noted or when a diagnosis of asthma is suspected, postbronchodilator spirometry determines whether there is reversibility of airflow limitation. Typically in asthma, airflow limitation is reversible, although a large component of airways edema and inflammation may need a course of inhaled or oral glucocorticoid therapy to achieve complete reversibility. Patients with a clinical suspicion of asthma and reversible airflow limitation on spirometry would be managed with a trial of specific therapy for asthma. Patients with a smoking history longer than 20 years and irreversible airflow limitation on spirometry are usually managed with a presumptive diagnosis of chronic obstructive pulmonary disease (COPD). However, other causes of irreversible airflow limitation should be considered if the patient does not respond to empiric therapy for asthma or COPD.

The chest radiograph may identify a pleural effusion, kyphoscoliosis, cardiomegaly, interstitial lung disease, or pulmonary vascular redistribution, as potential causes of dyspnea. A pleural effusion will need a directed evaluation as to the cause (e. g. , benign asbestos effusion, malignancy, trapped lung, rheumatoid effusion, infection, heart failure), usually including thoracentesis. Kyphoscoliosis identified on chest radiograph (and physical examination) is typically evaluated with full pulmonary function tests to determine the likelihood of hypercapnia. Interstitial lung disease is often evaluated further with measurement of lung volumes and diffusing capacity for carbon monoxide (DLCO) and by CT scan of the lungs to help characterize the underlying process. Heart failure suggested by the NT−proBNP and chest radiograph will need further evaluation with an echocardiogram to determine the cause.

11.7   Advanced testing in chronic dyspnea

Referral to a specialist is usually needed for patients who do not respond to treatment for the diagnosis deemed most likely by the initial evaluation and when diagnostic procedures such as a bronchoscopy, lung biopsy, cardiopulmonary exercise test, or pulmonary artery catheterization may be needed. The use of these tests to evaluate dyspnea is described in the table.

11.7.1   Suspected interstitial lung disease

The evaluation of interstitial lung disease that is suspected on the basis of pulmonary function testing and high resolution computed tomography (HRCT) may include additional laboratory testing, bronchoscopy with bronchoalveolar lavage, and lung or mediastinal lymph node biopsy, as described separately.

11.7.2   Pulmonary hypertension suggested by echocardiography

When elevated pulmonary artery pressures are suggested by Doppler echocardiography and are supported by an elevated brain natriuretic peptide (BNP) and oxygen desaturation on exertion, the next step is pulmonary artery catheterization to confirm elevated pulmonary artery systolic pressure (pulmonary arterial systolic pressure [PASP] >25 mmHg at rest) and exclude diastolic dysfunction (unlikely with pulmonary artery wedge pressure [PAWP] <15 mmHg).

11.7.3   Unclear cause of dyspnea on exertion

For patients who have dyspnea that is persistent and unexplained by the results of the above studies, additional testing may be warranted. At this point, it may be reasonable for the patient to engage in a conditioning program for two to three months to see whether dyspnea improves before proceeding with more invasive testing.

11.8 Chronic dyspnea with a normal evaluation

Occasionally patients with chronic dyspnea will go through a complete evaluation without identification of a cause. Others may have near normal testing, such that a slight decrease in peak oxygen uptake, anaerobic threshold, and peak heart rate are thought to be most consistent with deconditioning or obesity. While obese patients frequently report dyspnea, in a given individual it can be difficult to know how much dyspnea is attributable to obesity. For patients who report dyspnea but have normal or near normal testing, we explain the reassuring nature of testing in detail, advise a conditioning program, and ask the patient to return in 6–12 months for re-evaluation. The re-evaluation is important due to the infrequent situation in which a treatable cause of dyspnea is missed initially, but becomes apparent on subsequent testing.

Li Yi

Chapter 12

Hemoptysis

12.1　Epidemiology

Hemoptysis is defined as the expectoration of blood from the respiratory tract below the vocal cords. Most cases seen in the emergency department (ED) are mild episodes of small-volume hemoptysis, typically consisting of either bloodtinged sputum or minute amounts of frank blood and are most commonly caused by bronchitis. Although hemoptysis is commonly seen in the ED, only 1%-5% of hemoptysis patients have massive or life-threatening hemorrhage (generally accepted as 100-600 mL of blood loss in any 24-hour period), which can result in hemodynamic instability, shock, or impaired alveolar gas exchange and has a mortality rate approaching 80%.

12.2　Pathophysiology

Trace hemoptysis typically originates from tracheobronchial cap-illaries that are disrupted by vigorous coughing or minor bronchial infections. Conversely, massive hemoptysis nearly always involves disruption of bronchial or pulmonary arteries, the two sets of vessels that constitute the lung's dual blood supply. Bronchial arteries, which are direct branches from the thoracic aorta, are responsible for supplying oxygenated blood to lung parenchyma, and disruption of these vessels from arteritis, trauma, bronchiectasis or malignant erosion can result in sudden and pro-found hemorrhage. Although small in caliber, the bronchial circulation is a high-pressure system and the culprit in nearly 90% of the cases of massive hemoptysis requiring embolization.

Nearly all causes of hemoptysis have a common mechanism—vascular disruption within the trachea, bronchi, small-caliber airways, or lung parenchyma. Modes of vessel injury include acute and chronic inflammation (from bronchitis and arteritis), local infection (especially lung abscesses, TB, and aspergillosis), trauma, malignant invasion, infarction following a pulmonary embolus, and fistula formation (specifically aortobronchial fistulae).

Bronchiectasis, a chronic necrotizing infection resulting in bronchial wall inflammation and dilation, is one of the most common causes of massive hemoptysis. As tissue destruction and remodeling occur, rupture of nearby bronchial vessels can result in bleeding. Bronchiectasis can complicate chronic airway obstruction, necrotizing pneumonia, TB, or cystic fibrosis.

12.3　Diagnostic approach

12.3.1　Differential considerations

Nasal, oral, or hypo-pharyngeal bleeding sometimes contaminates the tracheobronchial tree, mimicking true hemoptysis. The clinician should closely inspect the nasopharynx and oral cavity to exclude this possibility. Gastric or proximal duodenal bleeding can similarly mimic hemoptysis, and differentiating a gastrointestinal (GI) source of bleeding is especially important because further evaluation and management of these two pathologies follow divergent pathways. Usually differentiation can be done by the patient and physician working together to differentiate coughing from vomiting. In unclear cases, inspection and pH testing may help to distinguish GI from tracheobronchial hemorrhage. Unless an active, brisk upper GI hemorrhage is present, the acidification of blood in the stomach results in fragmentation and darkening, producing specks of brown or black material often referred to as coffee-ground emesis. Pulmonary blood appears bright red or as only slightly darker clots and is alkaline.

12.3.2　Rapid assessment and stabilization

As a mitigating maneuver in patients with a known lateralizing source of bleeding, the "lung-down" position can be employed. For this position the patient is turned such that the bleeding lung is more dependent, promoting continued protection and ventilation of the unaffected lung and improved oxygenation. If intubation is required, a large diameter endotracheal tube should be used to facilitate emergent fiberoptic bronchoscopy. In selected cases of confirmed left-sided bleeding, a single-lumen right-mainstem intubation often can be successfully performed through advancement of the tube in the neutral position or use of a 90-degree rotational technique, during which the tube is rotated 90 degrees in the direction of desired placement and advanced until resistance is met. Left-mainstem intubations are more difficult but may be attempted when the bleeding site is on the right lung and simple lung-down positioning is not sufficient to stabilize the patient's airway and oxygenation.

12.4　Pivotal findings

12.4.1　History

Although patient reports of bleeding severity can be inaccurate, an estimate of the rate, volume, and appearance of expectorated blood should be obtained. Additional pertinent history includes prior episodes of hemoptysis or parenchymal pulmonary disorders, including bronchiectasis, recurrent pneumonia, chronic obstructive pulmonary disease, bronchitis, TB, and fungal infection. Inflammatory disorders that secondarily involve the lungs or pulmonary vasculature include Wegener's granulomatosis, Good-pasture's syndrome, and systemic lupus erythematosus, and a history of these should be elicited. Any risk factors for platelet dysfunction, thrombocytopenia, and coagulopathy should be noted, as should, conversely, any hypercoagulable states that might contribute to venous thromboembolic disease.

Primary or metastatic cancer can cause hemoptysis by erosion into pulmonary and bronchial vessels. Recent percutaneous or transbronchial procedures can cause immediate or delayed post-procedural bleeding, and any recent history of trauma should also be noted. A pertinent travel history to areas in which TB or pulmonary paragonimiasis is endemic is crucial.

12.4.2　Physical examination

After a primary survey and stabilization, a targeted examination may suggest the location and cause of bleeding but does so in less than 50% of cases. Focal adventitious breath sounds may indicate pneumonia or pulmonary abscess. A new heart murmur, especially in a febrile patient, may reflect endocarditis causing septic pulmonary emboli. Symptoms and signs of deep venous thrombosis should suggest pulmonary embolism. Ecchymoses and petechiae can indicate coagulopathy and thrombocytopenia, respectively.

12.4.3　Ancillary testing

Initial laboratory studies include a complete blood count, coagula-tion tests, and a type and screen or crossmatch. Renal function tests should be performed if vasculitis is suggested or contrast computed tomography (CT) is planned. Plain chest radiography screens for causes of hemoptysis (including infection and malignancy), although its sensitivity is poor. A prospective study of 184 consecutive patients with varying degrees of hemoptysis revealed that more than 40% of patients with a normal chest radiograph had positive findings on chest CT.

12.5　Diagnostic algorithm

12.5.1　Differential diagnosis

Potential causes of hemoptysis vary and include systemic illnesses as well as pulmonary parenchymal diseases. Table 12-1 includes the most common causes.

12.5.2　Management

Since the advent of high-resolution CT, radiologic evaluation has had an integral role in the evaluation and treatment of patients with hemoptysis. The challenge to the emergency physician is to rapidly assess the need for airway control before radiographic evaluation and hemodynamic stabilization. Unless the initial chest radiograph is diagnostic or the patient is hemodynamically unstable, a chest CT should be obtained. Further management decisions should be guided by the CT results and made in conjunction with pulmonary and thoracic surgery consultants.

12.5.3　Bronchoscopy

Early bronchoscopy facilitates both localization of bleeding and therapeutic intervention. Balloon and topical hemostatic tamponade, thermocoagulation, and injection of vasoactive agents can all effectively control arterial bleeding. Optimal timing for bronchoscopy remains conjectural; although stable patients with mild to moderate bleeding may benefit from early bronchoscopy, in unstable patients or those with brisk hemorrhage, bronchoscopy may facilitate airway management but is less likely to control bleeding.

12.5.4　Interventional angiography

Bronchial arterial embolization is an effective first-line therapy for massive hemoptysis and is the procedure of choice for patients either unable to tolerate surgery or in whom bronchoscopy has been unsuccessful. Hemostatic rates range from 91% –98%, but as many as 20% –50% of patients have early episodes of repeat bleeding. The risk of delayed bleeding may exist for up to 36 months. To guide therapy, initial localization of bleeding by bronchoscopy or CT is preferred.

12.5.5　Surgery

Emergency thoracotomy, in the operating room, is reserved for life-threatening hemoptysis or for persistent, rapid bleeding that is uncontrolled by bronchoscopy and percutaneous embolization. Pulmonary arterial hemorrhage from tumor necrosis represents a surgical emergency.

Table 12-1　Differential Diagnosis: Hemoptysis

Airway disease:
Bronchitis (acute or chronic) Bronchiectasis
Neoplasm (primary and metastatic) Trauma
Foreign body
Parenchymal disease:
Tuberculosis
Pneumonia, lung abscess Fungal infection Neoplasm
Vascular disease:
Pulmonary embolism Arteriovenous malformation Aortic aneurysm
Pulmonary hypertension
Vasculitis (Wegener's granulomatosis, systemic lupus erythematosus [SLE], Goodpasture's syndrome)
Hematologic disease:
Coagulopathy (cirrhosis or warfarin therapy) Disseminated intravascular coagulation Platelet dysfunction
Thrombocytopenia
Cardiac disease:
Congenital heart disease (especially in children) Valvular heart disease
Endocarditis
Miscellaneous:
Cocaine Postprocedural injury Tracheal-arterial fistula SLE

Gao Yanxia

Chapter 13

Bronchial Asthma

13.1 Introduction

The word asthma was used initially as a synonym for "breathlessness". The National Heart,Lung,and Blood Institute summarizes our current understanding of asthma as "a chronic inflammatory disorder of the airways in which many cells and cellular elements play a role in this inflammation causes recurrent episodes of wheezing, breathlessness,chest tightness,and coughing episodes are usually associated with widespread but variable airflow obstruction that is often reversible either spontaneously or with treatment. Asthma is thus a chronic inflammatory disease,and control of symptoms ultimately depends on ameliorating the inflammatory reaction that produces alterations in airway function and structure. Irreversible structural airway changes occurring in response to chronic airway inflammation may influence asthma therapies in emergency department(ED).

13.2 Epidemiology

In 2008,it was estimated that 38. 1 million Americans had been diagnosed with asthma by a health professional within their lifetime. The prevalence of asthma (defined as individuals who have been diagnosed and currently have asthma) in 2009 was 24. 6 million (17. 5 million adults and 7. 1 million children),and the asthma attack prevalence (the number of persons who had had at least one asthma attack in the previous year) was 12. 8 million,representing 52% of persons who had asthma.

13.3 Principles of disease

13.3.1 Pathophysiology

A variety of airway alterations occur in asthma,but airway inflammation is the final common pathway limiting airflow. Allergens and nonallergic stimuli induce bronchoconstriction via release of mediators and metabolic products from inflammatory cells. Compared with healthy individuals, patients with asthma show bronchial hyper-reactivity (hyper-responsiveness) in response to bronchoconstricting stimuli. Edema, inflammation, mucous production, and airway smooth muscle hypertrophy contribute to bronchoconstriction and hyper-reactivity and further airway obstruction and airflow limitation. Permanent structural airway changes (airway remodeling) may contribute to increased airway obstruction and hyper-responsiveness and decrease the response to therapy. The interaction of these features determines the clinical manifestations and severity of asthma and significantly influences the response to therapy. Evidence that inflammation is a component of asthma physiology was initially derived from autopsy findings in patients with fatal asthma. The airways revealed infiltration by neutrophils, eosinophils, and mast cells and the presence of subbasement membrane thickening, loss of epithelial cell integrity, goblet cell hyperplasia, and mucous plugs. Antemortem bronchial biopsy findings in patients with even mild degrees of asthma also demonstrate inflammatory changes in the central and peripheral airways that correlate with disease severity. Inflammatory and chemotactic cytokines produced by both resident airway and recruited inflammatory cells are identified in bronchoalveolar lavage washings and pulmonary secretions.

13.3.2   Genetics and asthma

It is likely that asthma is not a single disease, but a syndrome with various phenotypes. The natural history of asthma is highly variable. Most asthma begins in childhood and resolves with age. Remissions of variable duration may occur, whereas others experience progressive severe disease. Many aspects of asthma have identifiable genetic associations. Family history of both atopy and asthma are associated with lower rates of remission. Environmental influences (e. g. , allergens, pollutants, tobacco, and occupational exposures) are associated with asthma, and the interaction of genetic variability and environmental factors may allow prediction of future disease risk, expression, and severity.

13.3.3   Pathology

The pathology of the asthmatic airway reflects the inflammatory process is described earlier. Mucous gland hyperplasia and viscous mucous plugs in the smaller airways are present. Airway secretions reveal increased numbers of inflammatory cells. Airway epithelial damage and remodeling are evident. In contrast to patients with mild to moderate asthma, patients with acute severe asthma have extensive mucous hyperplasia, subepithelial thickening, and infiltration of inflammatory cells (particularly eosinophils). Necropsies of patients with status asthmaticus reveal grossly inflated lungs that may fail to collapse on opening of the pleural cavities. Histologic examination reveals luminal plugs consisting of inflammatory cells, desquamated epithelial cells, and mucus. Marked thickening of the airway basement membrane, submucosal inflammatory cells, increased deposition of connective tissue, mucous gland hyperplasia, and hypertrophy of airway smooth muscle are also observed.

13.4   Clincial features

13.4.1   Symptoms

Most patients with acute asthma have a constellation of symptoms, including cough, dyspnea, and wheezing. Cough often begins early in the attack, may be the sole manifestation of the disease in cough-variant asthma and elder patients, can be associated with sputum production, and is probably the result of subepithelial vagal stimulation. Nocturnal worsening is common, with most patients reporting cough or wheeze at least once per week. Nighttime mortality is higher than in the general population. Although increased airway resistance, diminished flow rates, and increased bronchial hyperactivity are contributing factors, asthmatic patients who come to the ED with nocturnal asthma attacks have disease severity similar to that of other asthmatics. Up to 40% of asthmatic women experience premenstrual worsening of symptoms, which peak 2-3 days before menses and are associated with more severe disease; ED visits increase during the preovulatory and perimenstrual intervals. There are interindividual differences in the dyspnea perceived by asthmatic subjects for the same level of airway narrowing.

13.4.2　Historical components

Slow-onset asthma with progressive deterioration over a period of at least 6 hours (usually days) occurs in over 80% of cases. This type has a female predominance, is triggered by upper respiratory tract infections, and has an airflow inflammation mechanism that results in a slower response to treatment. Sudden-onset asthma with rapid deterioration in less than 6 hours occurs in less than 20% of cases. This type has a male predominance, is triggered by respiratory allergens, exercise, and psychosocial stress, and has a bronchospastic cause resulting in more severe airway obstruction with a faster response to therapy.

13.4.3　Physical assessment

Patients with mild acute asthma usually speak in sentences, those moderate asthma in phrases, and those with severe asthma in words. Although alterations in mentation indicate severe asthma, restlessness and agitation do not reliably indicate hypoxia or hypercapnia. Patients who sit upright have severe airway obstruction; cyanosis is uncommon because of the left shift of the oxyhemoglobin dissociation curve produced by respiratory alkalosis. Diaphoresis can be seen secondary to the work of breathing, but if profound may be preterminal. Tachypnea and tachycardia are associated with severe obstruction, but a lower rate does not rule out severe asthma. The respiratory rate correlates poorly with PFT and indicates severe obstruction if it is higher than 40 breaths/min.

13.5　Diagnostic strategies

13.5.1　Pulmonary function tests

The severity of airflow obstruction can not be accurately assessed from symptoms and physical examination alone. Physicians initially tend to underestimate the degree of airway obstruction in acute asthma. Therefore routine PFT should be part of ED assessment and monitoring. The forced expiratory volume in 1 second from maximal inspiration (FEV_1) or the PEFR in liters per second, starting with fully inflated lungs and sustained for at least 10 msec, may be used. Both measurements require the patient's cooperation for maximal effort and are effort dependent. Whenever it is possible, the best of three consecutive values should be recorded. Any patient who could not perform a pulmonary function test should be considered to have severe airway obstruction. Although FEV_1 can be adequately measured in most acutely ill asthmatics to meet modified ATS performance goals, most ossessments ssessments in the ED use single-patient-use portable peak flow meters because PEFR is easier to measure.

13.5.2   Arterial blood gas analysis

Equilibration of oxyhemoglobin saturation occurs within 3–4 minutes of initiation or alteration of supplemental oxygen during an acute asthma attack. Stimulated hyperventilation leads to a modest fall in the partial pressure of carbon dioxide in arterial blood ($PaCO_2$). As airway obstruction increases, the $PaCO_2$ normalizes (PFT values 15% –25% predicted) and then increases (PFT values <15% predicted) with worsening hypoxemia. Because neither pretreatment nor post–treatment arterial blood gases (ABGs) correlate with PFTs or predict clinical outcome, ABG determination is rarely clinically useful in acute asthma exacerbations unless oxygen saturation can not be obtained reliably via pulse oximetry.

13.5.3   Other blood testing

Laboratory tests are rarely helpful in evaluating the patient with an acute asthma attack. Leukocytosis is common with acute asthma exacerbation but is not of discriminatory value in detecting acute superimposed pulmonary infection. Corticosteroids and catecholamines demarginate polymorphonuclear leukocytes after 1–2 hours, and patients on chronic steroid therapy may have normal or significantly elevated white blood cell (WBC) counts.

13.5.4   Radiology studies

A chest radiograph is of little value in most acute asthma exacerbations and should be restricted to patients with a complicating cardiopulmonary process, such as pneumonia, pneumothorax, pneumomediastinum, or congestive heart failure. Also, patients who do not respond to optimal therapy and require hospital admission have a higher likelihood of radiographically identifiable, unsuspected, clinically significant pulmonary complications of asthma.

13.5.5   Electrocardiogram and cardiac monitoring

The electrocardiogram (ECG) is selectively helpful in assessing patients with chest pain or a history of significant cardiovascular disease, in whom the asthma attack may be a physiologic stress test. In patients with severe asthma, the ECG may show a right ventricular strain pattern that reverses with improvement in airflow. Older patients, especially those with coexistent heart disease or with severe exacerbation, require continuous cardiac monitoring to detect dysrhythmias.

13.5.6   Future monitoring strategies

Noninvasive monitoring of bronchial inflammation may customize the ED assessment of acute asthma. This may include measurement of biologic biomarkers, such as cytokine profiles in the blood, evaluation of LTE4 in the urine, and the monitoring of exhaled pentane, hydrogen peroxide, NO, or carbon monoxide levels. Of these measurements, exhaled NO, a marker of airway inflammation, shows the most promise, as studies show that FENO can be measured in the ED with good reproducibility, and levels measured after 6 hours of care are associated with better asthma control after discharge.

13.5.7   Assessment summary

The severity of airflow obstruction can not be accurately judged by patients' symptoms, physical examination findings, and laboratory test results. Serial measurements of airflow obstruction (FEV_1 or PEFR) are key components of disease assessment and response to therapy.

13.6 Management of acute exacerbations

Home and First-Responder Strategies Subacute lack of asthma control (more than four outpatient visits or more than five short-acting beta 2-agonist prescriptions per year) is associated with increased risk of acute asthma exacerbation. Thus patients should be provided a plan to monitor their symptoms, signs, and PEFR to recognize early deterioration in the event of an exacerbation. Early therapy can prevent progression to severe attacks. Home management includes increased use of inhaled beta 2-agonists, early administration of systemic corticosteroids (not simply doubling the dose of current ICSs), and specific instructions regarding emergency care.

13.6.1 Management of acute asthma in the emergency department

The rapidity of reversal of the acute airflow obstruction is directly predictive of the outcome. Effective bronchodilation often results in a decreased need for hospitalization with significant cost.

13.6.2 Oxygen administration

All patients should receive supplemental oxygen titrated to maintain arterial oxygen saturation above 90% (above 95% in pregnant women and those with coexistent heart disease) rather than at predetermined concentrations or flow rates. Continuous oxygen saturation monitoring is essential during the acute phase. Humidification of the inspired air-oxygen mixture is not essential, although studies suggest that active airway rehydration should be revisited.

13.6.3 Adrenergic medication controversies in use

Epidemiologic studies reported an association between death and near death from asthma and the use of inhaled beta 2-agonists. The use of more than one canister per month doubles the risk for each additional monthly canister used. This relationship does not imply causality, but may be a marker for severe disease, particularly if anti-inflammatory treatment is underused. Guidelines for chronic use of inhaled beta 2-agonists, however, recommend limited daily use in a rescue-only mode. One form of albuterol is a racemic mixture of equal amounts of R and S isomers.

13.6.4 Short-acting inhaled beta 2-agonist choice and administration schedule

Racemic albuterol has remained the main beta 2-agonist used in the ED for more than 30 years. It is more beta 2-selective, is longer acting, and has fewerless side effects than other previously available drugs such as metaproterenol or isoetharine. Patients with more severe obstruction with a poor response to initial therapy should receive higher dosage schedules and possible continuous administration. Evidence to support the use of intravenous beta-agonists in ED patients with severe acute asthma is lacking; the potential risks are warranted only when inhaled therapy is not feasible. Epinephrine is used cautiously in patients older than 40 years or those with suspected cardiovascular disease, because it might provoke myocardial ischemia.

13.6.5 Long-acting beta 2-agonists (labas) and acute disease

Salmeterol is a long-acting (12 hours) beta 2-agonist that is an effective additional medication for management of symptoms that are not adequately well controlled by regular and adequate doses of effective controller medications such as inhaled steroids. It has an onset of action of 20 minutes and thus is not a rescue medication. Regular use of this drug without concomitant use of inhaled steroids results in greater hospitalizations and asthma−related deaths, resulting in a black box warning on the package insert.

13.6.6   Corticosteroids

Corticosteroids inhibit recruitment of inflammatory cells and release of proinflammatory mediators and cytokines. Corticosteroids activate cytoplasmic glucocorticoid receptors to regulate the transcription of certain target genes, resulting in the synthesis of new proteins.

Many studies clearly demonstrate that oral corticosteroids are as beneficial as intravenous corticosteroids in the ED. The initial oral dose is usually 60 mg of prednisone. If intravenous methylprednisolone is used, the dose is 40−80 mg/d in one or two divided doses until the switch to oral therapy or until PEFR reaches 70% of predicted or personal best. Continuing therapy with oral prednisone or prednisolone is given in an adult at the dose of 40−80 mg/d, usually as a single dose.

Gao Yanxia

Chapter 14

Chronic Obstructive Pulmonary Disease with Acute Exacerbation

14.1 Introduction

Chronic obstructive pulmonary disease (COPD) is a common respiratory condition characterized by airflow limitation. It affects more than 5% of the population and is associated with high morbidity and mortality. It is the third-ranked cause of death in the United States, killing more than 120,000 individuals each year. As a consequence of its high prevalence and chronicity, COPD causes high resource utilization with frequent clinician office visits, frequent hospitalizations due to acute exacerbations, and the need for chronic therapy.

14.2 Definitions

The definition of COPD and its subtypes (emphysema, chronic bronchitis, and chronic obstructive asthma) and the interrelationships between the closely related disorders that cause airflow limitation provide a foundation for understanding the spectrum of patient presentations.

14.2.1 COPD

The Global Initiative for Chronic Obstructive Lung Disease (GOLD), a project initiated by the National Heart, Lung, and Blood Institute (NHLBI) and the World Health Organization (WHO), defines COPD as follows: "COPD is a common, preventable, and treatable disease that is characterized by persistent respiratory symptoms and airflow limitation that is due to airway and/or alveolar abnormalities usually caused by significant exposure to noxious particles or gases. The chronic airflow limitation that characterizes COPD is caused by a mixture of small airways disease (e.g., obstructive bronchiolitis) and parenchymal destruction (emphysema), the relative contributions of which vary from person to person. Chronic inflammation causes structural changes, small airways narrowing, and destruction of lung parenchyma. A loss of small airways may contribute to airflow limitation and mucociliary dysfunction, a characteristic feature of the disease. "

14.2.2　Chronic bronchitis

Chronic bronchitis is defined as a chronic productive cough for three months in each of two successive years in a patient in whom other causes of chronic cough (e. g. , bronchiectasis) have been excluded. It may precede or follow development of airflow limitation. This definition has been used in many studies, despite the arbitrarily selected symptom duration.

14.2.3　Emphysema

Emphysema is a pathological term that describes some of the structural changes sometimes associated with COPD. These changes include abnormal and permanent enlargement of the airspaces distal to the terminal bronchioles that is accompanied by destruction of the airspace walls, without obvious fibrosis (i. e. , there is no fibrosis visible to the naked eye). Exclusion of obvious fibrosis is intended to distinguish the alveolar destruction due to emphysema from that due to the interstitial pneumonias.

14.3　Pathology

The predominant pathologic changes of COPD are found in the airways, but changes are also seen in the lung parenchyma and pulmonary vasculature. In an individual, the pattern of pathologic changes depends on the underlying disease (e. g. , chronic bronchitis, emphysema, α_1 antitrypsin deficiency), possibly individual susceptibility, and disease severity. While radiographic methods do not have the resolution of histology, high resolution computed tomography can assess lung parenchyma, airways, and pulmonary vasculature.

14.3.1　Airways

Airways abnormalities in COPD include chronic inflammation, increased numbers of goblet cells, mucus gland hyperplasia, fibrosis, narrowing and reduction in the number of small airways, and airway collapse due to the loss of tethering caused by alveolar wall destruction in emphysema. Among patients with chronic bronchitis who have mucus hypersecretion, an increased number of goblet cells and enlarged submucosal glands are typically seen. Chronic inflammation in chronic bronchitis and emphysema is characterized by the presence of CD8+ T-lymphocytes, neutrophils, and CD68+ monocytes/macrophages in the airways.

14.3.2　Lung parenchyma

Emphysema affects the structures distal to the terminal bronchiole, consisting of the respiratory bronchiole, alveolar ducts, alveolar sacs, and alveoli, known collectively as the acinus. These structures in combination with their associated capillaries and interstitium form the lung parenchyma. The part of the acinus that is affected by permanent dilation or destruction determines the subtype of emphysema.

(1) Proximal acinar (also known as centrilobular) emphysema refers to abnormal dilation or destruction of the respiratory bronchiole, the central portion of the acinus. It is commonly associated with cigarette smoking, but can also be seen in coal workers' pneumoconiosis.

(2) Panacinar emphysema refers to enlargement or destruction of all parts of the acinus. Diffuse panacinar emphysema is most commonly associated with α_1 antitrypsin deficiency, although it can be seen in

combination with proximal emphysema in smokers.

(3) In distal acinar (also known as paraseptal) emphysema, the alveolar ducts are predominantly affected. Distal acinar emphysema may occur alone or in combination with proximal acinar and panacinar emphysema. When it occurs alone, the usual association is spontaneous pneumothorax in a young adult.

(4) Pulmonary vasculature.

Changes in the pulmonary vasculature include intimal hyperplasia and smooth muscle hypertrophy/hyperplasia thought to be due to chronic hypoxic vasoconstriction of the small pulmonary arteries.

14.4   Clinical features

The most important risk factor for chronic obstructive pulmonary disease is cigarette smoking. Other exposures including passive smoke and biomass fuel use also play roles.

The amount and duration of smoking contribute to disease severity. Thus, a key step in the evaluation of patients with suspected COPD is to ascertain the number of pack years smoked (packs of cigarettes per day multiplied by the number of years), as the majority (about 80%) of patients with COPD in the United States have a history of cigarette smoking. A smoking history should include the age of starting and the age of quitting, as patients may underestimate the number of years they smoked. With enough smoking, almost all smokers will develop measurably reduced lung function.

The exact threshold for the duration/intensity of cigarette smoking that will result in COPD varies from one individual to another. In the absence of a genetic/environmental/occupational predisposition, smoking less than 10–15 pack years of cigarettes is unlikely to result in COPD.

There are three typical ways in which patients with COPD present.

• Patients who have an extremely sedentary lifestyle but few complaints require careful questioning to elicit a history that is suggestive of COPD. Some patients unknowingly avoid exertional dyspnea by shifting their expectations and limiting their activity.

• Patients who present with respiratory symptoms generally complain of dyspnea and chronic cough. The dyspnea may initially be noticed only during exertion. However, it eventually becomes noticeable with progressively less exertion or even at rest. The chronic cough is characterized by the insidious onset of sputum production, which occurs in the morning initially, but may progress to occur throughout the day.

• Patients who present with episodes of increased cough, purulent sputum, wheezing, fatigue, and dyspnea that occur intermittently, with or without fever. Diagnosis can be problematic in such patients. The combination of wheezing plus dyspnea may lead to an incorrect diagnosis of asthma.

Physical examination

The findings on physical examination of the chest vary with the severity of the COPD.

• Early in the disease, the physical examination may be normal, or may show only prolonged expiration or wheezes on forced exhalation.

• As the severity of the airway obstruction increases, physical examination may reveal hyperinflation, decreased breath sounds, wheezes, crackles at the lung bases, and/or distant heart sounds.

• Patients with end-stage COPD may adopt positions that relieve dyspnea, such as leaning forward with arms outstretched and weight supported on the palms or elbows. This posture may be evident during the examination or may be suggested by the presence of callouses or swollen bursae on the extensor surfaces of forearms. Other physical examination findings include use of the accessory respiratory muscles of the neck and shoulder girdle, expiration through pursed lips, paradoxical retraction of the lower interspaces during inspiration, cyanosis, asterixis due to severe hypercapnia, and an enlarged, tender liver due to right heart failure. Neck vein distention may also be observed because of increased intrathoracic pressure, especially during expiration.

● Yellow stains on the fingers due to nicotine and tar from burning tobacco are a clue to ongoing and heavy cigarette smoking.

14.5   Evaluation

Evaluation for COPD is appropriate in adults who report dyspnea, chronic cough, chronic sputum production or have had a gradual decline in level of peak activity, particularly if they have a history of exposure to risk factors for the disease (e. g. , cigarette smoking, indoor biomass smoke). All patients are evaluated with spirometry and selected patients have laboratory testing and imaging studies.

14.5.1   Laboratory

No laboratory test is diagnostic for COPD, but certain tests are sometimes obtained to exclude other causes of dyspnea and comorbid diseases.

Assessment for anemia is an important step in the evaluation of dyspnea. Measurement of plasma brain natriuretic peptide (BNP) or N-terminal pro-BNP (NT-proBNP) concentrations is useful as a component of the evaluation of suspected heart failure (HF). Blood glucose, urea nitrogen, creatinine, electrolytes, calcium, phosphorus, and thyroid stimulating hormone may be appropriate depending on the degree of clinical suspicion for an alternate diagnosis.

Among stable COPD patients with normal kidney function, an elevated serum bicarbonate may indirectly identify chronic hypercapnia. In the presence of chronic hypercapnia, the serum bicarbonate is typically increased due to a compensatory metabolic alkalosis. Abnormal results must be confirmed with arterial blood gas measurement.

14.5.2   Pulmonary function tests

Pulmonary function tests (PFTs), particularly spirometry, are the cornerstone of the diagnostic evaluation of patients with suspected COPD. In addition, PFTs are used to determine the severity of the airflow limitation, assess the response to medications, and follow disease progression. When evaluating a patient for possible COPD, spirometry is performed pre and post bronchodilator administration to determine whether airflow limitation is presented and whether it is partially or fully reversible. Airflow limitation that is irreversible or only partially reversible with bronchodilator is the characteristic physiologic feature of COPD.

The most important values measured during spirometry are the forced expiratory volume in one second (FEV_1) and the forced vital capacity (FVC). The postbronchodilator ratio of FEV_1/FVC determines whether airflow limitation is presented; the postbronchodilator percent predicted value for FEV_1 determines the severity of airflow limitation.

The indications for measuring ABGs [e. g. , PaO_2, $PaCO_2$, and acidity (pH)], which must be considered in the clinical context, include the following.

● Low FEV_1 (e. g. , <50% predicted).

- Low oxygen saturation by pulse oximetry (e. g. ,<92%).
- Depressed level of consciousness.
- Acute exacerbation of COPD.
- Assessment for hypercapnia in risk patients 30–60 minutes after initiation of supplemental oxygen.

In patients with mild to moderate COPD, arterial blood gases usually reveal mild or moderate hypoxemia without hypercapnia. As the disease progresses, the hypoxemia becomes more severe and hypercapnia may develop. Hypercapnia becomes progressively more likely when the FEV_1 approaches or falls below one liter. Blood gas abnormalities worsen during acute exacerbations and may also worsen during exercise and sleep.

Chest radiography and computed tomography (CT) are typically performed in patients with COPD when the cause of dyspnea or sputum production is unclear and during acute exacerbations to exclude complicating processes (e. g. , pneumonia, pneumothorax, heart failure). Imaging is not required to diagnose COPD. However, in patients with severe COPD, CT scanning identifies individuals with predominantly upper lobe disease who may be candidates for lung volume reduction surgery.

14.6　Diagnosis

The presence of symptoms compatible with COPD are suggestive of the diagnosis, especially if there is a history of exposure to triggers of COPD (e. g. , tobacco smoke, occupational dust, indoor biomass smoke), a family history of chronic lung disease, or presence of associated comorbidities. The diagnosis of COPD is confirmed by the following.

- Spirometry demonstrating airflow limitation [i. e. , a forced expiratory volume in one second/forced vital capacity (FEV_1/FVC) ratio less than 0. 7 or less than the lower limit of normal (LLN) PLUS an FEV_1 less than 80% of predicted] that is incompletely reversible after the administration of an inhaled bronchodilator.
- Absence of an alternative explanation for the symptoms and airflow limitation the differential diagnosis of COPD is discussed below.
- The Global Initiative for COPD (GOLD) guidelines suggest repeating spirometry on a separate occasion to demonstrate persistence of airflow limitation (FEV_1/FVC <0. 7 or less than the LLN) for patients with an initial FEV_1/FVC between 0. 6 and 0. 8.

After confirming the presence of COPD, the next step is to consider the cause. For the majority of patients, the etiology is long–term cigarette smoking. However, it is important to review with the patient whether underlying asthma, workplace exposures, indoor use of biomass fuel, a prior history of tuberculosis, or familial predisposition is contributory, because mitigation of ongoing exposures may reduce disease progression.

14.7　Staging

The initial Global Initiative for Chronic Obstructive Lung Disease (GOLD) guidelines used the forced expiratory volume in one second (FEV_1; expressed as a percentage of predicted) to stage disease severity. However, the FEV_1 only captures one component of COPD severity: two patients with the same percent predicted FEV_1 can have a substantially different exercise tolerance and prognosis. Other aspects of disease, such as the severity of symptoms, risk of exacerbations, and the presence of comorbidities, are important to the patient's experience of the disease and prognosis and are included in newer staging systems, such as the revised GOLD classification.

14.8   Management of COPD exacerbations

14.8.1   Home management of COPD exacerbations

Home management of chronic obstructive pulmonary disease (COPD) exacerbations generally includes intensification of bronchodilator therapy and initiation of a course of oral glucocorticoids; oral antibiotics are added based on individual characteristics.

14.8.1.1   Beta adrenergic agonists

Inhaled short-acting beta adrenergic agonists (e. g. , albuterol, levalbuterol) are the mainstay of therapy for an acute exacerbation of COPD because of their rapid onset of action and efficacy in producing bronchodilation. For patients being managed at home, these medications are usually administered by a metered dose inhaler (MDI) with a spacer device and may be combined with a short acting anticholinergic agent.

14.8.1.2   Anticholinergic agents

Ipratropium bromide, an inhaled short-acting anticholinergic agent (also known as a short-acting muscarinic agent) is an effective bronchodilator for exacerbations of COPD and is often used in combination with inhaled short-acting beta adrenergic agonists

14.8.1.3   Oral glucocorticoid therapy

Systemic glucocorticoid therapy appears to have a light but beneficial effect in outpatients with exacerbations of COPD. Occasional patients may benefit from a higher dose or a longer course depending on the severity of the exacerbation and response to prior courses of glucocorticoids.

14.8.1.4   Antibiotics

To try to maximize the benefit of antibiotic therapy, many clinical practice guidelines recommend antibiotic therapy only for those patients who are most likely to have bacterial infection or are most ill.

14.8.2   Hospital management of COPD exacerbations

Similar to at-home management, the major components of in-hospital management of exacerbations of chronic obstructive pulmonary disease (COPD) include reversing airflow limitation with inhaled short-acting bronchodilators and systemic glucocorticoids, treating infection, ensuring adequate oxygenation, and averting intubation and mechanical ventilation.

In-hospital monitoring typically includes frequent assessment of respiratory status, heart rate and rhythm, and also fluid status. Arterial blood gas measurement is performed to look for respiratory acidosis, confirm the accuracy of pulse oxygen saturation, and to monitor known hypercapnia.

14.8.2.1   Oxygen therapy

Supplemental oxygen is a critical component of acute therapy. Because of the risk of prompting worsened hypercapnia with excess supplemental oxygen, administration of supplemental oxygen should target a pulse oxygen saturation (SpO_2) of 88% – 92% or an arterial oxygen tension (PaO_2) of approximately

60-70 mmHg.

There are numerous devices available to deliver supplemental oxygen during an exacerbation of COPD.

- Venturi masks are the preferred means of oxygen delivery because they permit a precise delivered fraction of inspired oxygen (FiO_2). Venturi masks can deliver an FiO_2 of 24% ,28% ,31% ,35% ,40% ,or 60%.

- Nasal cannula can provide flow rates up to 6 L per minute with an associated FiO_2 of approximately 40% (calculator 1). They are more comfortable and convenient for the patient,especially during oral feedings.

- When a higher FiO_2 is needed,simple facemasks can provide an FiO_2 up to 55% using flow rates of 6-10 L per minute. However,variations in minute ventilation and inconsistent entrainment of room air affect the FiO_2 when simple facemasks (or nasal cannula) are used.

- Non-rebreathing masks with a reservoir,one-way valves,and a tight face seal can deliver an inspired oxygen concentration up to 90% ,but are generally not needed in this setting.

Adequate oxygenation must be assured,even if it leads to acute hypercapnia. Hypercapnia is generally well tolerated in patients whose arterial carbon dioxide tension ($PaCO_2$) is chronically elevated. However, mechanical ventilation may be required if hypercapnia is associated with depressed mental status,profound acidemia,or cardiac dysrhythmias.

14.8.2.2 Beta adrenergic agonists

As noted above,inhaled short-acting beta adrenergic agonists are the mainstay of therapy for an exacerbation of COPD because of their rapid onset of action and efficacy in producing bronchodilation. These medications may be administered via a nebulizer or a metered dose inhaler (MDI) with a spacer device and may be combined with a short acting muscarinic agent.

14.8.2.3 Anticholinergic agents

As noted above,the evidence is conflicting regarding the use of inhaled short-acting anticholinergic agent in combination with inhaled short-acting beta adrenergic agonists to treat exacerbations of COPD. Nonetheless these agents are typically used together for patients who require hospital-based treatment of a COPD exacerbation.

14.8.2.4 Systemic glucocorticoids

Systemic glucocorticoids,when added to the bronchodilator therapies described above,improve symptoms and lung function,and decrease the length of hospital stay. Oral glucocorticoids are rapidly absorbed (peak serum levels achieved at one hour after ingestion) with virtually complete bioavailability and appear equally efficacious to intravenous glucocorticoids for treating most exacerbations of COPD. The optimal dose of systemic glucocorticoids for treating a COPD exacerbation is unknown. The Global Initiative for Chronic Obstructive Lung Disease (GOLD) guidelines advise using the equivalent of prednisone 40 mg once daily for the majority of COPD exacerbations. Frequently used regimens range from prednisone 30-60 mg,once daily,to methylprednisolone 60-125 mg,two to four times daily,depending on the severity of the exacerbation.

14.8.2.5 Antibiotics and antiviral agents

Most clinical practice guidelines recommend antibiotics for patients having a moderate to severe COPD exacerbation that requires hospitalization. The optimal antibiotic regimen for the treatment of exacerbations of COPD has not been determined. We use a "risk stratification" approach when selecting initial antibiotic therapy,providing a broader antibiotic regimen for patients at risk for resistant organisms. The rationale,diagnosis, and treatment of infection in exacerbations of COPD, including antibiotic selection, are discussed separately.

14.8.2.6   Supportive care

Supportive care for patients hospitalized with an exacerbation of COPD may include one or more of the following therapies.

● Cigarette smoking cessation Hospitalization may provide an opportunity for smoking patients to move towards cigarette smoking cessation.

● Thromboprophylaxis Hospitalization for exacerbations of COPD increases the risk for deep venous thrombosis and pulmonary embolism.

● Nutritional support oral nutritional supplementation may have some benefits to improve pulmonary function during COPD exacerbations.

14.8.2.7   Palliative care

Given the high one-year mortality rate after hospitalization for a COPD exacerbation, it may be appropriate to consider a palliative care referral during or shortly after a hospitalization for COPD. Palliative care assessment can help explore the patient's understanding of their illness and prognosis, assess and manage symptoms, discuss the patient's goals of care and advance care planning, and help plan end-of-life care.

14.8.2.8   Mechanical ventilations

Ventilatory support may be needed for patients with more severe exacerbations of COPD, such as those characterized by severe dyspnea with clinical signs of respiratory muscle fatigue, increased work of breathing, or both, and also respiratory acidosis [arterial pH $\leqslant$ 7. 35 and arterial tension of carbon dioxide ($PaCO_2$) $\geqslant$45 mmHg ($\geqslant$6 kPa)]. Prior to initiating ventilatory support, it is important to review existing advance directives and ensure that ventilatory support is consistent with the patient's goals of care.

(1) Noninvasive ventilation

Noninvasive ventilation (NIV, also known as noninvasive positive pressure ventilation or NPPV) refers to mechanical ventilation delivered through a noninvasive interface, such as a face mask, nasal mask, or nasal prongs. It improves numerous clinical outcomes and is the preferred method of ventilatory support in many patients with an exacerbation of COPD. Most commonly, NIV is initiated in the emergency department, intensive care unit, or a speciali respiratory unit to enable close monitoring, although this has not been formally studied and varies among hospitals.

(2) Invasive ventilation

Invasive mechanical ventilation should be administered when patients fail to NIV, do not tolerate NIV, or have contraindications to NIV. Invasive mechanical ventilation for acute respiratory failure due to a COPD exacerbation is discussed separately.

14.9   Prevention

A number of medications, such as tiotropium, combination inhaled glucocorticoid and long-acting beta agonist (LABA), roflumilast, and N-acetylcysteine (NAC), can help to reduce the frequency of COPD exacerbations, although the evidence for roflumilast and NAC is less convincing than for the other two. The effect of long-term therapy with these agents on exacerbation frequency is discussed separately.

14.9.1   Pulmonary rehabilitation

While pulmonary rehabilitation is associated with a number of benefits in terms of exercise tolerance and quality of life, the effect on COPD exacerbations and rehospitalization is less clear and may be dependent on timing relative to hospitalization.

14.9.2   Action plan

A COPD exacerbation "action plan" may help patients mitigate the severity of exacerbations. Approximately two-thirds of patients know when an exacerbation of COPD is imminent because symptoms tend to be similar from one exacerbation to another. An action plan encourages early intervention by giving patients guidelines on how to recognize an exacerbation, how to change their medication regimen accordingly, and when to contact their healthcare provider.

Gao Yanxia

Chapter 15

Pneumothorax

15.1 Primary spontaneous pneumothorax (PSP) and secondary spontaneous pneumothorax(SSP)

Primary spontaneous pneumothorax occurs in people without preceding trauma and without an underlying history of clinical lung disease, but recent researches found that many patients who have primary spontaneous pneumothorax may already have subclinical lung disease, such as pleural blebs.

Secondary spontaneous pneumothorax occurs in people with a wide variety of parenchymal lung diseases. Patients have underlying pulmonary pathology that alters normal lung structure where air enters the pleural space.

15.1.1 Epidemiology

PSPs frequently occurs in tall and thin men aged 20–40 years, the peak incidence age is in the early 20s. PSP is rarely observed in people older than 40 years. The age–adjusted incidence of PSP is 7.4–18 cases per 100,000 persons per year for men and 1.2–6 cases per 100,000 persons per year for women. The male–to–female ratio of age–adjusted rates is 6.2 : 1.

More than 10% of patients may be asymptomatic or with only mild symptoms, it is likely that the incidence for spontaneous pneumothorax is underestimated.

15.1.2 Pathophysiology

In normal respiration, the pleural cavity has a negative pressure. It is −12 to −10 mmHg in inspiration and −4 mmHg in expiration. As the chest wall expands outward, the surface tension between the parietal and visceral pleura expands the lung outward. At the meantime, the intrinsic elastic recoil of the lung tissue tending to collapse inwards. The integrity of the pleural cavity is the key to keep negative pressure. If the pleural cavity is invaded by gas from a ruptured bleb, the lung collapses until equilibrium is achieved or the rupture is sealed. As the pneumothorax enlarges, the lung becomes smaller. The main physiologic consequence of this process is a decrease in vital capacity and partial pressure of oxygen.

15.1.3   Clinical manifestations

Most spontaneous pneumothoraces are asymptomatic. Young and otherwise healthy persons can tolerate the main physiologic consequences of a decrease in vital capacity and partial pressure of oxygen fairly well, with minimal changes in vital signs and symptoms, patient is severe and needs immediate treatment when shortness of breath or even dyspnea is presented, because of decreased lung reserve. Anxiety, cough, and vague presenting symptoms (e. g. , general malaise, fatigue) are less commonly observed.

The physical examinations are different depending on the severity of spontaneous pneumothorax. The typical signs may include: tachycardia which is the most common finding, the heart rate may rise to more than 120 beats/min, distant or absent breath sounds (unilaterally decreased or absent lung sounds is a common finding), hyperresonance on percussion, decreased tactile fremitus and adventitious lung sounds (e. g. , crackles, wheeze; an ipsilateral finding).

15.1.4   Supplementary examination

15.1.4.1   Chest radiography

We should use a systematic approach to evaluate the chest radiograph for pneumothorax. First of all, we need to make sure that there is no rotation, followed by comparing the symmetry and shape of the chest cage, and looking at the relative lengths of the ribs in the middle lung fields on each side on the anteroposterior (AP) or posteroanterior (PA) views.

Finding of pneumothorax on chest radiographs may include the following.

(1) An ipsilateral lung edge may be seen parallel to the chest wall. And a linear shadow of visceral pleura with lack of lung markings peripheral to the shadow may be observed, indicating collapsed lung.

(2) In supine patients, deep sulcus sign (very dark and deep costophrenic angle) with radiolucency along costophrenic sulcus indicates the occult pneumothorax; the anterior costophrenic recess becomes the highest point in the hemithorax and a depressed costophrenic angle.

(3) If the pneumothorax does not reexpand, small pleural may present and increase in size.

(4) Mediastinal shift toward the contralateral lung is rare.

(5) Airway or parenchymal abnormalities.

15.1.4.2   Computed Tomography of Chest

Chest CT is the most reliable imaging test for the diagnosis of pneumothorax, but it is not recommended for routine use in spontaneous pneumothorax. CT can help to distinguish between a large bulla and a pneumothorax, indicate underlying emphysema or emphysemalike changes (ELCs), determine the exact size of the pneumothorax, confirm the diagnosis of pneumothorax in patients with head trauma who are mechanically ventilated, detect occult/small pneumothoraces and pneumomediastinum.

15.1.4.3   Ultrasonography

Prehospital, portable ultrasonography may provide diagnostic and therapeutic benefit when conducted by a proficient examiner and may be quicker and more accurate than radiography for distinguishing free pleural effusion in time-sensitive evaluations.

Ultrasonography is increasingly used in the acute care setting as a readily available bedside tool, especially in the intensive care unit (ICU) and emergency department (ED) settings.

15.1.5   Diagnosis and differential diagnosis

According to the symptoms, signs and supplementary examinations most doctors may make a quick diagnosis, but who need to differentiate it from the following diseases:

(1) Pulmonary embolism

Pulmonary embolism is a blockage of the pulmonary circulation by a substance that has moved from elsewhere in the body through the bloodstream. Its clinical manifestation is similar with spontaneous pneumothorax, but the examination of X-ray or CT is normal, computed tomographic pulmonary angiography (CTPA) may find the blockage of the pulmonary artery.

(2) Acute myocardial infarction

Myocardial infarction is myocardial necrosis caused by ischemia. Its symptom also include chest pain, it may be differentiated by ECG, and cardiac-specific markers of myocardial damage. The CT or X-ray is commonly normal.

(3) Pneumonia

Pneumonia is an inflammation of the distal airways, alveoli, an interstitium of the lung that could be associated with pathogenic microorganisms, It is easy to be differentiated by elevated blood white cells count, inflammation associated markers, chest X-ray and CT scan.

15.1.6　Treatment

The first step is inhaling oxygen.

If the compression of lung is smaller than 15% and the patient is asymptomatic, observation could be the treatment of choice.

If the compression of lung is smaller than 15% (or estimated as small) and the patient is symptomatic but hemodynamically stable, needle aspiration is the treatment of choice.

If the compression of lung is greater than 15% (or estimated as large) aspiration using a pigtail catheter left to low suction or water seal is recommended. Strong suction should not be used with a spontaneous pneumothorax because of an often-delayed presentation, and thus, an increased risk of reexpansion pulmonary edema.

15.1.7　Prognosis

About 30% of patients with spontaneous pneumothorax experiences recurrence after either observation or tube thoracostomy for the first episode.

15.2　Iatrogenic and traumatic pneumothorax

Iatrogenic pneumothorax is a traumatic pneumothorax that results from injury to the pleura, with air entered the pleural cavity secondary to diagnostic or therapeutic medical intervention.

Traumatic pneumothorax is caused by a blunt trauma or penetrating trauma that disrupts the parietal or visceral pleura.

15.2.1　Epidemiology

Iatrogenic and traumatic pneumothoraces occur more frequently than spontaneous pneumothoraces, and the rate of iatrogenic pneumothorax is increasing in ICU as intensive care treatment modalities have become increasingly dependent on central venous catheter placement, positive-pressure ventilation, and other causes that potentially induce iatrogenic pneumothorax.

Iatrogenic pneumothorax may cause substantial morbidity and, rarely death. The incidence of iatrogenic pneumothorax is 5-7 per 10,000 hospital admissions.

15.2.2 Pathophysiology

The pathophysiology is nearly the same as spontaneous pneumothorax, but is induced by trauma or clinical operations.

15.2.3 Clinical manifestations

The clinical manifestations varies depend on the extent of the lung collapse. From chest pain, shortness of breath to dyspnea, cyanosis and even death.

15.2.4 History

Patients have the history of trauma and clinical procedures such as pleural biopsy, thoracentesis, subclavian or internal jugular vein catheter placement and so on.

15.2.5 Physical examinations

Depending on the extend of the pneumothorax, from mild tachycardia to diminished breath sounds, decreased tactile fremitus, decreased movement and jugular vein extension.

15.2.6 Supplementary examination

Chest X-ray, CT, ultrasonography and Arterial blood gas (ABG) analysis measures the degrees of hypoxemia, hypercarbia, and academia. But ABG analysis shouldn't neither replace physical diagnosis nor delay the treatment while awaiting results if symptomatic pneumothorax is suspected. However, ABG analysis may be useful in evaluating hypoxia and hypercarbia and respiratory acidosis.

15.2.7 Diagnosis and differential diagnosis

It is not hard to make diagnosis when patient has the symptoms and signs of pneumothorax and a chest trauma and clinical operations. The details of differential diagnosis could be seen in spontaneous pneumothorax.

15.2.8 Treatment

First of all, follow the ABCs (airway, breathing, circulation) consequence while assessing vital signs and oxygen saturation, especially in patients with thoracic trauma. Evaluate the patency of the airway and the adequacy of the ventilation. Assess the circulatory status and the integrity of the chest wall. Carefully evaluate the function of cardiovascular system.

Keep the patient's hemodynamic stable. All patients should receive supplemental oxygen to increase oxygen saturation.

Aspiration is the technique of choice for iatrogenic pneumothoraces, because of low recurrence rate. Tube thoracostomy is reserved for very symptomatic patients.

In general, traumatic pneumothoraces should be treated with insertion of a chest tube, particularly if the patient can not be closely observed.

The process of lung reexpansion and healing is not immediate and may be complicated by pulmonary edema. Therefore, a chest tube is usually left in place until the clinical conditions are met.

The patients who have a small (<15%), minimally symptomatic pneumothorax may be admitted, observed closely, and rechecked by using serial chest radiographs.

15.2.9　Prognosis

The prognosis of iatrogenic and traumatic pneumothorax is good, recurrence is rare after appropriate treatment.

15.3　Tension pneumothorax

A tension pneumothorax is a life-threatening condition when air is trapped in the pleural cavity under positive pressure. When tension pneumothorax occurs, the mediastinal structures may be displaced and the cardiopulmonary function is compromised. Prompt recognition of this condition is life-saving, both outside the hospital and in ICU.

15.3.1　Epidemiology

Tension pneumothorax is a complication in approximately 1% -2% of the cases of idiopathic spontaneous pneumothorax. The actual incidences of tension pneumothorax both outside of a hospital setting and in the intensive care unit (ICU) are unknown.

15.3.2　Pathophysiology

At anytime when a disruption involves the visceral pleura, parietal pleura, or the tracheobronchial tree, the tension pneumothorax may occur. In tension pneumothorax, the injured tissue forms a one-way valve, allowing air inflow into the pleural space with inhalation and prohibiting air outflow. The volume of this nonabsorbable intrapleural air increases with each inspiration because of the one-way valve effect. As a result, the pressure of the affected pleural cavity rises continuously.

As the pressure increases, the ipsilateral lung collapses, which causes hypoxia. Further pressure increase cause the mediastinum to shift toward the contralateral side and impinge on and compress both the contralateral lung and impair the venous return to the right atrium. Both hypoxia and decreased venous return impair cardiac function. It is most evident in trauma patients who are hypovolemic with reduced venous blood return to the heart.

15.3.3　Clinical manifestations

Signs and symptoms of tension pneumothorax are usually more severe than those seen with a simple pneumothorax. Symptoms of tension pneumothorax may include chest pain (90%), dyspnea (80%), anxiety, fatigue, or acute epigastric pain.

15.3.4　History

Besides the history of trauma, a high index of suspicion for tension pneumothorax is in patients on mechanical ventilation with acute onset of hemodynamic instability, difficult ventilation with high inspiratory pressures, and worsening hypoxemia and/or hypercapnia, even with a functioning chest tube in place.

Other great risk of a tension pneumothorax include those with COPD who are using ventilators; those with acute respiratory distress syndrome (ARDS); and those receiving a high tidal volume (>12 mL/kg).

15.3.5 Physical examinations

On examination, breath sounds are absent on the affected hemothorax and the trachea deviates away from the affected side. The thorax may also be hyperresonant; jugular venous distention and tachycardia may present. Hypotension and hypoxia may also occur as the cardiopulmonary system is compromised. If on mechanical ventilation, the airway pressure alarms are triggered.

15.3.6 Supplementary examination

Ultrasonography in the emergency setting is being increasingly used as an adjunct to the physical examination when there is doubt regarding the diagnosis. Chest radiography or CT should be used only in those instances when the clinician is in doubt regarding the diagnosis and when the patient's clinical condition is hemodynamically stable. Obtaining such imaging tests when the diagnosis of tension pneumothorax is not in question causes an unnecessary and potentially lethal delay in the treatment.

15.3.7 Diagnosis and differential diagnosis

The diagnosis of a tension pneumothorax should largely be based on the history and physical examination findings.

Always consider pneumothorax in the differential diagnosis of major trauma. In the patient with blunt trauma and mental status changes, hypoxia, and acidosis, symptoms of a tension pneumothorax may be masked by associated and similarly potentially lethal injuries.

15.3.8 Treatment

A tension pneumothorax is a life-threatening condition and requires immediate action (e. g. , needle thoracostomy or chest tube insertion). If a hemothorax is associated with the pneumothorax, additional chest tubes may be needed to assist drainage of blood and clots, but the clinicians should start from the ABCs (airway, breathing, circulation) consequence while assessing vital signs and oxygen saturation, especially in patients with thoracic trauma.

Tension pneumothorax is usually diagnosed under difficult conditions, with a simple emergency procedure as treatment (i. e. , needle decompression). Make sure no contraindications exist for the placement of an emergency decompression catheter into the thorax. Previous thoracotomy, previous pneumonectomy, and presence of a coagulation disorder, for example, are relative contraindications, because failure to treat tension pneumothorax expectantly can result in patient death.

Yin Wen

Chapter 16

Acute Respiratory Distress Syndrome

Acute respiratory distress syndrome (ARDS) is a clinical syndrome of severe dyspnea of rapid onset, hypoxemia, and diffuse pulmonary infiltrates leading to respiratory failure. ARDS is caused by diffuse lung injury from many underlying medical and surgical disorders. The lung injury may be direct, as it occurs in toxic inhalation, or indirect, as it occurs in sepsis (Table 16−1). The clinical features of ARDS are listed in Table 16−2. By expert consensus, ARDS is defined by three categories based on the degrees of hypoxemia. These stages of mild, moderate, and severe ARDS are associated with mortality risk and with the duration of mechanical ventilation in survivors. The annual incidence of ARDS is estimated to be as high as 60 cases/100,000 population. Approximately 10% of all intensive care unit (ICU) admissions involve patients with acute respiratory failure, of which, 20% of them meet the criteria for ARDS.

Table 16−1 Clinical disorders commonly associated with ARDS

Direct lung injury	Indirect lung injury
Pneumonia	Sepsis
Aspiration of gastric contents	Severe trauma
Pulmonary contusion	Multiple bone fractures
Near−drowning	Flail chest
Toxic inhalation injury	Head trauma
	Burns
	Multiple transfusions
	Drug overdose
	Pancreatitis
	Postcardiopulmonary bypass

Table 16−2 Diagnostic criteria for ARDS

Severity: Oxygenation	Onset	Chest radiograph	Absence of left atrial hypertension
Mild: 200 mmHg< $PaO_2/FiO_2 \leqslant 300$ mmHg	Acute or interstitial infiltrates	Bilateral alveolar or no clinical evidence of increased left atrial pressure	PAWP ≤ 18 mmHg
Moderate: 100 mmHg< $PaO_2/FiO_2 \leqslant 200$ mmHg			
Severe: $PaO_2/FiO_2 \leqslant$ 100 mmHg			

16.1 Etiology

While many medical and surgical illnesses have been associated with the development of ARDS, most cases (>80%) are caused by several clinical disorders: severe sepsis syndrome and/or bacterial pneumonia (40%–50%), trauma, multiple transfusions, aspiration of gastric contents, and drug overdose. Among patients with trauma, the most frequently reported surgical conditions in ARDS are pulmonary contusion, multiple bone fractures, and chest wall trauma/flail chest, whereas head trauma, near–drowning, toxic inhalation, and burns are rare causes. The risks of developing ARDS are increased in patients with more than one predisposing medical or surgical condition.

16.2 Clinical course and pathophysiology

The natural history of ARDS is marked by three phases, exudative, proliferative and fibrotic that each has clinical and pathologic characteristics.

16.2.1 Exudative phase

In this phase, alveolar capillary endothelial cells and type I pneumocytes (alveolar epithelial cells) are injured, with consequent loss of the normally tight alveolar barrier to fluid and macromolecules (Figure 16–1). Edema fluid riching in protein is accumulated in the interstitial and alveolar spaces. Significant concentrations of cytokines (e. g. , interleukin 1, interleukin 8, and tumor necrosis factor α) and lipid mediators are presented in the lung in this acute phase. In response to proinflammatory mediators, leukocytes (especially neutrophils) traffic into the pulmonary interstitium and alveoli. In addition, condensed plasma proteins aggregate in the air spaces with cellular debris and dysfunctional pulmonary surfactant to form hyaline membrane whorls. Pulmonary vascular injury also occurs early in ARDS, with vascular obliteration by microthrombi and fibrocellular proliferation.

Alveolar edema predominantly involves dependent portions of the lung, with diminished aeration and atelectasis. Collapse of large sections of dependent lung markedly decreases lung compliance. Consequently, intrapulmonary shunting and hypoxemia develop and the work of breathing increases, leading to dyspnea. The pathophysiologic alterations in alveolar spaces are exacerbated by microvascular occlusion that results in reductions in pulmonary arterial blood flow to ventilated portions of the lung (and thus in increased dead space) and in pulmonary hypertension. Thus, in addition to severe hypoxemia, hypercapnia secondary to an increase in pulmonary dead space is prominent in early ARDS.

The exudative phase encompasses the first 7 days of illness after exposure to a precipitating ARDS risk factor, with the patient experiencing the onset of respiratory symptoms. Although usually presenting within 12–36 hours after the initial insult, symptoms can be delayed by 5–7 days. Dyspnea develops, with the sensation of rapid shallow breathing and inability to get enough air. Tachypnea and increased work of breathing frequently result in respiratory fatigue and ultimately in respiratory failure. Laboratory tests are generally nonspecific and are primarily indicative of underlying clinical disorders. The chest radiograph usually reveals alveolar and interstitial opacities involving at least three–quarters of the lung fields. While characteristic for ARDS, these radiographic findings are not specific and can be indistinguishable from cardiogenic pul-

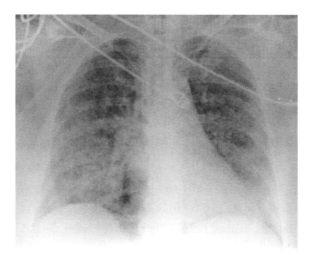

Figure 16-1   A representative anteroposterior chest X-ray in the exudative phase of ARDS shows diffuse interstitial and alveolar infiltrates that can be difficult to distinguish from left ventricular failure

monary edema. Unlike the latter, however, the chest X-ray in ARDS rarely shows cardiomegaly, pleural effusions, or pulmonary vascular redistribution. Chest CT in ARDS reveals extensive heterogeneity of lung involvement(Figure 16-2).

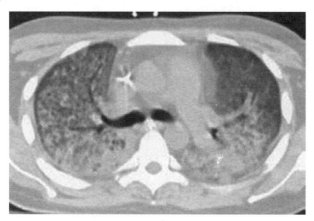

Figure 16-2   A representative CT scan of the chest during the exudative phase of ARDS, in which dependent alveolar edema and atelectasis predominate

Because the early features of ARDS are nonspecific, alternative diagnoses must be considered. In the differential diagnosis of ARDS, the most common disorders are cardiogenic pulmonary edema, diffuse pneumonia, and alveolar hemorrhage. Less common diagnoses to consider include acute interstitial lung diseases, acute immunologic injury, toxin injury, and neurogenic pulmonary edema.

16.2.2   Proliferative phase

This phase of ARDS usually lasts from day 7 to day 21. Most patients recover rapidly and are liberated from mechanical ventilation during this phase. Despite this improvement, many patients still experience dyspnea, tachypnea, and hypoxemia. Some patients develop progressive lung injury and early changes of pulmonary fibrosis during the proliferative phase. Histologically, the first signs of resolution are often evident in this phase, with the initiation of lung repair, the organization of alveolar exudates, and a shift from a neutrophil-to a lymphocyte-predominant pulmonary infiltrate. As part of the reparative process, type II pneumocytes proliferate along alveolar basement membranes. These specialized epithelial cells synthesize new pulmonary surfactant and differentiate into type I pneumocytes.

16.2.3 Fibrotic phase

While many patients with ARDS recover lung function 3-4 weeks after the initial pulmonary injury, some enter a fibrotic phase that may require long-term support on mechanical ventilators and/or supplemental oxygen. Histologically, the alveolar edema and inflammatory exudates of earlier phases are now converted to extensive alveolar-duct and interstitial fibrosis. Marked disruption of acinar architecture leads to emphysema-like changes, with large bullae. Intimal fibroproliferation in the pulmonary microcirculation causes progressive vascular occlusion and pulmonary hypertension. The physiologic consequences include an increased risk of pneumothorax, reductions in lung compliance, and increased pulmonary dead space. Patients in this late phase experience a substantial burden of excess morbidity (Figure 16-3).

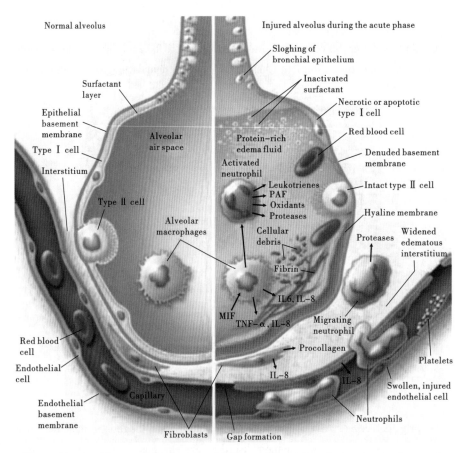

Figure 16-3 The normal alveolus (left) and the injured alveolus in the acute phase of acute lung injury and the acute respiratory distress syndrome (right)

16.3　Diagnosis

The acute respiratory distress syndrome (ARDS) was defined in 1994 by the American European Consensus Conference (AECC); since then, issues regarding the reliability and validity of this definition have emerged. Using a consensus process, a panel of experts convened in 2011 (an initiative of the European Society of Intensive Care Medicine endorsed by the American Thoracic Society and the Society of Critical Care Medicine) developed the Berlin Definition, focusing on feasibility, reliability, validity, and objective evaluation of its performance (Table 16-3).

Table 16-3　The Berlin definition of acute respiratory distress syndrome

Timing	Within 1 week of a known clinical insult or new or worsening respiratory symptoms
Chest imaginga	Bilateral opacities not fully explained by effusions, lobar/lung collapse, or nodules
Origin of edema	Respiratory failure not fully explained by cardiac failure or fluid overload need objective assessment to exclude hydrostatic edema if no risk factor present
Oxygenation	
Mild	PaO_2/FiO_2　200-300 mmHg with PEEP or CPAP$\geqslant$5 cmH_2O
Moderate	PaO_2/FiO_2　100-200 mmHg with PEEP$\geqslant$5 cmH_2O
Severe	PaO_2/FiO_2　0-100 mmHg with PEEP$\geqslant$5 cmH_2O

CPAP: continuous positive airway pressure; FiO_2: fraction of inspired oxygen.

PaO_2, partial pressure of arterial oxygen; PEEP, positive end-expiratory pressure.

16.4　Treatment

16.4.1　General principles

Recent reductions in ARDS mortality rates are largely the result of general advances in the care of critically ill patients. Thus, caring for these patients requires close attention to the recognition and treatment of underlying medical and surgical disorders (e. g. , sepsis, aspiration, trauma); the minimization of procedures and their complications; prophylaxis against venous thromboembolism, gastrointestinal bleeding, aspiration, excessive sedation, and central venous catheter infections; prompt recognition of nosocomial infections; and provision of adequate nutrition.

16.4.2　Management of mechanical ventilation

Patients meeting clinical criteria for ARDS frequently become fatigued from increased work of breathing and progressive hypoxemia, requiring mechanical ventilation for support.

16.4.3　Ventilator-induced lung injury

Despite its life-saving potential, mechanical ventilation can aggravate lung injury. Experimental models have demonstrated that ventilator-induced lung injury appears to require two processes: repeated alveolar overdistention and recurrent alveolar collapse. As is clearly evident from chest CT, ARDS is a heterogeneous disorder, principally involving dependent portions of the lung with relative sparing of other regions. Because compliance differs in affected versus more"normal"areas of the lung, attempts to fully inflate the consolidated lung may lead to overdistention of and injury to the more normal areas. Ventilator-induced injury can be demonstrated in experimental models of acute lung injury, with high-tidal-volume (VT) ventilation resulting in additional, synergistic alveolar damage.

16.4.4　Prevention of alveolar collapse

In ARDS, the presence of alveolar and interstitial fluid and the loss of surfactant can lead to a marked reduction of lung compliance. Without an increase in end-expiratory pressure, significant alveolar collapse can occur at end-expiration, with consequent impairment of oxygenation. In most clinical settings, positive end-expiratory pressure (PEEP) is empirically set to minimize FiO_2(inspired O_2 percentage)and maximize PaO_2(arterial partial pressure of O_2). On most modern mechanical ventilators, it is possible to construct a static pressure-volume curve for the respiratory system. The lower inflection point on the curve represents alveolar opening. The pressure at this point, usually 12-15 mmHg in ARDS, is a theoretical"optimal PEEP" for alveolar recruitment. Titration of the PEEP to the lower inflection point on the static pressure-volume curve has been hypothesized to keep the lung open, improving oxygenation and protecting against lung injury. Three large randomized trials have investigated the utility of PEEP-based strategies to keep the lung open. In all of the three trials, improvement in lung function was evident but overall mortality rates were not altered significantly. Until more data become available on the clinical utility of high PEEP, it is advisable to set PEEP to minimize FiO_2 and optimize PaO_2. Measurement of esophageal pressures to estimate transpulmonary pressure may help identify an optimal PEEP in some cases.

16.4.5　Fluid management

Increased pulmonary vascular permeability leading to interstitial and alveolar edema fluid rich in protein is a central feature of ARDS. In addition, impaired vascular integrity augments the normal increase in extravascular lung water that occurs with increasing left atrial pressure.

Maintaining a low left atrial filling pressure minimizes pulmonary edema and prevents further decrements in arterial oxygenation and lung compliance, improves pulmonary mechanics, shortens ICU stay and the duration of mechanical ventilation, and is associated with a lower mortality in both medical and surgical ICU patients. Thus, aggressive attempts to reduce left atrial filling pressures with fluid restriction and diuretics should be an important aspect of ARDS management, limited only by hypotension and hypoperfusion of critical organs such as the kidneys.

16.4.6　Neuromuscular blockade

In severe ARDS, sedation alone can be inadequate for the patient ventilator synchrony required for lung-protective ventilation. This clinical problem was recently addressed in a multicenter, randomized, placebo-controlled trial of early neuromuscular blockade (with cisatracurium besylate) for 48 hours. In severe ARDS, early neuromuscular blockade increased the rate of survival and ventilator-free days without increasing ICU acquired paresis. These promising findings support the early administration of neuromuscular blockade if needed to facilitate mechanical ventilation in severe ARDS; however, these results must be replicated prior to their widespread application in clinical practice.

16.4.7   Glucocorticoids

Many attempts have been made to treat both early and late ARDS with glucocorticoids, with the goal of reducing potentially deleterious pulmonary inflammation. Few studies have shown any benefit. Current evidence does not support the use of high dose glucocorticoids in the care of ARDS patients.

16.4.8   Other therapies

Clinical trials of surfactant replacement and multiple other medical therapies have proved disappointing. Inhaled nitric oxide and inhaled epoprostenol sodium can transiently improve oxygenation but do not improve survival or decrease the time on mechanical ventilation.

16.4.9   Recommendations

Many clinical trials have been undertaken to improve the outcome of patients with ARDS; most have been unsuccessful in modifying the natural history of ARDS. While results of large clinical trials must be judiciously applied to individual patients, evidence-based recommendations are summarized in Table 16-4, and an algorithm for the initial therapeutic goals and limits in ARDS management are provided in Figure 16-4.

Table 16-4   Evidence-based recommendations for ARDS therapies

Treatment	Recommendation
Mechanical ventilation	
Low tidal volume	I
Minimized left atrial filling pressures	II
High PEEP or open lung	III
Prone position	III
Recruitment maneuvers	III
High-frequency ventilation	IV
ECMO	III
Early neuromuscular blockade	I
Glucocorticoid treatment	IV
Surfactant replacement, inhaled epoprostenol, IV and other anti-inflammatory therapy	

I . recommended therapy based on strong clinical evidence from randomized clinical trials.

II . recommended therapy based on supportive but limited clinical data.

III . recommended only as alternative therapy on the basis of indeterminate evidence.

IV . not recommended on the basis of clinical evidence against efficacy of therapy.

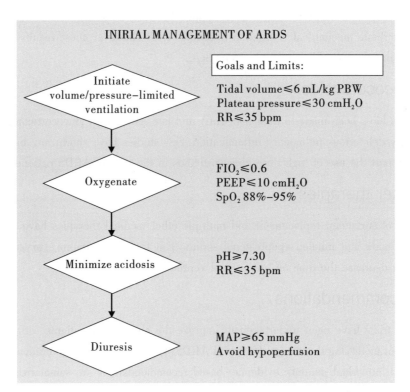

INIRIAL MANAGEMENT OF ARDS

Figure 16-4 **Algorithm for the initial management of ARDS**

Clinical trials have provided evidence-based therapeutic goals for a stepwise approach to the early mechanical ventilation, oxygenation, and correction of acidosis and diuresis of critically ill patients with ARDS.

16.5 Prognosis

The major risk factors for ARDS mortality are nonpulmonary. Advanced age is an important risk factor. Patients >75 years of age have a substantially higher mortality risk (60%) than those <45(20%). Moreover, patients >60 years of age with ARDS and sepsis have a threefold higher mortality risk than those <60. Other risk factors include preexisting organ dysfunction from chronic medical illness in particular, chronic liver disease, cirrhosis, chronic alcohol abuse, chronic immunosuppression, sepsis, chronic renal disease, failure of any nonpulmonary organ, and increased APACHE III scores.

Patients with ARDS arising from direct lung injury (including pneumonia, pulmonary contusion, and aspiration); Table 16-1 are nearly twice as likely to die as those with indirect causes of lung injury, while surgical and trauma patients with ARDS especially those without direct lung injury have a higher survival rate than other ARDS patients. An early (within 24 h of presentation) elevation in pulmonary dead space (>0.60) and severe arterial hypoxemia (PaO_2/FiO_2, <100 mmHg) predict increased mortality risk from ARDS; however, there is surprisingly little additional value in predicting ARDS mortality from other measures of the severity of lung injury, including the level of PEEP (≥ 10 cmH$_2$O), respiratory system compliance (≤ 40 mL/cmH$_2$O), the extent of alveolar infiltrates on chest radiography, and the corrected expired volume per minute (≥ 10 L/min).

16.6   Functional recovery in ARDS survivors

While it is common for patients with ARDS to experience prolonged respiratory failure and remain dependent on mechanical ventilation for survival, it is a testament to the resolving powers of the lung that the majority of patients recover nearly normal lung function. Patients usually recover maximal lung function within 6 months. One year after endotracheal extubation, more than one-third of ARDS survivors have normal spirometry values and diffusion capacity. Most of the remaining patients have only mild abnormalities in pulmonary function.

Yin Wen

Chapter 17

Pulmonary Embolism

Pulmonary embolism(PE)is a blockage of pulmonary arteries or its branches by a substance that has travelled from elsewhere in the body through the bloodstream. PE most commonly results from deep vein thrombosis (a blood clot in the deep veins of the legs or pelvis) that breaks off and migrates to the lung, a process termed venous thromboembolism (VTE). Non-thrombotic PE etiologies include fat embolism after pelvic or long bone fracture, tumor embolism, bone marrow embolism, air embolism and so on. The obstruction of the blood flow through the lungs and the resultant pressure on the right ventricle of the heart lead to the symptoms and signs of PE.

17.1 Epidemiology

VTE encompasses deep vein thrombosis (DVT) and PE. It is the third most frequent cardiovascular disease with an overall annual incidence of 100-200 per 100,000 inhabitants.

The epidemiology of PE is difficult to determine because it may remain asymptomatic, or its diagnosis may be an incidental finding: in some cases, the first presentation of PE may be sudden death. There is no accurate epidemiological data on pulmonary embolism in China.

17.2 Predisposing factors

DVT and PE have common risk factors, namely the risk factors of VTE. VTE is extensive collection of predisposing environmental and genetic factors. The two most common autosomal dominant genetic mutations are factor V Leiden, which causes resistance to the endogenous anticoagulant, activated protein C(which inactivates clotting factors V and VIII), and the prothrombin gene mutation, which increases the plasma prothrombin concentration. Antithrombin, protein C, and protein S are naturally occurring coagulation inhibitors. Deficiencies of these inhibitors are associated with VTE, but are rare. Antiphospholipid antibody syndrome is the most common acquired cause of thrombophilia and is associated with venous or arterial thrombosis. Other common predisposing factors include cancer, obesity, cigarette smoking, systemic arterial hypertension, chronic obstructive pulmonary disease, chronic kidney disease, blood transfusion, long-haul air travel, air pollution, oral contraceptives, pregnancy, postmenopausal hormone replacement, surgery, and trauma.

17.3   Pathophysiology

When deep venous thrombi detach from their site of formation, they embolize to the vena cava, right atrium, and right ventricle, and lodge in the pulmonary arterial circulation, thereby causing acute PE. Many patients with PE have no evidence of DVT because the clot has already embolized to the lungs. Acute PE interferes with both the circulation and gas exchange. Right ventricular (RV) failure due to pressure overload is considered the primary cause of death in severe PE. Pulmonary artery pressure increases only if more than 30%–50% of the total cross–sectional area of the pulmonary arterial bed is occluded by thromboemboli. Anatomical obstruction and vasoconstriction lead to an increase in pulmonary vascular resistance and a proportional decrease in arterial compliance. The abrupt increase in pulmonary vascular resistance results in RV dilation, which alters the contractile properties of the RV myocardium via the Frank–Starling mechanism. The increase in RV pressure and volume leads to an increase in wall tension and myocyte stretch. RV contraction time is prolonged, while neurohumoralactiction leads to inotropic and chronotropic stimulation. Together with systemic vasoconstriction, these compensatory mechanisms increase pulmonary vascular bed, and thus temporarily stabilize systemic blood pressure (BP). The extent of adaptation is limited, since a non–preconditioned, thin–walled right ventricle (RV) is unable to generate a mean pulmonary artery pressure above 40 mmHg.

17.4   Clinical symptoms

PE may escape prompt diagnosis since the clinical signs and symptoms are non–specific (Table 17–1). The most common symptom is unexplained breathlessness.

Table 17–1   Clinical characteristics of patients with suspected PE in the emergency department

Feature	PE confirmed (n=1,880)	PE not confirmed (n=1,880)
Dyspnoea	50%	51%
Pleyritic chest pain	39%	28%
Cough	23%	23%
Substernal chest pain	15%	17%
Fever	10%	10%
Haemoptysis	8%	4%
Syncope	6%	6%
Unilateral leg pain	6%	5%
Signs of DVT (unilateral extremity swelling)	24%	18%

17.5 Diagnosis

Low clinical likelihood of DVT if point score is 0; moderate likelihood if score is 1-2; High likelihood if score is 3 or greater (Table 17-2).

PE is known as "the Great Masquerader". Diagnosis is difficult because symptoms and signs are non-specific (Table 17-3).

Table 17-2 Clinical decision rules of DVT

Clinical variable	DVT score
Active cancer	1
Paralysis, paresis, or recent cast	1
Bedridden for >3 days; major surgery <12 weeks	1
Tenderness along distribution of deep veins	1
Entire leg swelling	1
Unilateral calf swelling >3 cm	1
Pitting edema	1
Collateral superficial nonvaricose veins	1
Alternative diagnosis at least as likely as DVT	-2

Table 17-3 Clinical decision rules of PE

Clinical Variable	PE score
Signs and symptoms of DVT	3.0
Alternative diagnosis less likely than PE	3.0
Heart rate >100/min	1.5
Immobilization >3 days; surgery within 4 weeks	1.5
Prior PE or DVT	1.5
Hemoptysis	1.0
Cancer	1.0

High clinical likelihood of PE if point score exceeds 4.

17.5.1 D-dimer

The plasma D-dimer quantified via enzyme-linked immunosorbent assay rises in the presence of DVT or PE because of the breakdown of fibrin by plasmin. Elevation of D-dimer indicates endogenous although often clinically ineffective thrombolysis. The sensitivivy of the D-dimer test is >80% for DVT (including isolated calf DVT) and >95% for PE. The D-dimer is less sensitive for DVT than for PE because the DVT thrombus size is smaller. A normal D-dimer is a useful 'rule out' test.

17.5.2   In blood gas analysis

Hypoxaemia is considered a typical finding in acute PE. Hypocapnia is also often present.

17.5.3   Elevated cardiac biomarkers

Serum troponin and plasma heart−type fatty acid−binding protein levels increase because of RV micro-infarction. Myocardial stretch causes release of brain natriuretic peptide or NT−pro−brain natriuretic peptide.

17.5.4   Electrocardiogram

The most frequently cited abnormality, in addition to sinus tachycardia, is the $S_1 Q_{III} T_{III}$ sign: an S wave in lead I, a Q wave in lead III, and an inverted T wave in lead III. This finding is relatively specific but insensitive. RV strain and ischemia cause the most common abnormality, T−wave inversion in leads V_1 to V_4.

17.5.5   Chest roentgenography

A normal or nearly normal chest X−ray often occurs in PE. Well−established abnormalities include focal oligemia (Westermark's sign), a peripheral wedged−shaped density above the diaphragm (Hampton's hump), and an enlarged right descending pulmonary artery (Palla's sign).

17.5.6   Echocardiography

Echocardiography is not a reliable diagnostic imaging tool for acute PE because most patients with PE have normal echocardiograms. However, echocardiography is a very useful diagnostic tool for detecting conditions that may mimic PE, such as acute myocardial infarction, pericardial tamponade, and aortic dissection.

17.5.7   Venous ultrasonography

Venous ultrasonography of the deep venous system relies on loss of vein compressibility as the primary criterion for DVT. When a normal vein is imaged in cross−section, it readily collapses with gentle manual pressure from the ultrasound transducer. This creates the illusion of a 'wink'. With acute DVT, the vein loses its compressibility because of passive distention by acute thrombus. The diagnosis of acute DVT is even more secure when thrombus is directly visualized. It appears homogeneous and has low echogenicity (Figure 17−1).

Patients with a low−to−moderate likelihood of DVT or PE should undergo initial diagnostic evaluation with D−dimer testing alone without obligatory imaging teses. However, patients with a high clinical likelihood of VTE should skip D−dimer testing and undergo imaging as the next step in the diagnostic algorithm.

17.5.8   Chest CT

CT of the chest with intravenous contrast is the principal imaging test for the diagnosis of PE. Since the introduction of multi−detector computed tomographic (MDCT) angiography with high spatial and temporal resolution and quality of arterial opacification, computed tomographic (VT) angiography has become the method of choice for imaging the pulmonary vasculature in patients with suspected PE. Sixty−order branches can be visualized with resolution superior to that of conventional invasive contrast pulmonary angiography (Figure 17−2).

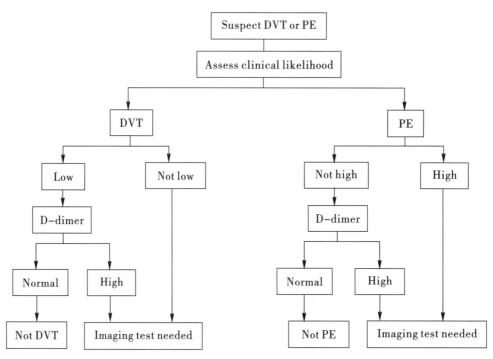

Figure 17-1　Algorithm for diagnostic imaging

17.5.9　Lung scanning

Lung scanning has become a second-line diagnostic test for PE, used mostly for patients who can not tolerate intravenous contrast. The perfusion scan defect indicates absent or desreased blood flow, possibly due to PE. Abnormal ventilation scans indicate abnormal nonventilated lung, thereby providing possible explanations for perfusion defects other than acute PE, such as asthma and chronic obstructive pulmonary disease.

17.5.10　Magnetic resonance（MR）（contrast-enhanced）imaging

When ultrasound is equivocal, MR venography with gadolinium contrast is an excellent imaging modality to diagnose DVT. MR pulmonary angiography may detect large proximal PE, but it is not reliable for smaller segmental and subsegmental PE.

17.5.11　Pulmonary angiography

Pulmonary angiography is invasive diagnostic modalities. Chest CT with contrast has virtually replaced invasive pulmonary angiography as a diagnostic test.

17.6　Treatment

17.6.1　Haemodynamic and respiratory support

Acute RV failure with resulting low systemic output is the leading cause of death in patients with high-risk PE.

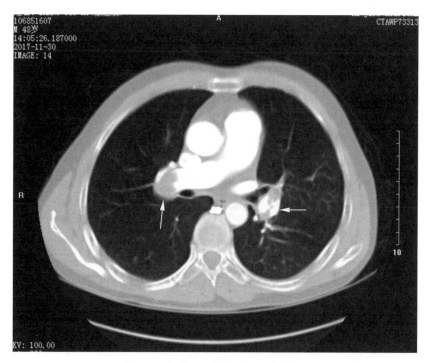

Figure 17-2　**Pulmonary embolism**

White arrows show filling defects in both pulmonary arteries, indicating pulmonary embolism.

17.6.2　Anticoagulation

Effective anticoagulation is the foundation for successful treatment of DVT and PE. The standard duration of anticoagulation should cover at least 3 months. Within this period, acute-phase treatment consists of administering parenteral anticoagulation [unfractionated heparin (UFH) , LMWH or fondaparinux] over the first 5-10 days. LMWH or fondaparinux are preferred over UFH for initial anticoagulation in PE, as they carry a lower risk of inducing major bleeding and heparin-induced thrombocytopenia (HIT). Parenteral heparin should overlap with the initiation of a vitamin K antagonist (VKA) ; alternatively, it can be followed by administration of one of the new oral anticoagulants : dabigatran or edoxaban. If rivaroxaban or apixaban is given instead, oral medicine treatment with one of these agents should be started directly or after a 1- 2 day administration of UFH, LMWH or fondaparinux.

17.6.2.1　Unfractionated heparin

UFH is dosed to achieve a target activated partial thromboplastin time (APTT) of 60-80 seconds. The most common method is using an initial bolus of 80 U/kg, followed by an initial infusion rate of 18 U/(kg · h). The major advantage of UFH is its short half-life, which is especially useful in patients in whom hour-to-hour control of the intensity of anticoagulation is desired.

17.6.2.2　Low-Molecular-Weight Heparins

These fragments of UFH exhibit less binding to plasma proteins and endothelial cells and consequently have greater bioavailability, a more predictable dose response, and a longer half-life than does UFH. No monitoring or dose asjustment is needed unless the patient is markedly obese or has chronic kidney disease.

17.6.2.3 Fondaparinux

An anti-Xa pentasaccharide, is administered subcutaneously as a weight-based once-daily. No laboratory monitoring is required. Fondaparinux is synthesized medicine and, unlike LMWH or UFH. It does not cause heparin-induced thrombocytopenia. The dose must be adjusted downward for patients with renal dysfunction.

17.6.2.4 Warfarin

This vitamin K antagonist prevents carboxylation activation of coagulation factors II, VII, IX, and X. The full effect of warfarin requires at least 5 days, even if the prothrombin time, used for monitoring, becomes elevated more rapidly. If warfarin is initiated as monotherapy during an acute thrombotic illness, a paradoxical exacerbation of hypercoagulability increases the likelihood of thrombosis. Overlapping UFH, LMWH, fondaparinux, or parenteral direct thrombin inhibitors with warfarin for at least 5 days will nullify the early procoagulant effect of warfarin. In an average-size adult, warfarin is often initiated in a dose of 5 mg. The prothrombin time is standardized by calculating the international normalized ratio (INR), which assesses the anticoagulant effect of warfarin. The target INR is usually 2.5, with a range of 2.0-3.0.

17.6.2.5 Novel oral anticoagulants

Novel oral anticoagulants are administered in a fixed dose, which establish effective anticoagulation within hours of ingestion, require no laboratory coagulation monitoring, and have few of the drug-drug or drug-food interactions that make warfarin so difficult to dose. Rivaroxaban, a factor Xa inhibitor, is approved for treatment of acute DVT and acute PE as monotherapy. Apixaban is likely to receive similar approval for oral monotherapy. Dabigatran, a direct thrombin inhibitor, and edoxaban, a factor Xa inhibitor, are likely to be approved for treatment of VTE after an initial course of parenteral anticoagulation.

17.6.2.6 Duration of anticoagulation

For DVT isolated to an upper extremity or calf that has been provoked by surgery, trauma, estrogen, or an indwelling central venous catheter or pacemaker, 3 months of anticoagulation usually are sufficed. For an initial episode of provoked proximal leg DVT or PE, 3-6 months of anticoagulation are considered sufficient. Among patients with idiopathic, unprovoked VTE, the recurrence rate is high after cessation of anticoagulation. American College of CHEST Physicians (ACCP) guidelines recommend considering anticoagulation for an indefinite duration with a target INR between 2 and 3 for patients with idiopathic VTE. An alternative approach after the first 6 months of anticoagulation is to reduce the intensity of anticoagulation and to lower the target INR range to between 1.5 and 2.

17.6.3 Thrombolytic treatment

Thrombolytic treatment of acute PE restores pulmonary perfusion more rapidly than anticoagulation with UFH alone. The early resolution of pulmonary obstruction leads to a prompt reduction in pulmonary artery pressure and resistance, with a concomitant improvement in RV function. The haemodynamic benefits of thrombolysis are confined to the first few days; in survivors, differences are no longer apparent at one week after treatment. Commonly used thrombolytic drugs include urokinase (UK), streptokinase (SK) and recombinant tissue plasminogen activator (rtPA).

17.6.4 Inferior vena caval (IVC) filters

The two principal indications for insertion of an IVC filter are active bleeding that precludes anticoagulation and recurrent venous thrombosis despite intensive anticoagulation.

17.6.5   Pulmonary embolectomy

The risk of major hemorrhage with systemically administered fibrinolysis has prompted a renaissance of interest in surgical embolectomy, an operation that had almost become extinct. More rapid referral before the onset of irreversible multisystem organ failure and improved surgical technique have resulted in a high survival rate.

Yin Wen

Chapter 18

Vomiting and Diarrhea

Vomiting and diarrhea are among the most common complaints of patients presenting to emergency departments. They are mainly seen in gastrointestinal dysfunction, such as acute gastroenteritis and ileus. Therefore, many patients complaining of vomiting and diarrhea have a cause of other diseases, such as uremia, myocardial infarction, alcohol or drug poisoning, motion sickness, migraine, neuropathic gluttony, severe pain, etc. Emergency physicians must consider not only the gastrointestinal emergencies manifested as vomiting or diarrhea but also the non-gastrointestinal emergencies manifested as gastrointestinal dysfunction.

18.1 Vomiting

18.1.1 Pathophysiology

Vomiting is a complex, highly coordinated activity involving the gastrointestinal tract, the central nervous system and the vestibular system. Vomiting is controlled by two different medullary centers, the emetic center on the dorsal side of the lateral reticular structure and the chemoreceptor trigger zone on the dorsal side of the fourth ventricle. Three stages of vomiting have been described as nausea, retching and emesis. The process begins with the relaxation of the fundus, the contraction of the pylorus, followed by the strong contraction of powerful abdominal muscles simultaneously.

18.1.2 Etiology

There are many causes of vomiting, involving almost all organs and systems. The most common cause in emergency is digestive disorder. The causes of nervous system, endocrine system and poisoning are also common seen. Asking the right history of the patient will help to uncover the etiology.

18.1.3 Clinical manifestations

The cause of vomiting is various, with different premonitory symptoms, the time of the vomiting, frequency, the definition of the vomitus and the accompanying symptoms. A intense vomiting can lead to a series of clinical consequences, so it is important to give an early evaluation of patients and deal with emergency. Vomiting may result in the following complications: low blood volume, metabolic alkalosis, low potassium, Mallory – Weiss tear (esophageal and cardiac linear tear) , Boerhaave syndrome (esophageal rupture) , and aspiration.

18.1.4   Diagnosis

There are hundreds of causes of vomiting, which can generally be found by detailed medical history collection and physical examination.

18.1.4.1   History of diseases

(1) Present history

1) Composition of vomitus: hematemesis is seen with gastritis, peptic ulcer disease, gastric and esophageal tumors, and Mallory–Weiss tears. Nonbilious emesis occurs with gastric outlet obstruction, as in patients with pyloric strictures secondary to ulcer disease or infants with pyloric stenosis.

2) Accompanying symptoms: vomiting may be accompanied by salivation, defecation, tachycardia, bradycardia, atrial fibrillation or paroxysmal rapid ventricular arrhythmia. Vomiting is one of the signs of increased intracranial or intraocular pressure. If nausea and vomiting are accompanied by chronic headache, intracranial lesions should be suspected. In female patients, obstetric and gynecologic causes of vomiting should always be considered. In a pregnant woman, epigastric pain and vomiting accompanying hypertension may indicate preeclampsia.

(2) Personal history

Including alcoholism and other drug addiction.

(3) Previous medical history

The digestive system diseases and surgical history should be emphasized. There is also a history of nutrition and medication should be collected.

18.1.4.2   Physical examination

If jaundice, enlarged lymph nodes, abdomen mass, and bloody stools are found, it may help determine the cause. The vital sign should be monvtered in patients with dehydration, dizziness, weakness, or signs of intoxication should be record by the vital signs. Severely volume–depleted patients require immediate intervention, lest circulatory collapse be imminent. The physical examinations of nervous system include cranial nerves, fundoscope and gait.

18.1.4.3   Laboratory inspection

Determine the appropriate laboratory examination according to the medical history and physical examination findings.

(1) Blood routine: the increased haematocrit and hemoglobin indicates the blood concentration. And there is no specific change in white blood cells.

(2) Electrolytes: severe and prolonged vomiting may cause hypochloremia, hypokalemia and metabolic alkalosis. The patients with symptoms longer than 3 days, who need intravenous fluids, should be tested for electrolytes.

(3) Serum urea nitrogen and creatinine: the ratio of serum urea nitrogen to creatinine exceeds 20 : 1 indicates severe dehydration.

(4) Serum amylase: when serum amylase and lipases are increased, it indicates the possibility of pancreatitis.

(5) Urine test: fertile women are required to have a urine pregnancy test. If nitrite, white blood cells and bacteria are found in the urine, it indicates urinary infection. Ketone body indicates diabetic ketosis, while hematuria may result from urinary calculus.

(6) Blood drug concentration test: it is necessary to take a blood drug concentration test for those patients taking theophylline, digoxin and salicylic acid, especially for the elderly.

(7) Chest and abdominal radiography: chest and abdominal radiography can assist in the determination of the presence or absence of pneumoperitoneum, pneumonia, or intestinal obstruction.

Electrocardiogram: the patients suspected of coronary ischemia should be examined.

18.1.5　Treatment

18.1.5.1　Rapid assessment and treatment

Regardless of cause, initial management of the acute vomiting patients is the same. Firstly, take a quick evaluation of the vital signs, to assess whether the patient's hemodynamic state is stable. The patient with circulatory collapse secondary to severe dehydration, aggressive volume repletion must be given immediately upon arrival. Two large-bore intravenous catheters should be placed, and crystalloid should be administered aggressively in order to restore circulation quickly.

18.1.5.2　Further treatment

For patients with less acute conditions, treatment hinges on making the correct diagnosis.

(1) General treatment: decreased intake is the main cause of dehydration and malnutrition in patients with vomiting, so gastric tube should be placed in patients with persistent vomiting.

(2) Etiological treatment: etiological treatment is fundamental to relieving nausea and vomiting.

(3) Expectant treatment: the effect of antiemetics varies from person to person. Antihistamines and phenothiazine are commonly used. Antihistamines have promethazine (12.5-25 mg, iv, im, po or rectally q 6 h), diphenhydramine aminophylline (20mg, im q 8 h). Phenothiazide has complex effects, mainly by antagonizing dopamine receptors in the chemoreceptor trigger zone. Prochlorazine is commonly used (5-10 mg, iv, im, po q 4 h or 25 mg rectally q 6 h).

18.2　Diarrhea

18.2.1　Pathophysiology

Relative to the patient's normal condition, diarrhea is defined as the increasement of volume and frequency of stool, or feces are watery. There are four basic mechanisms of diarrhea: increased intestinal secretion, decreased intestinal absorption, increased osmotic load, and abnormal intestinal motility.

Diarrhea can be classified as acute and chronic, with a disease course of less than 4 weeks called acute diarrhea, while over 4 weeks called chronic diarrhea. According to the characteristics, diarrhea can be divided into: infiltration, secretion, inflammatory and abnormal dynamic diarrhea.

18.2.2　Clinical manifestations

Strictly speaking, diarrhea is presented when the daily stool weight exceeds 200 g. Practically speaking, however, diarrhea is presented when the patient discharges more stools of lesser consistency, more frequently. Once a true diarrheal illness is confirmed, the physician's focus should change to ascertain the cause of the diarrhea. Part of patients also suffer from some accompanying symptoms, such as fever, abdominal pain, headache or vomiting.

18.2.3   Diagnosis

After initial evaluation and treatment, the acquirement of history, physical examination and laboratory examination can help further identify the cause of diarrhea.

18.2.3.1   History

(1) Volume, frequency and characteristics of defecation: it is important to ask the beginning and duration of diarrhea, accompanying symptoms such as vomiting, fever, abdominal pain, stress, and neurological symptoms.

(2) The relationship of diarrhea with other symptoms. A large number of watery diarrhea followed by the occurrence of spasmodic pain indicates the possibility of gastroenteritis. Abdominal pain after defecation may indicate surgical lesions. Make sure whether diet aggravates diarrhea.

(3) Define the diarrhea: is it bloody or melanotic? Is it associated with the ingestion of certain foods, such as milk or sorbitol?

(4) What is the effect of diarrhea treatment? Is there any previous history of medication and surgery therapies? Is there previous history of HIV infection, diabetes, gastrointestinal bleeding, malignant tumors, abdominal surgery or endocrine disease? Medications commonly have diarrhea as a side effect or sequel. Is the patient taking medication that may have contributed to the diarrhea (e. g., antibiotics, lithium, chemotherapy, colchicine, and laxatives)?

(5) Special situations in personal and family history. Has the patient traveled outside or to the countryside recently? Rural hiking places the patient at risk for Giardia, particularly if water purification procedures were not strictly followed. Sexual and occupational histories are also important. A patient's sexual preference or occupation may be the physician's only clue to a diagnosis of gay bowel disease or organophosphate poisoning.

18.2.3.2   Physical examination

(1) Assessment of circulating volume: as with a diarrhea patient, the examination begins with the vital signs. The assessment of hydration status occurs shortly after the physician arrives at the bedside. Like the history, a careful physical examination can help the differential diagnosis.

Only by doing a thyroid examination can the physician discover a thyroid mass that may be contributing to diarrhea.

(2) Abdominal and rectal examinations: abdominal and rectal examinations are critical. Especially in the elderly, fecal impaction may result in diarrhea as liquid stool passes around the impaction. Special attention should be given to the presence or absence of surgical scars, tenderness, masses, or peritoneal signs. Checking the stool for the presence or absence of blood is also important, since bloody diarrhea can be caused by inflammation, infection, or ischemia. An elderly patient with bloody diarrhea and abdominal pain out of proportion to the physical examination may have mesenteric ischemia.

18.2.3.3   Laboratory inspection

Most diarrhea is self-limiting, so laboratory tests and diagnostic tests are of limited value.

(1) Fecal occult blood test and fecal leukocytes: it is not appropriate to use leukocytes in defecate smear examination primarily to speculate that patients suffering from gastroenteritis and to decide whether to use antibiotics, because it has no specificity for bacterial colitis but only supports the diagnosis. Inflammatory diarrhea with fecal leukocytes and erythrocytes may be caused by many factors, including bacteria, parasites and many non-infectious factors, such as chemotherapy, radiotherapy, allergic reactions, autoimmune

diseases and inflammatory bowel disease. In feces and urine erythrocytes are not necessarily existed with leukocytes at the same time. Only erythrocytes existed in the feces without leukocytes often hint amoeba, malignant tumor, hemorrhoids, heavy metal poisoning, perforation, intestinal ischemia and gastrointestinal bleeding, etc.

(2)Clostridium difficile toxin assay: clostridium difficile diarrhea is most commonly seen during antibiotic use. If the patient complains of recent use of antibiotics, this examination should be considered. Twenty-five to forty percent of cases do not develop diarrhea until 12 weeks after antibiotic use.

(3)Escherichia coli O157:H7 toxin: in endemic areas and suspected haemorrhagic uremia syndrome patients may be considered for this examination.

(4)Fecal bacterial culture: patients with fever, poisoning, immunosuppression, advanced age, prolonged course of disease and ineffective traditional treatment must undergo fecal bacterial culture.

(5)Detection of fecal parasites and parasitic eggs: not recommended for routine examination except for the following cases: reports of chronic diarrhea, parliamentary tourism history, contact with the baby in the nursery and HIV infected persons.

(6)Urine test: urine test should be conducted when urinary system infection or pregnancy is suspected.

18.2.4 Treatment

18.2.4.1 Rapid assessment and initial treatment: management

The evaluation and treatment of a patient with diarrhea should begin with the assessment of the vital signs. Diarrhea of any type can cause circulatory collapse. Attention should be paid to evidence of hemodynamic instability, such as low blood pressure, tachycardia, wet, cold, pale skin, oliguria, shortness of breath, and changes in mental state. Rehydration of severely dehydrated patients should begin immediately after large-bore intravenous access is achieved, meanwhile looking for the signs of systemic diseases such as fever, abdominal pain, dehydration, bloody stool, muscle pain, headache, loss of appetite, etc.

18.2.4.2 Further treatment

According to the severity of dehydration, initial treatment for patient includes support for care and assessment of dehydration.

Patient with mild to moderate dehydration is recommended to take oral rehydration therapy. Mildly dehydrated patients should aim to drink 30-50 mL/kg over the next 4 hours. For moderate dehydration, patients should drink 100 mL/kg over the next 4 hours. Patients with significant dehydration should be given intravenous saline or lactate lindgren's solution. Children are recommended a supplement normal saline at a dose of 20 mL/kg.

Thereafter, treatment is dictated by the differential diagnosis.

Noninfectious diarrhea: almost all true diarrheal emergencies are of noninfectious origin, such as gastrointestinal bleeding, adrenal insufficiency, thyroid storm, toxicologic exposures, acute radiation syndrome, and mesenteric ischemia. The emergency physician must be ever mindful of them because patients with those conditions require intensive treatment and hospitalization.

Infectious diarrhea: viruses cause the vast majority of infectious diarrheas, followed by bacterial and parasitic organisms. Treatment of infectious diarrhea involves antibiotic therapy, antimotility agents, restoration of fluid balance, and avoidance of agents that worsen diarrhea.

Li Xiaogang

Chapter 19

Abdominal Pain

Abdominal pain is a common complaint in emergency department (ED) and often diagnostically challenging. The nature and quality of abdominal pain may be difficult for the patient to convey. Physical examination findings are variable and can be misleading. The location and severity of the pain may change over time.

19.1 Pathophysiology

Abdominal pain is traditionally divided into three categories: visceral, parietal, and referred. The causes may be inflammatory, mechanical, vascular, neoplastic, congenital and trauma. The common causes of abdominal pain are as displayed in Table 19-1.

Table 19-1 Common causes of abdominal pain

Causative disorder or condition	Etiology	Presentation	Physical examination	Useful test(s)
Gastric, esophageal, or duodenal inflammation	Infection, exogenous sources	Epigastric, localized Pain	Epigastric tenderness without rebound or guarding	Testing for Helicobacter pylori, stool routine
Acute appendicitis	Crapulent, exces-sive drinking	Epigastric or periumbilical pain	Tenderness, rebound	CT is sensitive and specific, Leukocyte count usually elevated
Biliary tract disease	Gallstones, cholecystitis	Crampy pain, nausea or postprandial pain	tenderness, rebound, and jaundice	Lipase and liver function tests, ultrasound
Ureteral colic	Family history, gout, Proteus infection.	flank pain radiating to groin, nausea	Tenderness on renal region	Hematuria, CT
Diverticulitis	Infection, perforation, peritonitis, abscesses	Stool frequency change, fever, nausea	Fever, pain without rebound	CT is often diagnostic
Acute gastroenteritis	Travel, immunocompromise	Diarrhea, nausea and Vomiting	Fever, peritoneal signs	Heme-positive stools
Constipation	Idiopathic or hypokinesis secondary	Abdominal pain; change the habits of bowel movement	peritoneal signs, hard stool or impaction	Radiographs
Nonspecific abdominal pain	Unknown	Chronic, recurrent pain	No peritoneal signs, Rectal examination	Variable and oftencan be done

(1) Visceral pain results from stimulation of autonomic nerves invested in the visceral peritoneum surrounding internal organs. It is often the earliest manifestation of a particular disease process. Distention of hollow organs by fluid or gas and capsular stretching of solid organs from edema, blood, cysts, or abscesses are the most common stimuli. This discomfort is poorly characterized and difficult to localize. If the involved organ is affected by peristalsis, the pain often is described as intermittent, crampy, or colicky. In general, visceral pain is perceived from the abdominal region that correlates with the embryonic somatic segment.

(2) Parietal or somatic abdominal pain is caused by irritation of fibers that innervate the parietal peritoneum. Because parietal afferent signals are sent from a specific area of peritoneum, parietal pain can be localized to the dermatome directly above the site of the painful stimulus. As the underlying disease process evolves, the symptoms of visceral pain give way to the signs of parietal pain, with tenderness and guarding. As localized peritonitis develops further, rigidity and "rebound" appear.

(3) Referred pain is defined as pain felt at a distance from its source because peripheral afferent nerve fibers from many internal organs enter the spinal cord through nerve roots that also carry nociceptive fibers from other locations. This makes interpretation of the location of noxious stimuli difficult for the brain. Both visceral pain and somatic pain can manifest as referred pain. Two examples of referred pain are the epigastric pain associated with an inferior myocardial infarction and the shoulder pain associated with blood in the peritoneal cavity irritating the diaphragm. Lower lobe pneumonias can cause referred abdominal pain secondary to diaphragmatic irritation. Finally, some metabolic disorders and toxidromes may manifest with abdominal pain.

19.2 Clinical features

(1) Abdominal topography

This topographic configuration is particularly relevant to the broad spectrum of undifferentiated abdominal pain seen in emergency practice. It incorporates both the early (visceral, poorly localized) and late (parietal, better localized) pain of an evolving intraabdominal pathologic process, as well as the more generalized pain associated with toxic-metabolic derangements. Although one can not exclude a particular diagnosis based solely on the location of abdominal pain or tenderness, localization and pain migration also are helpful components of the pain history.

(2) Historical features

A careful and focused history is central to unlocking the puzzle of abdominal pain. Historical data can be conveniently divided into attributes of pain, associated symptoms, and past history.

(3) Pain attributes

The severity and descriptive nature of the pain are the most subjective aspects of the pain history. The principal characteristics of abdominal pain include location, quality, severity, onset, duration, aggravating and alleviating factors, and change in any of these variables over time.

(4) Associated symptoms

These can be subdivided into one of the four main organ systems that are involved in intraabdominal pain.

1) Gastrointestinal symptoms

Anorexia, nausea, and vomiting (unless bloody) are among the least helpful symptoms for specific diagnosis.

2) Genitourinary symptoms

The hallmark of abdominal pain of genitourinary (GU) origin is the alteration in micturition—e. g. , dysuria, frequency, urgency, hematuria, incomplete emptying, or incontinence.

3) Gynecologic symptoms

Distinguishing gastrointestinal symptoms from gynecologic causes of acute abdominal pain is one of the most challenging clinical dilemmas in emergency practice. A thorough gynecologic history is indicated, including menses, mode of contraception, fertility, sexual activity, sexually transmitted diseases, vaginal discharge, recent dyspareunia, and a past gynecologic history, including pregnancies, deliveries, abortions, ectopic pregnancies, cysts, fibroids, pelvic inflammatory disease, and laparoscopy.

4) Vascular symptoms

History of myocardial infarction (MI), other ischemic heart disease or cardiomyopathy, atrial fibrillation, anticoagulation, congestive heart failure, peripheral vascular disease, or a family history of aortic aneurysm are all pertinent historical features in patients.

19.3　Diagnosis

19.3.1　Physical examination

The patient's general appearance—including facial expression, diaphoresis, pallor, and degree of agitation—provides information about the severity of pain. Although this is helpful in determining the immediacy of need for analgesia, severity of abdominal pain bears no necessary relationship to illness severity.

(1) Vital signs. Obtaining a core temperature is important, careful counting of rate and observation of depth of respirations can provide crucial information about tachypnea or hyperpnea. Pulse and blood pressure should include orthostatic changes if there is any reason to suspect intravascular volume contraction.

(2) Abdomen inspection. The abdomen should be inspected for distention (with air or fluid), rigid, visible peristalsis, scars, and masses.

(3) Auscultation. It appears that only hyperactive obstructive bowel sounds have some clinical utility. Although not sensitive, peristaltic noises coinciding with colic in small–bowel obstruction can be heared. Diffuse increased bowel sounds could be heard in gastroenteritis. Silent abdomen or occasional tinkling sounds in late bowel obstruction or diffuse peritonitis.

(4) Palpation. The vast majority of clinical information obtained from examination of the abdomen is acquired through gentle palpation.

(5) Rebound tenderness, often regarded as the clinical criterion standard of peritonitis, has several important indications. Enlargement of the liver or spleen and other masses, including a distended bladder, should be sought. The examiner should also examine for hernias, particularly those that are tender, suggesting incarceration or strangulation.

19.3.2 Ancillary testing

(1) Complete blood count. Complete blood counts frequently are ordered for patients with abdominal pain, but findings seldom are contributory to a diagnosis. Despite the association of elevated WBC counts with many infectious and inflammatory processes, the WBC count is neither sufficiently sensitive nor sufficiently specific to be considered as a discriminatory test to help establish or rule out a serious cause for the pain.

(2) Abdominal plain film. Plain radiography of the abdomen has limited usefulness in the evaluation of acute abdominal pain. Bowel obstruction, paralytic ileus, and caecal and sigmoid volvulus have typical findings. A paucity of bowel gas may be the only clue to mesenteric infarction.

(3) CT scanning. CT of the abdomen has become the imaging modality of choice with nonobstetric, nonbiliary abdominal pain. It allows visualization of both intraperitoneal and extraperitoneal structures and has a high degree of accuracy. Incidental findings are common on CT scans and may lead to a diagnosis. CT scan results often lead to a change in diagnosis. The proper execution and interpretation of CT studies will reduce mortality, and medical expenses.

(4) Abdominal ultrasound is the preferred imaging modality for cholelithiasis, obstructive uropathy, suspected abdominal aortic aneurysm and abdominal masses. It can also be used to quickly evaluate patients for free intraperitoneal fluid and volume status. Ultrasound assessment should be part of the initial examination and is very important in guiding treatment and disposition.

(5) Urinalysis and testing for pregnancy are perhaps the most time-and cost-effective ancillary testing. Results can be obtained quickly, and lead to early diagnosis and further evaluation. It is necessary to interpret urinalysis results within the context of the patient's clinical picture. Pyuria, with or without bacteriuria, often is presented in a variety of conditions besides a simple urinary tract infection.

(6) Liver enzymes and coagulation studies are helpful only in a small subset of patients with suspected liver disease. If pancreatitis is suspected, the most useful diagnostic result is serum lipase elevated to at least double the normal value, because it is more specific and more sensitive than serum amylase for this process. Measurement of serum amylase is of no value if a serum lipase level is available.

19.4　Differential diagnosis

The differential considerations with abdominal pain include a significant number of potentially life-or organ-threatening entities, particularly in the setting of a hemodynamically unstable or toxic-appearing patient. The approach to the differential diagnosis of abdominal pain generally is based on the location of maximum tenderness. When the very broad differential list is compartmentalized by both history and physical examination, ancillary testing should proceed to either confirm or support the clinical suspicion.

Women of reproductive age with abdominal pain should take pregnancy testing early. A known pregnancy or a positive result on urine or serum pregnancy testing associated with abdominal pain should be considered to represent an ectopic pregnancy.

19.5　Treatment

19.5.1　General strategies

The main therapeutic goals in managing acute abdominal pain are physiologic stabilization, mitigation of symptoms (e. g. , emesis control, pain relief) , and expeditious diagnosis, with consultation if required. Categories for disposition may include surgical versus nonsurgical consultation and management, admission for observation, and discharge to home with follow-up evaluation. Physiologically compromised patients should be brought to a treatment area immediately, and resuscitation initiated. Sepsis or protracted severe volume loss (emesis, diarrhea) can lead to shock; prompt resuscitation is required. Leaking abdominal aortic aneurysm, perforated viscus, advanced peritonitis, mesenteric infarction and strangulated bowel should be sent to surgery.

19.5.2　Disposition

(1) Hypotension

In abdominal pain with relative hypotension, management depends upon the presumed etiology. In the absence of heavy gastrointestinal bleeding, teatment is isotonic crystalloid. Hypotension results from abdominal sepsis, appropriate antibiotics and isotonic crystalloid, pressors may be necessary to sustain blood pressure.

(2) Analgesics

Analgesia is usually withheld from patients with acute abdominal pain until a firm treatment plan is formulated. There is no evidence to support withholding analgesics from patients with acute abdominal pain to preserve the accuracy of subsequent abdominal examinations. Because there have been major advances in diagnostic technology, which is largely independent of the patient's degree of evolving pain and tenderness, and there have been parallel advances in therapeutic technology, including the universal availability of antibiotics and sophisticated intra-and perioperative monitoring. Analgesia will help clinical assessment by reducing distress and anxiety.

(3) Antiemetics

Antiemetics may obviate the need for insertion of a nasogastric tube, whose therapeutic value in abdominal pain has never been convincingly demonstrated. Although metoclopramide (Reglan) appears to be a more effective antiemetic, prochlorperazine (Compazine) is theoretically preferred for control of vomiting in acute abdominal pain because it is less likely to increase motility.

(4) Antibiotics

Antibiotics are indicated in suspected abdominal sepsis and in most patients with localized and all patients with diffuse peritonitis. If intra-abdominal infection is suspected, broad-spectrum anti-biotic therapy should be initiated promptly.

Li Xiaogang

Chapter 20

Gastrointesinal Hemorrhage

Gastrointesinal hemorrhage (GIH) or Gastrointestinal bleeding (GIB) is a common problem in emergency medical practice and should be considered potentially life-threatening until proven otherwise.

Hospitalization for nonvariceal upper gastrointestinal hemorrhage (UGIH) is still common with an incidence of 100/100,000 adults/year. Mortality rates range between 8 and 14%. It is more common among males and markedly more common among the elderly. Lower GIB is somewhat less common, with an annual incidence of hospitalization of approximately 36/100,000 population. The rate of hospitalization is even higher in the elderly.

20.1 Pathophysiology

Causes of upper gastrointestinal bleeding

Upper GIB is defined as that originating proximal to the ligament of Treitz, whereas lower GIB originates more distally.

(1) Peptic ulcer disease

Peptic ulcer disease, including gastric, duodenal, and stomal ulcers, remains the most common etiology for upper GIH, encompassing approximately 60% of all cases. Duodenal ulcers, approximately 29% of the total, will rebleed in approximately 10% of cases, usually within 24–48 hours. Gastric ulcers, approximately 16% of all cases, are more likely to rebleed. Stomal ulcers are uncommon (less than 5% of all upper GI bleeds) and are present in only one-third of bleeding patients with a history of prior peptic ulcer surgery.

(2) Erosive gastritis and esophagitis

Erosive gastritis, esophagitis, and duodenitis together are responsible for approximately 15% of all cases of upper GIH. Irritative factors, such as alcohol, salicylates, and nonsteroidal anti-inflammatory agents, are predisposing factors.

(3) Esophageal and gastric varices

Esophageal and gastric varices result from portal hypertension and, in the United States, are most often a result of alcoholic liver disease. Although varices account for only about 6% of all cases of upper GIH, they are highly likely to rebleed and carry a high mortality rate.

（4）Mallory—weiss syndrome

The Mallory—Weiss syndrome is upper GIB secondary to a longitudinal mucosal tear in the cardioesophageal region. The classic history is repeated retching followed by bright red hematemesis, but coughing and seizures have also been reported as etiologic factors.

（5）Other etiologies

Stress ulcer, arteriovenous malformation, and malignancy are other etiologies of upper GIH. ENT（ear, nose, and throat）sources of bleeding can also masquerade as GIH. An aortoenteric fistula secondary to an aortic graft is an unusual but important cause of bleeding.

20.2　Causes of lower gastrointestinal bleeding

Acute lower GIB is defined as that occurring from the colon, rectum, or anus, and presenting as either hematochezia（bright red blood, clots or burgundy stools）or melena. Among patients with an established lower GI source of their bleeding, the most common etiology is hemorrhoids. Among nonhemorrhoidal bleeding, angiodysplasia and diverticular disease are most common, followed by adenomatous polyps and malignancies.

（1）Diverticulosis

Diverticular bleeding is usually painless and is thought be resulted from erosion into the penetrating artery of the diverticulum. Diverticular bleeding may be massive. Patients are often elderly with underlying medical illnesses that contribute to both the morbidity and the mortality rates.

（2）Angiodysplasia

Arteriovenous malformations（angiodysplasia）, usually at the right colon, are a common etiology of obscure lower GIB, particularly in the elderly population. They are thought to be more common in patients with hypertension and aortic stenosis.

（3）Other etiologies

Numerous other lesions may result in lower GIH. Although carcinoma and hemorrhoids are relatively common causes of bleeding, massive hemorrhage is unusual. Similarly, inflammatory bowel disease, polyps, and infectious gastroenteritis rarely cause severe bleeding. Finally, Meckel diverticulum is an unusual but important etiology.

20.3　Diagnosis

20.3.1　Medical history

Although the medical history may suggest the source of bleeding, it is often misleading. Most patients will complain hematemesis, hematochezia, or melena, but GIB may have more subtle presentations. Patients who present with hypotension, tachycardia, angina, syncope, weakness, confusion, or even cardiac arrest may harbor occult, underlying GIH.

We should focus on the circumstances surrounding the episode of bleeding when asking histoy. Severe vomiting before bleeding is indicative of a Mallory—Weiss tear. A long history of gastroesophageal reflux that has recently worsened might point toward a gastric or duodenal ulcer. Weight loss and a change in stool caliber are worrisome for colorectal cancer. Complaints of "weakness or light—headedness" when arising from a lying or seated position may indicate significant GIB. A careful medication history is also essential and should focus on NSAID and anticoagulant use.

20.3.2　Physical examination

Patients with significant GIB show signs of hypovolemic shock manifested by tachycardia and/or hypotension. Altered mental status, postural drops in blood pressure, or an increase in the pulse rate also indicate significant blood loss. A thorough examination of the nose and throat should be conducted to look for potential sources of swallowed blood that may mimic a GIB. The abdomen should be examined for the presence of a surgical process with emphasis placed on the presence of peritoneal signs (rebound and involuntary guarding). A rectal examination with fecal occult blood testing should be performed on every patient suspected of having a GIB. Examination of the extremities should focus on signs of shock (cool clammy extremities indicating peripheral vasoconstriction).

20.3.3　Laboratory data

In patients with significant GIB, the most important laboratory test is to type and crossmatch blood. Another important laboratory test is the complete blood count. Additionally, blood urea nitrogen (BUN), creatinine, electrolyte, glucose, and coagulation studies, as well as liver function studies, should be considered. The initial hematocrit level often will not reflect the actual amount of blood loss. Upper tract hemorrhage may elevate the BUN through digestion and absorption of hemoglobin. Coagulation studies, including prothrombin time, partial thromboplastin time, and platelet count, are of obvious benefit in patients taking anticoagulants or those with underlying hepatic disease. An electrocardiogram should be considered in the coronary artery disease age group. Silent ischemia can occur secondary to the decreased oxygen delivery accompanying significant GIB and supplemental oxygen is advised for such patients.

20.3.4　Diagnosis

Routine abdominal radiographs are often obtained in patients with GIB. In the absence of specific indications, they are of limited value. Similarly, routine admission chest X—rays for patients with acute GIH, even those admitted to the intensive care unit, have been shown to be of limited utility in the absence of known pulmonary disease or abnormal findings on lung exam. Barium contrast studies are similarly of limited diagnostic value in an emergency setting. Furthermore, barium limits the use of subsequent endoscopy or angiography.

Angiography can sometimes detect the site of bleeding, particularly in cases of obscure lower tract hemorrhage. Moreover, angiography permits therapeutic options such as transcatheter arterial embolization or the infusion of vasoconstrictive agents. However, to be diagnostic, angiography requires a relatively brisk bleeding rate (0.5—2.0 mL/min).

Technetium—labeled red cell scans have also been used to localize the site of bleeding in obscure hemorrhage. Such localization can be used to map the therapeutic approach, whether via angiography or operatively. Scintigraphy appears more sensitive than angiography and can localize the site of bleeding at a rate of 0.1 mL/min.

Another approach is endoscopy, which may be not only diagnostic, but through the use of endoscopic hemostasis, also therapeutic. In most circumstances, endoscopy is more accurate than arteriography or scintigraphy. The capsule endoscopy plays an important role in diagnosing etiologies of obscure GIB.

20. 4   Treatment

20. 4. 1   Primary

Rapid assessment and resuscitation should precede the diagnostic evaluation in unstable patients with severe bleeding. Some patients may require intubation to decrease the risk of aspiration. Patients with active bleeding resulting in hemodynamic instability should be admitted to an intensive care unit for resuscitation and close observation. Patients with active bleeding and coagulopathy should be considered for transfusion with fresh frozen plasma, and those with active bleeding and thrombocytopenia should be considered for transfusion with platelets. Blood transfusions generally should be administered to those with a hemoglobin level of 7 g/dL (70 g/L) or less; hemoglobin level should be maintained at 9 g/dL (90 g/L).

A nasogastric (NG) tube often brings discomfort to the patient, and it can not help the clinician to judge whether the patient needs endoscopic hemostasis. It can not effectively improve the endoscopy visual field, and has no definite value to improve the prognosis of the patients. Therefore, NG tube is not recommended now.

20. 4. 2   Secondary

(1) Endoscopy

Upper GI endoscopy is the most accurate technique for the identification of upper tract bleeding sites. It predicts morbidity, and, with the advent of therapeutic endoscopy, is associated with improved outcomes. Early therapeutic endoscopy, if available, should be considered the treatment of choice for significant upper GIB.

Esophageal varices can be endoscopically treated by either band ligation or injection sclerotherapy. Endoscopic variceal ligation is the endoscopic therapy of choice in the treatment of acute esophageal variceal hemorrhage and is recommended by both the American Association for the Study of Liver Diseases (AASLD) and the Baveno consensus. Sclerotherapy is only indicated when Endoscopic variceal ligation is not feasible.

In lower GIB, proctoscopy is often diagnostic in patients with anorectal sources of bleeding, such as hemorrhoids. If an anorectal source is suspected, the patient should be carefully evaluated for significant volume loss or more dangerous proximal sources of bleeding mimicking anorectal bleeding. Colonoscopy can be diagnostic in other forms of lower tract hemorrhage, such as diverticulosis or angiodysplasia, and may also allow ablation of bleeding sites by using the aforementioned technologies.

(2) Drug therapy

Infusions of somatostatin and its synthetic, longer-acting derivative, octreotide, have been shown to be effective in reducing bleeding from both varices and peptic ulcer disease. Octreotide has been shown to be as effective as sclerotherapy in acute variceal bleeding. Both agents, when used in addition to sclerotherapy, are more effective than sclerotherapy alone. These agents possess the advantages of vasopressin, with considerably fewer side effects. They should be considered useful adjuncts, either before endoscopy or when endoscopy is unsuccessful, contraindicated, or unavailable.

Vasopressin has been used in the past to control GIB, most commonly from varices. However, adverse reactions are common, including hypertension, dysrhythmias, myocardial and splanchnic ischemia, decreased cardiac output, and gangrene from local infiltration. Although the concomitant use of nitroglycerin has been shown to reduce the incidence of these side effects, the use of vasopressin has been largely supplanted by the use of somatostatin, octreotide, and therapeutic endoscopy.

Studies have also suggested that the proton-pump inhibitor (PPI) may be useful to reduce rebleeding, transfusion requirements, and the need for surgery in the treatment of bleeding peptic ulcers.

Other drugs may be of benefit in patients with GIH. For instance, antibiotic prophylaxis not only decreases the rate of infections but also improves survival. The AASLD guideline recommends short – term (maximum 7 days) antibiotic prophylaxis with oral norfloxacin in all cirrhotic patients admitted with GI hemorrhage (variceal or nonvariceal). B-blocker therapy has been shown to be beneficial in patients with varices, in preventing both initial variceal bleeds and rebleeding. Additionally, the treatment of Helicobacter pylori infection with antibiotics reduces the recurrence of peptic ulcer and rebleeding.

(3) Surgery

With patients who do not respond to medical therapy, and in whom endoscopic hemostasis fails, if available, emergency surgical intervention is indicated. Surgical consultation on any patient admitted to the hospital for GIB is prudent, in case uncontrollable rebleeding occurs. Current recommendation for those acute esophageal variceal hemorrhage patients who fail combination endoscopic pharmacological therapy is transjugular intrahepatic portosystemic shunt(TIPS) placement. Control of hemorrhage with rescue TIPS exceeds 85% but is associated with a high mortality.

20.4.3 Recurrent hemorrhage

Rebleeding after successful endoscopic therapy occurs in 10% –20% of patients. The risk of rebleeding and mortality can be calculated with a clinical decision rule such as the Rockall risk scoring system. If rebleeding occurs, a second attempt at endoscopic therapy is recommended. In patients at high risk of rebleeding, scheduled repeat endoscopy may reduce the rebleeding rate and be cost-effective. However, in patients who are not considered to be at high risk of rebleeding, a routine second-look endoscopy on the next day is not recommended.

20.5 Prevention

H. pylori infection and NSAIDs are the major causes of peptic ulcer bleeding in the United States; therefore, preventive strategies should focus on these etiologies. Smoking and alcohol use impair ulcer healing, and patients should be counseled about smoking cessation and moderation of alcohol use. In patients with a history of peptic ulcer bleeding, aspirin, clopidogrel, and NSAIDs should be avoided if possible. In patients taking aspirin who develop peptic ulcer bleeding, aspirin therapy with PPI therapy should be restarted as soon as the risk of cardiovascular complication is thought to outweigh the risk of rebleeding.

Li Xiaogang

Chapter 21

Gastric-intestinal Perforation

21.1　Introduction

The gastrointestinal traumatic injury of gastrointestinal perforation can come from disease that originates in other systems and invades the gastrointestinal system. Perforation of the esophagus, stomach, small intestine, large intestine, or rectum can result from a variety of causes that are traumatic or nontraumatic. Traumatic causes include blunt or penetrating trauma, such as gunshot wounds, stabbings, motor vehicle collisions (MVCs), and crush injuries. Nontraumatic causes include appendicitis, Crohn disease, cancer, diverticulitis, ulcerative colitis, blockage of the bowel, and chemotherapy. Gastrointestinal trauma can result in injury to the stomach, small bowel, colon, or rectum. This trauma can occur from blunt or penetrating injuries. The mechanism of injury will affect both the nature and the severity of any resulting injuries.

21.2　Anatomical background

The anatomic placement of abdominal organs can determine injury potential. The stomach is located in the left upper abdominal quadrant. Anatomically, it is located adjacent to the diaphragm, liver, colon, and abdominal wall anteriorly. Structures that are posterior to the stomach include the left kidney and adrenal gland, spleen, splenic artery, pancreas, transverse colon, megacolon, and left diaphragm. The gastric arteries provide blood supply to the stomach. The small bowel is anatomically divided into 3 distinct portions. These portions are the duodenum, jejunum, and ileum. The duodenum is predominantly retroperitoneal. The duodenum consists of 4 segments, an initial one of which is transverse. This first segment starts at the pylorus and ends at the common bile duct superiorly and gastroduodenal artery inferiorly. A second segment is inferior to the ampulla of Vater. A third segment is transverse to the superior mesenteric vein and artery. A fourth portion extends from where the duodenum emerges from the retroperitoneum and joins the jejunum. A large portion of the duodenum lies directly over the spinal column. The duodenum arterial supply arrives from the celiac artery. There is additional circulatory support from the right gastric artery. Venous drainage follows arterial pathways. The colon and rectum also occupy gastrointestinal space. The colon structures are transverse, ascending, and descending. The transverse colon is intraperitoneal and extends from the hepatic flexure to the splenic flexure. The ascending and descending colons are retroperitoneal. The rectum measures 12 – 15 cm and continues distally from the colon. The rectum is anterior to several bony structures. They are the sacral vertebrae and coccyx. It is posterior to the vagina in women and the bladder in men.

21.3　Trauma

Many gastrointestinal injuries result from MVCs. These injuries can occur from a vehicular collision with another vehicle, an animal, road debris, a pedestrian, or a stationary object (e. g. , utility pole, building, tree, roadway abutment). Airborne vehicle accidents can produce the same type of injuries caused by MVCs depending on the object of impact upon landing. Other causes of gastrointestinal injury include penetrating wounds that can occur from knife or other sharp penetrating object injuries and gunshot wounds. They can even occur from seatbelt use, especially those that fit across the pelvic area.

21.4　Penetrating gastrointestinal injuries

The severicy of penetrating would depends on the mechanism of injury. These wounds can be caused by foreign instruments, hand guns or long guns, and archery bows. Management varies based on injury mechanism and location, hemodynamic stability, neurologic status, associated injuries that accompany the gastrointestinal trauma, and institutional resources. Routine laparotomy can be one response to penetrating wound management. Nonoperative management of penetrating abdominal wounds was addressed by the Shaftan report. This report identified that of the 92% of patients studied with stab wounds operative intervention was initiated if the patient had primary peritoneal irritation manifested by abdominal tenderness, rebound tenderness, reduced or absent bowel sounds or secondary signs of blood per rectum, positive paracentesis, or hematemesis(Figure 21-1).

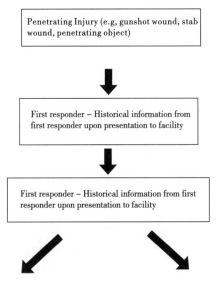

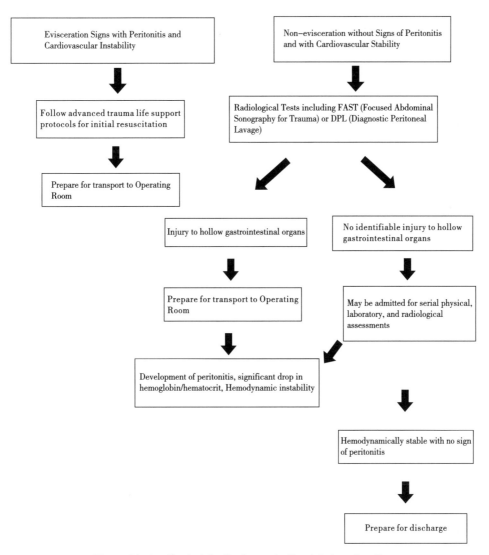

Figure 21-1   Gastrointestinal penetrating injuries algorithm

21.5   Seatbelt syndrome

Although there are benefits to wearing seatbelts, there are potential injuries that can result. There is increasing reported injury of gastrointestinal trauma from seatbelts. Injury results from the redistribution of forces that occur during impact. The collective term used for seatbelt-associated injuries is called "the seatbelt syndrome." This seatbelt syndrome is most often associated with use of a lap belt and identified by a bruising pattern that follows the course of the seatbelt itself across an individual's torso. The seatbelt sign has been validated as indicative of an increased risk of gastrointestinal injury.

21.6   Traumatic abdominal wall hernia

Gastrointestinal injury can include an acute traumatic abdominal wall hernia (TAWH). This type of herniation injury can occur from high impact or low impact to the abdominal wall. High–energy injuries can occur during MVCs or vehicle versus pedestrian accidents. Low–energy herniations can occur as a result of abdominal wall impact on a small (focused) blunt object.

TAWH occurs when there is perforation of the abdominal viscera with an intact outer abdominal wall. This type of injury is also referred to as a "handlebar hernia". This type of injury has been reported to occur with various types of accidents. TAWH can present as ecchymosis and/or a localized palpable hernia. An area of ecchymosis gastrointestinal traumatic injuries can surround the hernia and develop soon after the initial accident. Any quadrant of the abdomen can be involved (right upper, right lower, left upper, or left lower). The herniation can contain abdominal contents, such as the small bowel, transverse colon, ileum, sigmoid colon, or cecum.

Management of a TAWH involves early diagnosis and intervention. Evaluation should include history and thorough assessment, noting current conditions of the external abdominal wall and continued evaluation to observe for occurring changes (e. g. , ecchymosis and/or bulges). Diagnostic tests include imaging for validation of herniation presence and degree of involvement of gastrointestinal contents. With confirmed or highly suspected diagnosis of TAWH, surgical intervention can include laparotomy or laparoscopy. This intervention can vary by hernia location. The highest report of acute therapeutic surgical intervention occurred with anterior abdominal hernias.

Li Xiaogang

Chapter 22

Acute Intestinal Obstruction

22.1　Introduction

Through obstacles of intestinal contents caused by any cause are collectively referred to as intestinal obstruction and are one of the common surgical acute abdomen diseases. After the onset of intestinal obstruction, not only changes in the morphology and function of the intestinal tract, but also can lead to a series of systemic pathological changes, in serious cases can endanger the lives of patients.

22.1.1　Classification of acute intestinal obstruction

22.1.1.1　Classified by cause of obstruction

(1) Mechanical intestinal obstruction

This is the most common clinical type because of mechanical factors that cause the narrow and unclear intestinal lumen, which results in the inability of intestinal contents to pass through. Common causes include: ① extra-intestinal factors, such as adhesion and band compression, incarcerated hernia, tumor compression, etc; ② intestinal wall factors, such as intussusception, intestinal torsion, tumor, congenital malformations; ③ intestinal cavity factors, such as obstruction of aphids, foreign bodies, fecal matter, or gallstone blockage.

(2) Dynamic intestinal obstruction

It is divided into two types including paralysis and spasticity, due to nerve inhibition or toxin stimulation resulting in intestinal wall muscle movement disorder, but no organic intestinal stricture. Paralytic ileus is more common and occurs most often in patients undergoing abdominal surgery, abdominal trauma, or diffuse peritonitis due to severe changes in nerves, body fluids, and metabolism (e. g. , hypokalemia). Obstructive intestinal obstruction is rare and can occur in patients with acute enteritis, intestinal disorders, or chronic lead poisoning.

(3) Mesenteric vascular obstruction

Due to mesenteric vascular embolism or thrombosis, the intestinal blood flow obstacles the peristaltic capacriy of intestine lost, although the intestinal lumen is not obstractity, the contents of the intestines stop moving, it can also be summarized in the classification of dynamic intestinal obstruction. However, it can rapidly develop into intestinal necrosis, which is apparently different from intestinal paralysis in treatment.

22.1.1.2　Classified by the blood flow in the intestinal wall

Simple intestinal obstruction: only have the obstruction of the content of intestine to pass through, and there is no hemodynamic barrier in the intestine canal.

Strangulated intestinal obstruction: due to the compression state in the mesenteric vessels or small blood vessels in the intestinal wall, embolism or thrombosis in the lumen of the blood vessels, lead to corresponding intestinal acute ischemia, causing intestinal necrosis and perforation.

22.1.1.3　Classified by obstruction location

According to the classification of obstruction location, it is divided into high intestinal (jejunum) obstruction, low intestinal (ileum) obstruction and colonic obstruction. The latter is due to the role of ileocecal valve, the intestinal contents can only enter the colon from the small intestine, and can not be refluxed. Also known as "closed loop obstruction". Any obstruction at both ends of the bowel, such as a bowel twist, all belong to a closed loop obstruction. Acute complete intestinal obstruction occurs mostly as strangulated intestinal obstruction, while simple intestinal obstruction is chronic incomplete intestinal obstruction, can be transformed into each other. For example, simple intestinal obstruction can develop into strangulated intestinal obstruction if without treament in time; mechanical intestinal obstruction, if the obstruction lasts for excessive time, and the bowel over the obstruction excessively expanded, patients can appear clinical manifestations of paralytic ileus; chronic incomplete intestinal obstruction with inflammatory edema can develop the pathophysiology changes of acute complete high position obstruction. Theses changes can also occur in the late stage of low position obstruction.

22.1.2　Pathophysiology of acute intestinal obstruction

After the intestinal obstruction occurs, a series of complicated pathophysiological changes will appear in the intestine and the whole body.

22.1.2.1　Intestine

In acute complete obstruction, the bowel rapidly expands, the wall of the intestine becomes thinner, and the pressure in the intestine increases. The pressure in the normal small intestine is 0.27–0.53 kPa. When a complete intestinal obstruction occurs, the proximal pressure of the obstruction can increase to 1.33–1.87 kPa, and the maximal peristalsis can reach 4 kPa or higher. Intestinal wall venous return can be blocked, causs which capillaries and lymphatic fluid deposition, intestinal wall congestion, edema, fluid extravasation. At the same time, due to the lack of oxygen, cell energy metabolism is disorded, resulting in increased intestinal wall and capillary permeability, bleeding in the intestinal wall, and bloody exudate into the intestine and abdominal cavity. In closed intestinal obstruction, intestinal pressure can increase to a higher point. Initially, it was mainly manifested as obstruction of venous return, congestive and edema of the bowel wall, dark red color, followed by obstruction of arterial blood supply, thrombosis, loss of viability of the intestinal wall, and purple–black intestine. In addition, the wall of the intestine is thinned, and the ischemia and permeability are increased. Intestinal contents and a large amount of bacteria penetrate the abdominal cavity, causing peritonitis. Finally, the bowel can be broken and perforated due to ischemia and necrosis.

22.1.2.2　Systemic changes

(1) Water–electrolyte and acid–base imbalances

When the intestinal obstruction is relieved, the gastrointestinal secretion fluid can not be absorbed and returned to the systemic circulation and accumulates in the intestine. The intestinal wall continues to leak fluid into the intestine, causing loss of body fluid in the third gap. Large amounts of vomiting in high intestinal obstruction are more prone to dehydration. At the same time large amount of gastric acid and chloride ions are lost, so there is metabolic alkalosis; loss of a large number of alkaline digestive fluid plus poor tissue perfusion, acidic metabolites increased dramatically, can cause severe metabolic acidosis low intestinal obstruction.

(2)Blood volume decrease

Intestinal swelling can affect the blood supply of the intestinal wall, and large amount of plasma leaks into the intestine and abdominal cavity. If there is intestinal sparing, it will lose a lot of plasma and blood. In addition, increased protein breakdown during intestinal obstruction and decreased ability of the liver to synthesize proteins can aggravate the decrease in plasma protein and blood volume.

(3)Shock

Severe lack of water, blood concentration, hypovolemia, electrolyte imbalance, acid-base in balance, bacterial infection, poisoning, etc. , can cause shock. When the intestinal necrosis, perforation and peritonitis occurs, systemic poisoning is particularly serious. Finally, it can cause severe hypovolemic shock and toxic shock.

(4)Respiratory and cardiac dysfunction

Abdominal pressure increases when the intestines are inflated, and the diaphragm increases, affecting gas exchange in the lungs; abdominal pain and bloating can weaken abdominal respiration; increased abdominal pressure and insufficient blood volume can reduce the return flow of the inferior vena cava and reduce cardiac output.

22.2   Clinical manifestations

The clinical manifestations of intestinal obstruction caused by different reasons are various, but it's in common that the intestinal contents can not pass through the intestine. The common clinical manifestations are abdominal pain, vomiting, bloating and stopping the defecation. However, due to the type, cause, pathological nature, obstruction site and degree of intestinal obstruction, clinical manifestations have their own characteristics.

22.2.1   Symptom

(1)Abdominal pain

When mechanical obstruction occurs, abdominal pain occurs due to strong bowel movement above the obstruction site. After the peristalsis occurs, the abdominal pain is transiently relaxed due to the excessive fatigue of the intestinal muscles, and the abdominal pain is also disappeared. Therefore, the abdominal pain of the mechanical intestinal obstruction is the nature of paroxysmal colic. In addition to the abdominal pain, it is accompanied by a bowel sound of sorghum. When there is a gas accumulation in the intestine, the bowel sounds are over-water sounds or high-profile metallic sounds. Patients often feel that the gas in the intestine channeling and is obstructed in certain areas. Sometimes they can see bowel type and peristaltic waves. If the intermittent period of abdominal pain continues to shorten, it would result in severe and persistent abdominal pain, we should be alert that it would be the performance of strangulated intestinal obstruction.

(2) Vomiting

It is one of the main symptoms of mechanical obstruction. Vomiting at high obstruction occurrs earlier and shortly after obstruction, vomiting is more frequent, and the contents of sputum is mainly from stomach and duodenum. Vomiting of small lower bowel obstruction occurs later, initially with stomach contents and a longer quiescent period. The late vomit is intestinal contents accumulated in the intestines and fermented and rotted into feces. The vomiting of colonic obstruction does not occur until later period. Vomiting contents is brown or bloody, and it is a manifestation resulting from intestinal blood flow disorders. In paralytic ileus, vomiting is mostly spilled.

(3) Abdominal distension

After abdominal pain occurs, its degree is related to the obstruction site. Obstruction of the high intestinal obstruction is not obvious, but sometimes visible gastric type. Low intestinal obstruction and paralytic ileus have significant bloating throughout the entire abdomen. In patients with a thin abdominal wall, it can often be seen that the intestine expands above the obstruction and the bowel type appears. In the case of colonic obstruction, if the regrowth flap is well closed and the intestine stays above the obstruction can become closed, then the abdominal swelling is significant. Asymmetrical abdominal bulge is the characteristics of intestinal twist and other types of closed loop obstruction.

(4) Flatus and defecation stopped

Complete intestinal obstruction, intestinal contents can not pass the obstruction site, below the intestinal obstruction site, it presents an empty state, and clinical manifestations present as stoping exiting flatus and feces. However, in the early stage of obstruction, especially in the high position, gas and feces in the area under it can still be excreted. It should not be mistaken for intestinal obstruction or incomplete intestinal obstruction. Some strangulated intestinal obstruction, such as intussusception, mesenteric vascular embolization or thrombosis, can discharge bloody mucous—like feces.

22.2.2　Signs

There was no significant change in the general body condition of simple intestinal obstruction. Due to vomiting, dehydration and electrolyte imbalance, it can have dry lips, dry eye sockets, decreased skin elasticity weak pulse and so on in later period. Strangulated intestinal obstruction can have symptoms of systemic poisoning and shock.

(1) Abdominal visual examination

Intestinal type and peristaltic waves are often seen in mechanical intestinal obstruction; abdominal distention is more asymmetrical when the bowel is twisted; abdominal distention is severe if the paralytic ileus is obstructed.

(2) Abdominal palpation

Simple intestinal obstruction due to intestinal dilatation, may have mild tenderness, but no peritoneal irritation sign; strangulated intestinal obstruction, there may be fixed tenderness and peritoneal irritation, tender mass often indicating strangulated bowel.

(3) Abdominal percussion

When strangulated intestinal obstruction occurs, there is exudate in the abdominal cavity, and mobile dullness can be positive.

(4) Abdominal auscultation

Hyperactive bowel sounds, over—the—air sounds or metallic sounds are signs of mechanical obstruction, and bowel sounds weaken or disappear when paralytic ileus occurs.

22.2.3 Auxiliary inspection

(1)Laboratory tests

Early changes of simple intestinal obstruction are not obvious. As the disease progresses, white blood cell count, hemoglobin, and hematocrit can all increase owing to dehydration and blood concentration. We need to check blood gas analysis and changes in serum Na^+, K^+, Cl^-, urea nitrogen, and muscle drunk to understand the state of acid−base imbalances, electrolyte imbalance, and renal function status. High intestinal obstruction, frequent vomiting, a large number of gastric fluid loss can cause hypokalemia, hypochloremia and metabolic alkalosis; in the low intestinal obstruction, there may be general electrolyte and metabolic acidosis.

(2)X−ray examination

Generally 4−6 hours after bowel obstruction, X−ray examination shows gas in the intestine. Due to the different sites of intestinal obstruction, X−ray findings also have their own characteristics, the circular folds of the jejunal mucosa appear as fish bone punctures when inflated in the intestine; ileum dilatation have more interstinalis, can be seen step−like fluid level. Barium enema can be used for patients suspected of having a colonic obstruction. It can show the location and nature of colon obstruction. However, in the small bowel obstruction, avoid the use of gastrointestinal imaging methods, so as not to aggravate the condition.

22.3 Diagnosis

First, according to the common features of clinical manifestations of intestinal obstruction. We need to determine whether it is intestinal obstruction, and further determine the type and nature of obstruction, and finally be clear the location and causes of obstruction. These are indispensable steps in the diagnosis of intestinal obstruction.

22.3.1 Whether it is intestinal obstruction

Whether there is intestinal obstruction based on abdominal pain, vomiting, bloating, stop the defecation and abdominal visible bowel or peristaltic waves, bowel sounds hyperthyroidism, etc., generally we can make a diagnosis. However, sometimes patients may not have these typical performances, especially in the early stage of certain strangulated intestinal obstruction, and may be confused with acute gastroenteritis, acute pancreatitis, ureteral calculi, and others. In addition to medical history and detailed abdominal examinations, laboratory tests and X−rays can help the diagnosis.

22.3.2 Type and nature of obstruction

Mechanical obstruction or mechanical obstruction mechanical obstruction is a common type of intestinal obstruction, with the above typical clinical manifestations, early abdominal distension may not be significant. During the period of Paroxysmal intestinal obstruction there is no paroxysmal colic and other peristalsis hyperthyroidism performance, on the contrary, there exists weakened or inactive bowel movements, abdominal distension is significant, bowel sounds weaken or disappear, and more secondary to abdominal infection, retroperitoneal bleeding, abdominal surgery, intestinal inflammation, spinal cord injury, etc. Abdominal X−ray plain film is very valuable in differential diagnosis. Paralytic ileus shows that the large intestine and small intestine are all inflated. The expansion of flatulence in mechanical intestinal obstruction is limited to part of the intestinal tract above the obstruction. Even with late enteral strangulation and intestinal paralysis, the colon does not fully flatten.

With the following performance, the possibility of strangulated intestinal obstruction should be considered: ①the onset of abdominal pain is abrupt, initial severe pain is persistent, or there is persistent pain between paroxysmal aggravation, and sometimes low back pain. ②The condition develops rapidly, shock occurs early, and the improvement is not obvious after anti-shock treatment. ③Signs of peritonitis, body temperature rises, pulse rate increases, increased blood white cell count. ④Abdominal distension, abdominal bulge or touch tender mass (isolated ansa interstinalis). ⑤Vomiting occurs early and frequently, vomitus, gastrointestinal decompression fluid, and anal discharge are all bloody. Abdominal puncture can pump hemorrhagic fluid. ⑥Abdominal X-ray examination shows isolated enlarged ansa interstinalis. ⑦After active non-surgical treatment, there was no significant improvement in symptoms and signs.

22.3.3 High or low small intestinal obstruction

Vomiting of high intestinal obstruction occurs early and frequently, abdominal distention is not obvious; abdominal distention of low intestinal obstruction is obvious, vomiting occurs late sputum excreted; clinical manifestations of colonic obstruction and low intestinal obstruction are similar, because the ileocecal valve has a one-way valve role in the formation of closed loop intestinal obstruction, abdominal distention as the main symptoms, abdominal pain, vomiting, bowel sounds hyperthyroidism are less than small intestinal obstruction obviously, physical examination can be found in the abdomen Asymmetric bulging. X-ray examination helps identify. Low intestinal obstruction, expansion of the interstinalis in the middle of the abdomen, was "staircase-like" arrangement, colonic obstruction when the expansion of ansa interstinalis around the abdomen, visible bags of the colon, flatulence colon shadow suddenly interrupted in the obstruction site, cecal flatulence is the most visible. Barium enema or colonoscopy can further confirm the diagnosis.

22.4 Treatment

The principle of treatment is to correct the physiological disorder caused by intestinal obstruction and relieve the obstruction. The choice of treatment method should be based on the cause, nature, and location of the intestinal obstruction as well as the general condition and the severity of the disease.

22.4.1 Basic treatment

Regardless of the use of non-surgical treatment or surgical treatment, the basic treatment needs to be applied.

22.4.1.1 Gastrointestinal decompression

This is one of the main measures for the treatment of intestinal obstruction. The purpose of gastrointestinal decompression is to reduce gas and fluid accumulation in the gastrointestinal tract, reduce the swelling of the intestinal lumen, and facilitate the recovery of blood circulation in the intestinal wall, reducing the intestinal wall edema, so that some obstruction of intestinal obstruction due to bowel swelling and secondary complete obstruction can be eased, but also can make some distortion of theansa interstinalis to reduce the symptoms. Gastrointestinal decompression can also reduce the intra-abdominal pressure and improve the breathing and circulatory disturbances caused by the elevation of the diaphragm.

22.4.1.2 Correcting water-electrolyte imbalances and acid-base imbalances

Water-electrolyte imbalances and acid-base imbalances are the most significant physiological disorders of acute intestinal obstruction and should be corrected as soon as possible. Before the results of blood biochemical tests have not been obtained balanced salt solution should be given first (Lactated Ringer's solution). After the result of the measurement, the electrolyte should be added to correct the acid-base balance. In the absence of heart, lung and kidney dysfunction, the initial input of liquid may be slightly faster, but urine volume monitoring is needed, and if necessary, central venous pressure monitoring is performed to prevent fluid excess or deficiency. In the late stage of simple intestinal obstruction or strangulated intestinal obstruction, a large amount of plasma and blood often seep into the intestine or abdominal cavity, and plasma and whole blood need to be supplemented.

22.4.1.3 Anti-infection

After intestinal obstruction, blood circulation of the intestinal wall is obstructed, intestinal mucosal barrier function is impaired and intestinal bacterial translocation, or bacteria in the intestinal lumen directly penetrate the intestinal wall to produce infection within the abdominal cavity. Intestinal bacteria can also quickly reproduce. At the same time, elevation of the diaphragm affects the gas exchange and excretion of the lungs and is prone to lung infections. Therefore, antibiotics should be given to prevent or treat abdominal infections or lung infections during intestinal obstruction.

22.4.1.4 Other treatments

Bloating can affect the function of the lungs, and the patient should absorb oxygen. Somatostatin may be administered to reduce the secretion of gastrointestinal fluid in order to reduce the swelling of the gastrointestinal tract. General symptomatic treatments such as sedatives and spasmolytics may be given, but the use of analgesics should follow the principle of acute abdomen treatment.

22.4.2 Surgery

Most intestinal obstructions require surgery. The purpose of surgery is to relieve obstruction and remove the cause. The surgical method can be selected according to the patient's condition and the location and cause of the obstruction.

22.4.2.1 The simple surgery to relieve the obstruction

It includes adhesion lysis, intestinal excision to remove manure, worms, etc. , intussusception or torsion and repositioning.

22.4.2.2 Intestinal resection

Intestinal tumors, inflammatory stenosis, or local inactivation of the intestine has necrosis, we should do a bowel resection. For strangulated intestinal obstruction, it should strive to relieve obstruction before intestinal necrosis and restore intestinal blood circulation. If the following symptoms occur after the cause of the obstruction is relieved, it indicates that the bowel has no vitality: ①The intestine wall is purple and black and has collapsed. ②The intestinal wall loses its ability of tension and peristalsis; the intestine tube expands and responds to stimulation without contraction. ③The corresponding mesenteric end has no small arterial pulse. It is often difficult to determine the viability of the intestine during surgery. When it is not known whether the small intestine has any disturbance of blood flow, it is safe to remove it. However, when there is a long segment of the bowel, especially when the entire small intestine is twisted, rash removal will affect the patient's future survival. While correcting hypovolemia and oxygen supply, 1% procaine or phentolamine is injected into the roots of the mesenteric vessels to relieve vasospasm and the intestine can be returned to the abdominal cavity. After 15—30 minutes, if it still can not be determined, it can be repeated once; after confirming that there is no vitality, consider cutting off.

22.4.2.3   Intestinal short—circuit anastomosis

When the obstruction site is difficult to remove, such as extensive invasion of the tumor to the surrounding tissue, or adhesion is widely difficult to separate, but no intestinal necrosis phenomenon, in order to lift the obstruction, the proximal and distal intestine can be separated and short—circuited, set up the obstruction department. However, it should be noted that the proximal bowel, especially the obstruction, should not be too long to avoid blind loop syndrome.

22.4.2.4   Intestinal colostomy or extra—intestinal surgery

The lesions in the intestinal obstruction are complicated or the patient's condition is poor. Complex surgery is not allowed. This type of surgery can be used to relieve the obstruction. The expanded intestine at the proximal end of the obstruction to perform a gastrostomy to reduce the pressure and relieve the physiological disturbance caused by the high expansion of the intestine. Mainly applicable to low intestinal obstruction, such as acute colonic obstruction, due to the role of the ileocecal valve, closed obstruction caused by complete colonic obstruction, intestinal cavity pressure is high, the blood supply of the colon is not as rich as the small intestine, prone to bowel obstruction of wall blood flow, and colon bacteria, so the first phase of intestinal resection and anastomosis, often difficult to smooth healing. Therefore, a proximal obstruction (cecal or transverse colon) stoma can be used to relieve obstruction. If there has been intestinal necrosis or intestinal tumour, the necrotic bowel segment or tumour intestine segment can be removed, the two ends are externally made ostomy, and the second stage of surgery is followed to rebuild the continuity of the intestinal tract.

Chen Haiming

Chapter 23

Acute Pancreatitis

Acute pancreatitis is a common acute abdominal disease. According to pathological changes, the classification can be divided into edema and hemorrhagic necrotic acute pancreatitis, the former accounting for about 80% -90%. Clinical conditions are classified as light acute pancreatitis and severe acute pancreatitis, which accounts for about 10% -20%. The former is mild, self-limited, with good prognosis and mortality < 1%; the latter is a dangerous condition, often involving multiple organs throughout the body, with a mortality rate of 10% -30%.

23.1 Etiology

Acute pancreatitis has a variety of pathogenic risk factors, and domestic biliary disease is the majority, accounting for more than 50%, which is called biliary pancreatitis.

23.2 Pathogenesis and pathophysiology

The pathogenesis of acute pancreatitis is complicated and has not been fully elucidated. Most researchers believe that acute pancreatitis is the result of abnormal activation of pancreatic enzymes in the gland. Pancreatase activation induces the normal digestion of pancreatic parenchyma. Thus, the inflammatory cytokines are released by the adenocytic cells, such as tumor necrosis factor (TNF-α), IL-1, IL-2, IL-6 and anti-inflammatory media such as IL-10 and IL-1 receptor blockers, which can cause inflammatory cascade reactions. The cascade reaction of inflammation is self-limited in about 80% -90% of patients, but it can lead to local hemorrhage and necrosis of the pancreas, and even systemic inflammatory response syndrome can lead to multiple organ failure.

23.3 Pathology

The basic pathological changes are edema, hyperemia, hemorrhage and necrosis of the pancreas.

23.3.1 Acute edema pancreatitis

The pancreas is swollen and hard, congested, strained by the membrane, and fluid in the pancreas. The fatty tissue in the abdominal cavity, especially the large omentum, can be seen in the yellow–white saponified plaque (fatty acid calcium) of the granule or plaques. The peritoneal water is light yellow, and the interstitial hyperemia, edema and inflammatory cell infiltration are seen under the microscope. Sometimes localized fat necrosis can occur.

23.3.2 Acute hemorrhagic necrotizing pancreatitis

The lesions are characterized by hemorrhage and necrosis of the pancreas. The pancreas is swollen and dark purple, with a blurry leaf structure, black in the necrotic foci, and black in the whole pancreas. In the abdominal cavity, saponified plaques and fat necrotic lesions can be seen. In the abdomen or peritoneum, there is brown or dark red blood fluid or bloody cloudy fluid. Fat necrosis and glandular destruction are seen under the microscope. The interstitial small vessel wall also has necrosis, presenting patchy hemorrhage and inflammatory cell infiltration. A combined infection of late necrotic tissue can result in pancreatic or peripancreatic abscess.

23.4 Clinical manifestation

Due to different degree of lesion, the patient's clinical manifestation is very different.

23.4.1 Abdominal pain

Is the main symptom of the disease. It often occurs after a full meal and alcohol drinking, and the abdominal pain is intense, often on the left upper abdomen, and the left shoulder and the left side of the back. The gallbladder originates from the right upper abdomen and gradually shifts to the left. When the lesion is involved in the whole pancreas, the pain range is wider and radiates to the lower back.

23.4.2 Abdominal distension

It also exists with abdominal pain. It is the result of the stimulation of the abdominal nerve plexus, early reflex, secondary infection after retroperitoneal inflammatory stimulation. The more inflamed the retroperitoneal inflammation, the greater the abdominal distention. Peritoneal effusion can aggravate abdominal distension. The patient defecates and exhausts. Increased abdominal pressure can lead to abdominal syndrome.

23.4.3 Nausea and vomiting

This symptom can appear in the early stage, vomiting often violent and frequent. Vomit is gastroduodenum contents, occasionally brown color. Abdominal pain does not relieve after vomiting.

23.4.4 Peritonitis

In acute edema pancreatitis, tenderness is confined to the upper abdomen, often without obvious muscle tension. Acute haemorrhagic necrotizing pancreatitis is obvious, and there is muscle tension and rebound pain, which is wide or extended to full abdomen. The mobility dullness is mostly positive. The bowel sounds are attenuated or disappeared.

23.4.5 Other

Light acute edema pancreatitis is mild. Combined biliary tract infection is often accompanied by chills and fever. Persistent hyperthermia is one of the main symptoms of pancreatic necrosis associated with infection. Jaundice can occur if the stone is incarcerated or the head of the pancreas is enlarged. Patients with necrotizing pancreatitis can have fast pulse rate, a drop in blood pressure, and even shock. Early shock is mainly caused by low blood volume, and subsequent secondary infection complicated and difficult to correct. Breathing difficulties and cyanosis can occur with acute lung failure. The pancreatic necrosis is accompanied by infection, and edema, redness and tenderness can appear in the waist skin. The hemorrhage of the pancreas of a few serious patients can be infiltrated by the peritoneal pathway. In the waist, hypochondriac and lower abdomen can be seen, a large number of bluish purple stasis, called grey−turner; if it occurs in the umbilicus, it is called the Cullen sign. Gastrointestinal bleeding can have hematemesis and hematopoiesis. When plasma calcium decreases, the limbs can appear twitch. Severe cases can be characterized by DIC and central nervous system symptoms, such as sensory dullness, confusion and even coma.

23.5 Diagnosis

23.5.1 Laboratory examination

23.5.1.1 Serum enzynes

Serum, urine amylase assay is the most commonly used diagnostic method. Serum amylase began to increase in the hours of onset, and reached its peak in 24 hours, gradually dropping to normal after 4−5 days. The urine amylase began to rise in 24 hours, to peak at 48 hours, to slow down, and return to normal after 1−2 weeks. The serum amylase value is over 500 U/dL(normal value of 40−180 U/dL, Somogyi method), and the urine amylase is also significantly increased (80−300 U/dL, Somogyi method), to diagnostic value. The higher the amylase value, the greater the diagnostic accuracy. However, the magnitude of the increase is not positively correlated with the severity of the lesion.

It is important to note that of intestinal obstruction, choletitis, mesenteric ischemia, parotitis and macroamylase can also have elevated serum amylase. The serum lipase amylase is significantly increased (23− 300 U/L), and it is also an objective diagnostic indicator.

23.5.1.2 Other tests

They include leukocyte elevation, hyperglycemia, abnormal liver function, hypocalcemia, abnormal blood gas analysis, etc. It is helpful to diagnose based on increase the hemorrhagic exudate of peritoneal puncture and increase amylase value. Increased C−reaction protein (CRP) (Onset 48 hours>150 mg/mL) indicates the severity of the disease.

23.5.2 Imaging diagnosis

23.5.2.1 Abdominal ultrasound

The ultrasound is simple and easy, but due to the disturbance of gastrointestinal gas in the upper abdomen, the accuracy of diagnosis can be affected. Pancreatic enlargement and peripancreatic fluid accumulation are observed. When the pancreatic edema is shown to be uniform low echo, there is a strong echo prompting. There may be bleeding or necrosis. If bile duct stones are found, bile duct expansion, biliary pancreatitis is more likely.

23.5.2.2　Enhanced CT scan

It is the most diagnostic imaging examination. Not only can acute pancreatitis be diagnosed, but the pancreatic tissue necrosis can be identified. If the file is now in the background of the diffuse enlargement of the pancreas uneven texture, liquefaction and honeycomb low density area, can be diagnosed as pancreatic necrosis can also in omental bursa, peripancreatic, renal side before or after the clearance, even the place such as iliac fossa found after the colon the pancreatic fluid and necrotic infection signs. In addition, it also has diagnostic value for the disease such as pancreatic abscess and pseudocyst.

23.5.2.3　MRI

MRI can provide diagnostic information similar to CT. There is value in evaluating pancreatic necrosis, inflammation, and presence of free gas. MRCP is a clear indication of bile duct and pancreatic duct, which plays an important role in the diagnosis of recurrent pancreatitis and unexplained pancreatitis.

23.5.3　Clinically classified light acute pancreatitis

Edema pancreatitis, mainly manifested as upper abdominal pain, nausea and vomiting; peritonitis is limited to the upper abdomen and is light; increased blood and urine amylase; the timely treatment of liquid therapy can improve the mortality rate in the short term. Severe acute pancreatitis: mostly hemorrhagic necrotic pancreatitis, with the exception of the above symptoms, peritonitis is widespread and serious. The abdominal distension is obvious, the bowel sound attenuates or disappears. Ascites is bloody or purulent. Severe shock, multiple organ dysfunction and severe metabolic disorders. Laboratory examination could present: laboratory examination: leukocytosis ($>16 \times 10^9$/L), elevated blood glucose (>11.1 mmol/L), decreased serum calcium (<1.87 mmol/L), increased blood urea nitrogen or creatinine, and acidosis; PaO_2 decreased to should be considered as ARDS; even in DIC, mortality is high. There are many evaluation criteria for severe acute pancreatitis. The prognosis of Ranson is 3 positive, indicating severe acute pancreatitis. Acute physiology and chronic health scoring standard APACHE II. (acute physiology and chronic health evaluation II) $\geqslant 8$, Indicates severe acute pancreatitis, which is helpful for evaluation of disease and prognosis.

23.5.4　Clinical stages

23.5.4.1　Acute reaction period

Onset to about 2 weeks, patients can have shock, respiratory failure, renal failure, central nervous system dysfunction.

23.5.4.2　Systemic infection period

Two weeks to two months, systemic bacterial infection and deep fungal infection or both are major complications.

23.5.4.3　Residual infection period

After 2−3 months. It belongs to the postoperative special performance: if malnutrition occurs, there is abdominal cavity and posterior peritoneal cavity residual abscess, often drainage is not smooth, the sinus tract is not healed, there are some gastrointestinal fistula.

23.6   Local complications of acute pancreatitis

23.6.1   Necrosis of pancreas and peripancreatic tissue

It refers to the diffuse or focal necrosis of the pancreatic parenchyma, and the necrosis of fat in the pancreas, including the retroperitoneal space, according to whether or not infection is divided into infectious and aseptic pancreatic necrosis.

23.6.2   Pancreatic and peripancreatic abscess

The pancreas and (or) the surrounding tissue of the pancreas, which is caused by pancreatic tissue and (or) peripancreatic tissue necrosis, is caused by bacterial or fungal growth of the pus.

23.6.3   Pancreatic pseudocyst

The fluid accumulates around the pancreas through the pancreatic duct, which is damaged by the necrosis of the pancreas.

23.6.4   Gastrointestinal fistula

The digestion of pancreatic juice and the corrosion of infection can cause the necrosis and perforation of the gastrointestinal wall. The common site is the colon, the duodenum, and sometimes the stomach and jejunum.

23.6.5   Upper gastrointestinal hemorrhage

Because of the digestion and infection of the pancreatic juice, especially with fungal infections, there is sometimes a large hemorrhage after abdominal pain.

23.7   Treatment

According to the classification, stage and etiology of acute pancreatitis, appropriate treatment methods should be selected.

23.7.1   Non-surgical treatment

It is suitable acute pancreatitis systemic reaction stage, edema and uninfected blood necrotic pancreatitis.

23.7.1.1   Fasting and gastrointestinal decompression

Continuous gastrointestinal decompression may prevent vomiting, relieve abdominal distension, and reduce abdominal pressure.

23.7.1.2   Hydrating, preventing and treating shock

Intravenous infusion, supplementing electrolyte, rectifying acidosis, preventing and treating hypotension, maintaining circulatory stability and improving microcirculation are important inshock treatment. Intensive care should be carried out for critically ill patients, oxygen inhalation and maintenance of SaO_2 is greater than 95%.

23.7.1.3 Analgesic spasmolysis

In the case of definite diagnosis, antispasmodic analgesics are commonly used such as, anisodamine, atropine, etc. Although morphine can cause Oddi sphincter tension, it has no adverse effect on prognosis.

23.7.1.4 Inhibition of pancreatic secretion

Proton pump inhibitors or H_2 receptor blockers can indirectly inhibit pancreatic secretion; it is believed that somatostatin (such as octreotide) and trypsin inhibitor also inhibit pancreatic secretion.

23.7.1.5 Nutritional support

Nutrition is mainly dependent on total parenteral nutrition (TPN) during fasting period. When the condition is stable, the bowel function can be restored early to give the enteral nutrition.

23.7.1.6 Application of antibiotics

It can be empirically or targeted to use antibiotics when there is evidence of infection. Common pathogenic bacteria include escherichia coli, pseudomonas aeruginosa, klebsiella and proteus.

23.7.2 Surgical treatment

23.7.2.1 Surgical indications

The surgical indications include acute peritonitis can not exclude other acute abdomen, pancreatic and peripancreatic necrotic tissue secondary infection and the obstruction or biliary tract infection of the common bile duct which combined intestinal perforation, massive hemorrhage or pancreatic pseudocyst.

23.7.2.2 Surgical method

The most commonly used is necrotic tissue removal and drainage. Open surgery (either via abdominal or retroperitoneal incision) or endoscopic (nephroscope, etc.) can be used to remove drainage. Open operation by the arc or midline incision open, into omentum sac remove peripancreatic and retroperitoneal drainage, pus, and necrotic tissue, put more drainage tube after thoroughly flushed from the abdominal wall or the waist, so that postoperative lavage and drainage. If there are more incisions in the necrotic tissue, it can also be partially open, so that the necrotic tissue can be cleared repeatedly after the incision. At the same time, gastric orifice and jejunostomy (enteral nutrition channel) could be performed, and biliary drainage is performed as appropriate. After retroperitoneal approach, small incision in the side of the waist is required to enter the purulent cavity for necrotic tissue removal and drainage. If the secondary enteric fistula, the fistula can be placed outside or near the end of the intestinal canal. The formation of pseudo cysts may be performed as appropriate.

23.7.2.3 Treatment of biliary pancreatitis

The purpose of surgery is to remove stones in the bile duct, remove obstruction, and free drainage, depending on whether there are gallstones or bile duct stones. Cholecystolithiasis is the only one that can be removed during the initial hospitalization. The pancreas is in serious condition and needs to wait for the condition to be stable. Combined with bile duct stones, and the condition is more serious. It is not suitable for the patients to be able to undergo the emergency or early treatment of the ooddi sphincter incision, the removal of stones, and the drilling of bile duct drainage.

Chen Haiming

Chapter 24

Oliguria and Anuria

The output of 24-hour urine in healthy adults' is about 1,000-2,500 mL. If the output of 24-hour urine is less than 400 mL or the hourly urine output is less than 17 mL, it is called oliguria. If the output of 24-hour urine is less than 100 mL or complete anuria within 12 hours, it is called anuria or urine closure (anuria). The amount of urine is affected by many physiological and pathological factors.

24.1　Etiology

Patients with oliguria or anuria may be classified into prerenal, renal and post-renal depending on the causes of oliguria and anuria. Common causes are given in Table 24-1.

Table 24-1　Classification of oliguria or anuria

Classification	Causes
Pre-renal	
Low blood volume	Loss of body fluid through the skin, kidneys, gastrointestinal tract, or hemorrhage: extensive burns, blood loss, dehydration, vomiting, diarrhea, gastrointestinal decompression, excessive diuresis, hyperthermia, serous effusion; Redistribution of body fluids: peritonitis, pancreatitis, various shocks, etc.
Reduced cardiac output	Congestive heart failure, acute pulmonary edema, valvular heart disease, pericardial tamponade, etc.
Other causes	Allergies, sepsis, hypoproteinemia, nephrotic syndrome, liver failure, hemolysis, crush syndrome, etc.
Renal	
Vascular	Renal vascular embolism, systemic vascular disease (thrombotic thrombocytopenic purpura, DIC, scleroderma, malignant hypertension), and a dramatic decrease in adrenal cortical blood flow (see Non-steroidal anti-inflammatory drugs)
Glomerular lesions	Primary glomerular disease (emergent glomerulonephritis), autoimmune disease (systemic lupus erythematosus), bacterial endocarditis, systemic vasculitis, etc.

Continued to Table 24-1

Classification	Causes
Tubulointerstitial lesions	Ischemic acute tubular necrosis, toxic tubular damage (drugs, exogenous toxicants), drug-induced interstitial nephritis, renal parenchymal injury, or oppression (kidney neoplasms, acute uric acid nephropathy, ethylene glycol poisoning, etc.
Post-renal	
Intrarenal and ureteral lesions	Blood clots, stones, retroperitoneal fibrosis, deposition of uric acid/oxalate crystals, renal papillary necrosis, and exogenous tumor compression
Bladder, prostate and urethra	Tumors, stones, blood clots, benign prostatic hyperplasia/tumor, urethral stricture, redundant prepuce, neurogenic bladder dysfunction
Drug influence	Sulfamethoxazole, methotrexate, acyclovir, etc.

24.2　Clinical features

24.2.1　Clinical manifestations

In addition to the original disease manitestation, oliguria and anuria is mainly associated with the changes of protein, serum creatinine concentration, ion and acid-base balance and other factors. Most patients began to have oliguria or anuria after pioneering symptoms such as fatigue, and edema. The main symptoms are as follows.

24.2.1.1　The digestive system

Oliguria and anuria is accompanied by nausea, vomiting, anorexia, hiccups and diarrhea.

24.2.1.2　Respiratory system

Oliguria and anuria is is associcted with deep and fast breathing, frequent shortness of breath, and even Kussmaul breathing. Due to the retention of metabolites and low immune-competence with infection, respiratory infections are common, manifested as bronchitis, pneumonia, pleural effusion and pleural effusion.

24.2.1.3　Circulatory system

Blood pressure rises, and severe cases can show hypertensive encephalopathy. When pericarditis occurs, left chest is severely painful and often accompanied by pericardial friction and even pericardial tamponade. Cardiac enlargement, various arrhythmias and heart failure may occur late.

24.2.1.4　The blood system

The majority of patients with oliguria and auuria suffer from anemia, which is usually normal cell size or pigment anemia, which is exacerbated by decreased renal function. And patients with oliguria and auuria may also sutler from subcutaneous hemorrhage, epistaxis, menorrhagia, and gastrointestinal bleeding.

24.2.1.5　The nervous system

Patients with oliguria and anuria may sufler from dizziness, irritability, severe disturbances in consciousness, convulsions, flapping tremors and myoclonus, etc. , there is lack of concentration, insomnia or drowsiness, peripheral neuropathy, autonomic symptoms.

24.2.1.6   Skin manifestations

Patients with oliojuna and anuria may suffer from pale complexion, edema, dry skin, scaling, dullness, and hyperpigmentation. Intractable skin pruritus is more common, sometimes with ecchymosis, due to itching and decreased resistance, prone to cause skin purulent infections.

24.2.1.7   Gonadal dysfunction

Patients with olisuria and anuria may suffer from hypothyroidism and hypogonadism which for men they may have loss of libido and impotence for women they may have amenorrhea, infertility.

24.2.2   Auxiliary inspection

It is of great value for the etiological diagnosis of oliguria and anuria.

24.2.2.1   Urine examination

The urine specific gravity of prerenal oliguria or anuria is higher than that of acute tubular necrosis. The urine specific gravity of acute tubular necrosis is generally lower than 1.014. If urine contains a large number of pathological components, it suggests that it's renal oliguria, such as urine sodium quantification >30 mmol, urine protein qualitative positive (++++ range). Urine sediment microscopic examination can see thick granular tube type, red/white blood cells, etc.

24.2.2.2   Renal function tests

Blood urea nitrogen and creatinine are increased in most of one cases. Blood urea nitrogen/blood creatinine ≤10 is a diagnostic index for multiple numbers. In addition, urinary urea/blood urea <15 (normal urinary urea 200−600 mmol/24 h, urine/blood urea ratio>20), urinary creatinine/creatinine ≤ 10 also have diagnostic significance.

24.2.2.3   Blood tests

Red blood cells, hemoglobin and platelets are decreases, leukocytes are increase. It often accompanied with high serum potassium, low serum sodium, high serum magnesium, high serum phosphorus, low serum calcium, etc. Carbon dioxide binding force is also reduced. It may also accompanied with impaired glucose tolerance, elevated triglyceride levels, increased low density lipoproteins, etc.

24.2.2.4   Determination of filtered sodium excretion fraction

There is a certain significance for the etiological diagnosis of oliguria and anuria. If the value is greater than 1, it suggests that it is acute tubular necrosis and is found in non−oliguric acute tubular necrosis or urinary tract obstruction. If the value is less than 1, it suggests that it is prerenal azotemia or acute glomerulonephritis.

24.2.2.5   Determination of central venous pressure(CVP)

The identification of prerenal and acute tubular necrosis is significant to sure cup, and it also has a role in guiding treatment.

24.2.2.6   Imaging examination

The choice of urinary tract X−rays (such as plain radiographs), ultrasound, CT, and cystoscopy can help determine the etiological diagnosis of oliguria and couria.

24.2.2.7   Kidney diagram

Kidney diagram is more sensitive than venous pyelography in assessing the degree of renal function damage which is caused by urinary tract obstruction. It is a reliable and simple method for diagnosing post urinary oliguria such as urinary tract obstruction and has a high detection rate. The kidney graph can also provide renal function status at an early stage, which is helpful for judging the curative effect and mastering the development of the disease.

24.3 Diagnosis

Oliguria or anuria can be diagnosed based on an accurate calculation of the urine volume within a limited time, but the etiological diagnosis that causes oliguria or anuria is a prerequisite for treatment. In order to identify oliguria, two aspects must be clarified: on the one hand, whether it is caused by prerenal deficiency, which is caused by insufficient perfusion of the kidney or by post-renal obstruction; on the other hand, whether it is caused by acute deterioration of renal function or acute renal dysfunction in patients with chronic kidney disease.

There are three key points for the diagnosis. Firstly, a detailed and accurate understanding of the medical history is needed; secondly, all the diagnosis should be based on clinical and laboratory methods. Thirdly, the basic theory of pathophysiology is analyzed to determine the location and etiology of the lesion. If it is necessary, a biopsy of the kidney can be performed to confirm the diagnosis.

24.4 Emergency treatment

24.4.1 Emergency treatment

Priority should be given to the treatment of life-threatening fluids with excess or deficiency, hyperkalemia, etc. We should check general vital signs and central venous pressure to assess whether blood volume is adequate. If blood volume is insufficient, rehydration should be done in time. If blood volume is overloaded, emergency hemofiltration or dialysis should be considered and oxygen, furosemide, nitrate drugs should be given.

24.4.2 Hyperkalemia treatment

Ten percent of calcium gluconate at 10-20 mL intravenously can be given, which can be repeated after one hour according to requirement; 50% glucose 50 mL plus 10 U of insulin should be given within 15 - 30 minutes; if condition allows dialysis treatment can often achieve better results.

24.4.3 Etiology treatment

We should complete relevant tests as soon as possible to clarify the cause of oliguria or anuria and take appropriate measures. ①Prerenal disease: treatment of the cause, such as blood volume, correction of dehydration and shock, improvement of circulation, treatment of heart failure, etc. ②Renal parenchymal disease: according to the original disease to give different treatments, adequate use of diuretic drugs can be administrated on the premise of adequate blood volume. ③Post-renal disease: obstructive causes are clearly identified and the obstruction is relieved in time. Patients with indications for surgery should be treated as soon as possible.

24.4.4   Symptomatic treatment

If there is urinary retention, catheterization should be promptly treated, and if necessary, urethral catheter should be indwellinged.

24.5   Patient placement

Patients with persistent unexplained oliguria and urine should stay in observation room for care. Patients with systemic symptoms (fever, chills, stubborn vomiting, etc.) should be admitted to the hospital. Patients who need additional diagnosis and treatment (azotemia, systemic infections, water and electrolyte disturbances, etc.) also need to be admitted to hospital for further treatment. Patients with urinary retention and be discharged if obstruction is disappeared after they were inserted urethral catheter and asymptomatic. Then follow-up is needed weekly to urology clinic.

Li Peiwu, Zhang Yao

Chapter 25

Acute Kidney Injury

25.1 Concept

Acute kidney injury(AKI) is a clinical syndrome in which the ability of the kidney to remove metabolic waste rapidly decreases due to various causes. The main clinical manifestations are the accumulation of nitrogen metabolites, the disturbance of water and electrolyte acid−base balance, and changes in urine output. The glomerular filtration rate (GFR) is widely accepted as the best overall index of kidney function. However, GFR is difficult to measure and is commonly estimated from the serum level of endogenous filtration markers, such as creatinine. Although urine output is both a reasonably sensitive functional index for the kidney as well as a biomarker of tubular injury, the relationship between urine output and GFR, and tubular injury is complex.

25.2 Morbidity

AKI is a common clinical syndrome which could occurr at various clinical departments and the severe patients could have with multiple system complications. The morbidity is 3% −10% in general hospitals and 30% −60% in ICU. Mortality in high−risk AKI patients are as high as 30% −80%. About 50% of surviving patients are left with permanent renal dysfunction, and some need lifetime hemodialysis.

25.3 Etiology

The causes of AKI are diverse and can be divided into three categories based on the anatomical site of the etiology: prerenal, renal and postrenal. Acute tubular necrosis (ATN) is the most common kind of AKI, which is usually caused by ischemia or nephrotoxicity.

25.3.1　Prerenal AKI

Prerenal AKI refers to ischemic renal injury caused by insufficient blood flow of kidneys caused by various causes, which is also called as prerenal azotemia, accounting for about 55% of the AKI. It is classified into four stages: innitiation period, progressing period, persistent period and recovery period.

The causes of prerenal AKI is various, including the reduction in effective blood volume(shock, vomiting, diarrhea, gastrointestinal fluid loss due to extra-intestinal fistulae; diuretic, high body temperature, skin fluid loss caused by burns, and hemorrhage-induced loss of blood volume), reduced cardiac output(congestive heart failure, pulmonary embolism), vasodilation of the whole body(hepatorenal syndrome, sepsis), renal hemodynamics changes (non-steroidal anti-inflammatory drugs, hypercalcemia, ACEI).

25.3.2　Renal AKI

Renal AKI is caused by nephron, interstitial and vascular damage caused by various reasons. Renal tubular epithelial cell damage (such as ATN) caused by renal ischemia and nephrotoxic substances is the most common.

Causes of renal AKI include acute tubular necrosis (hypotension, shock, sepsis, ischemic acute tubular necrosis due to respiratory arrest, and nephrotoxicity caused by aminoglycosides, contrast agents, and rhabdomyolysis, etc.), Acute interstitial nephritis (penicillin, rifampicin, non-steroidal anti-inflammatory drugs, furosemide and other drug-induced; bacterial, viral, tuberculosis and other infections; SLE, Sjogren syndrome and other systemic diseases; multiple myeloma and other tumor-related), acute glomerulonephritis (post-streptococcal glomerulonephritis; endocarditis glomerulonephritis; acute glomerulonephritis and systemic blood vessels Inflammation) and renal vascular disease (renal artery: thrombosis, atherosclerotic plaque, aortic dissection; renal vein: thrombosis).

25.3.3　Postrenal AKI

Postrenal AKI is caused by acute urinary tract obstruction, and obstruction can occur at any position from renal pelvis to urethra. Common causes include stones, tumors, prostatic hypertrophy, renal papillary necrosis, blood clots, retroperitoneal diseases, and neurogenic bladder.

25.4　Pathogenesis

25.4.1　Prerenal AKI

Prerenal AKI is the most common reason, caused by insufficient blood flow to the kidneys, this indicates that renal dysfunction is mainly caused by systemic factors that reduce GFR. Common causes include: ①effective hypovolemia; ②decreased cardiac output; ③systemic vasodilation; ④renal artery contraction; ⑤impaired renal autoregulatory response; these etiologies can lead to the reducing of the extracellular fluid, or decreaseing the effective circulating blood although the amount of extracellular fluid is normal, or reducing of the glomerular capillary perfusion pressure, and then leading to insufficient perfusion of the kidney.

25.4.2　Renal AKI

The main pathological changes of renal AKI are in the kidney. According to the anatomy of the kidney and the injury site, renal ARF includes tubule, vascular and glomerulus. ATN is the most common among them.

Different initiating factors and continuous development factors can lead to varying degrees of ATN, among which poisoning and ischemia are the most common causes to lead to ATN. Both of them can be a single effect, such as nephrotoxic drugs or rhabdomyolysis; or it can also be a common cause of ATN.

25.4.2.1   Tubular factors

Ischemia and nephrotoxic drugs can cause apoptosis or necrosis of tubule epithelial cells and affect reabsorption of the proximal tubular. Simultaneously, exfoliated tubule epithelial cells can form tubular to block renal tubules leading to the intracolumn pressure increases, and GFR decreases. Severe tubular damage can lead to reversal of glomerular filtration, leakage through the damaged epithelium or basement membrane, leading to renal interstitial edema and renal parenchymal injury.

25.4.2.2   Vascular and inflammatory factors

Kidney ischemia can lead to vascular endothelial cell damage, vasomotor dysfunction, renal dysfunction, and inflammatory response, result in imbalance of vasoconstriction factor and relaxation factor, releaseing of inflammatory mediators, the increaseing of vasoconstriction factor, decreaseing of relaxation and inflammatory mediators work together on the renal blood vessels, leading to abnormal hemodynamics and blood redistribution, descreasing of renal blood flow and renal cortical blood flow, renal medulla congestion, leading to decreased GFR.

25.4.3   Postrenal AKI

Urinary obstruction is the most common cause of postrenal AKI outside the hospital. Renal AKI can occur when bilateral urinary tract obstruction or unilateral urinary tract obstruction occurs in patients with isolated kidneys. Common causes include prostatic hyperplasia that plugs the bladder neck, pelvic tumors, or retroperitoneal fibrosis, necrotic nipples, or large stones in ureters.

25.5   Clinic features

AKI clinic manifestation is various, which is related to different etiology and stage of disease. Hence, it includes primary disease, metabolic disorder and complications.

The typical clinical manifestations of ATN are three stages: initial stage, maintenance stage, and recovery stage.

25.5.1   Initial stage

Patient is undergoing with ischemia or nephrotoxicity attack, without renal parenchymal damage in evidence, which is usually absent of obvious clinical symptoms. AKI in this stage is preventable. It can last a couple of hours or days.

25.5.2   Maintenance stage

Maintenance stage is also called as oliguria stage. It has renal parenchyma damage and GFR is reduced below 5-10 mL/min. It can last for 7-14 days, or several months. Some patients would appear oliguria (<400 mL/d or anuria(<100 mL/d)). Urine output is more than 400 mL/d in some patient, which called as non-oliguric AKI, could always means better prognosis. However, urine output is whether or not decrease uremic symptom would appear with renal dysfuction. In addition. This period is prone to occur complications such as infection, cardiovascular disease and upper gastrointestinal bleeding(Table 25-1).

Table 25-1   Symtpms and signs in maintenance stage

System	Uremic manifestation
Digestive system	Anorexia, nausea, vomiting, diarrhea, mouth ulcers, gastrointestinal bleeding
Respiratory system	pulmonary edema, infection
Circulatory System	Hypertension, heart failure, arrhythmia
Neurology	Headache, dizziness, restlessness, disturbance of consciousness, coma
Hematology	Anemia, bleeding tendency
Electrolyte and acid-base disorder	Metabolic acidosis, hyperkalemia, hyponatremia, hypocalcemia, hyperphosphatemia

Hyperkalemia could have no clinical characteristic manifestations, severe case could occur atrioventricular block, Sinus arrest, intraventricular conduction delay or ventricular fibrillation. Electrocardiographic changes in hyperkalemia can occur before clinical manifestations, so ECG monitoring is particularly important. The hyperkalemia electrocardiogram feature include shortened ST segment, high T wave, widened QRS wave, disappeared P wave, and sinus conduction. When hyponatremia, hypocalcemia and acidosis present simultaneously, the electrocardiogram of hyperkalemia is more pronounced.

25.5.3   Recovery stage

Rcovery stage is also called as polyuria stage. While renal tubular epithelial cell is recovering and GFR is approaching to normal standard. Increased progressive urine output is a sign of renal function recovery, renal function does not immediately recover after polyuria, serum creatinine and urea nitrogen can still rise, hyperkalemia can occur early in polyuria, and hypokalemia is prone to occur at late stage of polyuria. In addition. This period is prone to occur complications such as infection, cardiovascular disease and upper gastrointestinal bleeding. Polyuria lasts for 1-3 weeks or longer. Symptoms disppeared, creatinine and urea nitrogen were close to normal, urine output returned to normal, compared with GFR, renal tubular epithelial cell function recovery is relatively delayed, and it often takes several months to recover. A small number of patients may have different degrees of renal structural and functional defect.

25.6   Laboratory test

25.6.1   Blood tests

Mild anemia, elevated serum creatinine and urea nitrogen, decreased pH and bicarbonate ion concentration, lower or normal serum sodium, lower serum calcium, and elevated serum phosphorus and elevated serum kalium.

25.6.2   Urine test

According to different etiology, urine test is different. It is an important distinguish examination between ATN and prerenal AKI(Table 25-2).

Table 25-2 Distinguish between ATN and prerenal AKI

Urine test	Prerenal AI	ATN
Urine specific gravity	>1.018	<1.012
Urine osmolality(mOsm/kg · H_2O)	>500	<250
(mmol/L)	<10	>20
Urinary sodium/serum sodium	>40	<20
Serum urea nitrogen(mg/dL)/serum creatinine(mg/dL)	>20	<10-15
Fractional sodium excretion	<1%	>1%
Renal failure index 1 *	<1	>1
Urinary sediment	hyaline cast	brown granular cast

1 * :renal failure index=urinary sodium/(urinary creatinie/serum creatinine).

25.6.3 Medical imaging

Ultrasound is preferred. Ultrasound or CT could show thinning of the renal or cortical tissue which suggests chronic renal dysfunction, and enlarged kidneys suggest AKI and acute inflammation, infiltrative lesions, and obstruction. Considerable asymmetry in the size of kidneys might indicate renal macro vascular disease.

25.6.4 Renal biopsy

After excluding pre-renal and post-renal etiology, if there is no contraindication to the diagnosis of renal AKI but no clear cause, renal biopsy should be performed as soon as possible so that targeted treatment can be given as soon as possible. In addition, biopsy can be used for the existing kidney disease and it is an important diagnostic method. But AKI and renal function can not be restored.

25.7 Definition

It is not hard to identify AKI by acute renal dysfunction(serum creatinine and urine output), clinical feature, laboratory examination and imaging.

In clinic, it is necessary to identify AKI, severity and complication which requiring urgent treatment at first. Next, it is important to find out whether there is any previous chronic kidney disease. Finally, search the cause of AKI(Table 25-3).

AKI is defined as any of the following.

(1)Increase in SCr by 0.3 mg/dL (or 26.5 μmol/L) with 48 hours; or

(2)Increase in SCr to 1.5 times of baseline, which is known or presumed to have occurred within the prior 7 days; or

(3)Urine volume is reduced to 0.5 mL/(kg · h).

Table 25-3　Staging of AKI

Stage	Serum creatinine	Urine output
1	1.5-1.9 times of baseline OR ≥0.3 mg/dL(≥26.5 mmol/L)	<0.5 mL/(kg·h)for 6-12 hours
2	2.0-2.9 times of baseline	<0.5 mL/(kg·h)for ≥12 hours
3	3.0 times of baseline OR increase in serum creatinine to ≥4.0 mg/dL (≥353.6 mmol/L) OR initiation of renal replacement therapy OR, In patients <18 years, decrease in eGFR to <35 mL/min per 1.73 m²	<0.3 mL/(kg·h)for ≥24 hours OR Anuria for ≥12 hours

25.8　Treatment

The principle of AKI treatment is to identify and correct reversible causes as soon as possible and to prevent further damage to the kidneys. Meanwhile, maintaining water, electrolyte and acid-base balance, actively preventing complications and receiving renal replacement therapy(RRT) in time is also necessary. All patients with AKI should stay in bed and get proper nutrition. Furthermore, adjusting the dose of the drug according to GFR should be noticed, while monitor plasma creatinie concentration.

25.8.1　Correcting the incentive as soon as possible

The effect of adequate rehydration on the prevention and treatment of prerenal and contrast agent kidney injury has been fully affirmed. In patients with congestive heart failure in the past, attention should be paid to the rehydration speed and cease nephrotoxic drugs in a timely manner. The obstruction of urinary tract for postrenal AKI patient should be lifted as soon as possible(Figure 25-1).

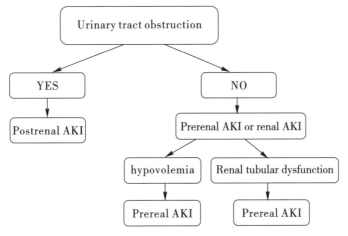

Figure 25-1　Etiology searching workflow

25.8.2　Proper nutrition

Patients with any stage of AKI should achieve a total energy intake of 20-30 kcal/(kg·d). To prevent or delay initiation of RRT, avoiding restriction of protein intake should be noticed. In noncatabolic AKI patients without need for dialysis should take 0.8-1.0 g/(kg·d) of protein; patients with AKI on RRT should take 1.0-1.5 g/(kg·d), and patients on continuous renal replacement therapy (CRRT) and hypercatabolic patients could take up to a maximum of 1. 7 g/(kg · d). In critically ill patients, insulin therapy targeting plasma glucose is 110–149 mg/dL (6. 1–8. 3 mmol/L).

25. 8. 3　Maintain fluid balance

The daily rehydration volume should be the dominant fluid loss plus intrinsic fluid loss minus endogenous water volume. The approximate daily fluid intake can be calculated by adding 500 mL of urine volume for the previous day. Diuretics is not recommended to treat AKI, and only should be used at controlling vlolume while it is useful.

25. 8. 4　Treatment of complication

25. 8. 4. 1　Hyperkalemia and metabolic acidosis

If serum potassium exceeds 6. 5 mmol/L, the presence of hyperkalemia indicated by the ECG must be corrected. Hemodialysis or peritoneal dialysis treatment is the most effective, when serum potassium higher than 6. 5 mmol/L being an indication for hemodialysis. In addition, when hyperkalemia is found, all potassium-containing foods should be stopped immediately and blood from the inventories should be avoided. Calcium gluconate should be given by intravenous injection firstly to antagonize the toxic effects of potassium i-ons on cardiomyocytes. At the same time, given 50% glucose solution 50–100 mL plus regular insulin 6–12 U intravenous injection should be given too, which can promote the transfer of potassium ions into the cell. For patients with metabolic acidosis, when the actual bicarbonate of plasma is lower than 15 mmol/L, 5% sodium bicarbonate 100–250 mL should be given intravenously, and the drip rate should be controlled according to the cardial function and the blood gas analysis should be dynamically monitored.

25. 8. 4. 2　Heart failure

When AKI is accompanied by heart failure, diuretics and digitalis have poor effects and are prone to digitalis poisoning. Hemodialysis is the preferred treatment.

25. 8. 4. 3　Infection

Infection is a common complication of AKI and the main cause of death in the oliguria period. According to bacterial culture and drug sensitivity test, we should choose the antibiotic which has no toxic to the kidney rationally and pay attention to adjust the dose.

25. 8. 5　Renal replacement therapy(RRT)

RRT indications: blood potassium higher than 6. 5 mmol/L, severe metabolic acidosis (pH<7. 2), a-cute pulmonary edema(diuretic effect is not satisfactory). With the extensive development of RRT, the number of cases directly dying from AKI has been significantly reduced, and the main cause of death is primary disease and complications. If the prerenal AKI and postrenal AKI etiology can be promptly relieved, the prognosis is relatively good. The prognosis of renal AKI is quite different, which is related to etiology and complication severe degrees.

25. 9　Prevention

Active treatment of primary disease, alerting people at high risk of AKI, timely detection and removation of risk factors and removal is the key to prevention and treatment of AKI(Table 25–4).

Table 25-4   Causes of AKI:exposures and susceptibilities for non-specific AKI

Exposures	Susceptibilities
Sepsis	Advanced age
Critical illness	Female gender
Circulatory shock	Black race
Burns	CKD
Trauma	Chronic diseases (heart, lung, liver)
Cardiac surgery (especially	Diabetes mellitus
with CPB)	Cancer
Major noncardiac surgery	Anemia
Nephrotoxic drugs	
Radiocontrast agents	
Poisonous plants and animals	
Pehydration or volume depletion	

Li Peiwu ,Zhang Yao

Chapter 26

Hypoglycemia

Hypoglycemia is most commonly caused by drugs used to treat diabetes mellitus or by exposure to other drugs, and alcohol. However, a number of other disorders, including critical organ failure, sepsis and inanition, hormone deficiencies, non-beta-cell tumors, insulinoma, and prior gastric surgery, may cause hypoglycemia.

26.1 Definition and diagnosis

26.1.1 Patients with diabetes

In patients with diabetes, hypoglycemia is defined as all episodes of an abnormally low plasma glucose concentration (with or without symptoms) that expose the individual to harm. People with diabetes should become concerned about the possibility of hypoglycemia at a self-monitored blood glucose level or continuous glucose monitoring level ≤70 mg/dL (3.9 mmol/L).

26.1.2 Patients without diabetes

In a person without diabetes, the presence of a hypoglycemic disorder can not be diagnosed with confidence solely on the basis of a low plasma glucose concentration. Although neurogenic and neuroglycopenic symptoms may be highly suggestive of hypoglycemia, they can not be ascribed to hypoglycemia with confidence unless the plasma glucose concentration is low at the same time and the symptoms are relieved when it is raised, the so-called Whipple's triad. Glucose levels<55 mg/dL (3.0 mmol/L) with symptoms that are relieved promptly after the glucose level is raised document hypoglycemia.

26.2 Causes of hypoglycemia in adults

(1) Drugs: insulin or insulin secretagogue; others.
(2) Critical illness: hepatic, renal, or cardiac failure; sepsis; inanition.

（3）Hormone deficiency：cortisol；glucagon and epinephrine.

（4）Non-islet cell tumor.

（5）Endogenous hyperinsulinism：insulinoma；functional beta-cell disorders；insulin autoimmune hypoglycemia（antibody to insulin or to insulin receptor）；insulin secretagogue；other.

（6）Accidental，surreptitious，or malicious hypoglycemia.

26.3　Clinical features

Neuroglycopenic symptoms of hypoglycemia are the direct result of central nervous system（CNS）glucose deprivation. They include behavioral changes，confusion，fatigue，seizure，loss of consciousness，and if hypoglycemia is severe and prolonged，death. Neurogenic symptoms of hypoglycemia are the result of the perception of physiologic changes caused by the CNS-mediated sympathoadrenal discharge triggered by hypoglycemia. They include adrenergic symptoms such as palpitations，tremor，and anxiety. They also include cholinergic symptoms such as sweating，hunger，and paresthesia. Clearly，these are non-specific symptoms. Their attribution to hypoglycemia requires a corresponding low plasma glucose concentration and their resolution after the glucose level is raised（Whipple's triad）.

Common signs of hypoglycemia include diaphoresis and pallor. Heart rate and systolic blood pressure are typically increased but may not be raised in an individual who has experienced repeated，recent episodes of hypoglycemia. Neuroglycopenic manifestations are often observable. Transient focal neurologic deficits occur occasionally. Permanent neurologic deficits are rare.

26.4　Management

26.4.1　Urgent treatment

Oral treatment with glucose tablets or glucose-containing fluids，candy，or food is appropriate if the patient is able and willing to take these. A reasonable initial dose is 20 g of glucose. If the patient is unable or unwilling，because of neuroglycopenia，to take carbohydrates orally，parenteral therapy is necessary. Intravenous glucose（25 g）should be given and followed by a glycose infusion guided by serial plasma glucose measurements. If intravenous therapy is not practical，subcutaneous or intramuscular glucagon（1 mg in adults）can be used，particularly in patients with T1DM. It acts by stimulating glycogenolysis. Glucagon is ineffective in glycogen-depleted individuals（e. g. ，those with alcohol-induced hypoglycemia）. It also stimulates insulin secretion and is therefore less useful in T2DM. These treatments raise plasma glucose concentrations only transiently，and patients should therefore be urged to eat as soon as is practical to replete glycogen stores.

26.4.2　Prevention of recurrent hypoglycemia

Prevention of recurrent hypoglycemia requires an understanding of the hypoglycemic mechanism. Offending drugs can be discontinued or their doses reduced. Hypoglycemia caused by a sulfonylurea can persist for hours or even days. Underlying critical illnesses can often be treated. Cortisol and growth hormone can be replaced if they are deficient. Surgical resection of an Insulinoma is curative; medical therapy with diazoxide or octreotide can be used if resection is not possible. Failing these treatments, frequent feedings and avoidance of fasting may be required.

Gao Yanxia

Chapter 27

Diabetic Ketoacidosis

Diabetic ketoacidosis (DKA) is one of the most serious acute complications of diabetes. DKA is characterized by ketoacidosis and hyperglycemia. DKA is the leading cause of morbidity and mortality in individuals with type 1 diabetes mellitus. Less commonly, it can occur in individuals with type 2 diabetes mellitus. DKA may be the initial symptom complex that leads to the diagnosis of type 1 diabetes mellitus.

27.1 Pathophysiology

DKA results from relative or absolute insulin deficiency combined with hormone excess (glucagon, catecholamine, cortisol and growth hormone). Both insulin deficiency and glucagon excess are necessary for DKA to develop. The decreased ratio of insulin to glucagon promotes gluconeogenesis, glycogenolysis and ketone body formation in the liver, as well as increases in substrate delivery from fat and muscle to the liver. Lack of insulin action means that cells can not use glucose in the blood. So cells need to get fuel from other sources. The increased level of glucagon and other hormones stimulates muscle and fat breakdown, causing a rise in plasma free fatty acids and a further increase in blood glucose (from glucogenic amino acids). The use of fatty acids as fuel results in the production of ketone bodies in plasma. These have two effects: lowering of blood pH (acidosis), nausea and vomiting. High blood glucose level exceeds the renal threshold and causes an osmotic diuresis. Together with nausea and vomiting, this diuresis causes dehydration. The acidosis may result in Kussmaul's respiration.

27.2 Clinical features and laboratory test

Nausea and vomiting are often common manifestations. Abdominal pain may be severe and can resemble acute pancreatitis or ruptured viscus. Hyperglycemia leads to glucosuria blood, volume depletion and tachycardia. Hypotension can occur because of blood volume depletion in combination with peripheral vasodilation. Kussmaul respirations and a fruity odor on the patient's breath (secondary to metabolic acidosis and increased acetone) are classic signs of the disorder. Lethargy and central nervous system depression may evolve into coma with severe DKA. Cerebral edema, an extremely serious complication of DKA, is seen most frequently in children. Occasionally, the serum glucose is only minimally elevated. Serum bicarbonate is frequently less than 10 mmol/L, and arterial blood pH ranges between 6.8 and 7.3, depending on the severity of the acidosis. Despite a total-body potassium deficit, the serum potassium at presentation may be mildly elevated secondary to the acidosis. Total body stores of sodium, chloride, phosphorus and magnesium are reduced in DKA but are not accurately reflected by their levels in the serum because of dehydration and hyperglycemia. Elevated blood urea nitrogen and serum creatinine reflect blood volume depletion.

27.3 Diagnosis

DKA is characterized by the triad of hyperglycemia, ketosis and metabolic acidosis. Metabolic acidosis is often the major finding. The serum glucose concentration is often approximately 350-500 mg/dL (19.4-27.8 mmol/L). However, serum glucose concentrations may exceed 900 mg/dL (50 mmol/L) in patients with DKA who are comatose. In certain settings, such as starvation, pregnancy, treatment with insulin prior to arrival in the emergency department, or use of SGLT2 inhibitors, the glucose level may be only mildly elevated.

The diagnostic criteria proposed by the American Diabetes Association (ADA) for mild, moderate, and severe DKA are shown in the table (Table 27-1).

Table 27-1　Typical laboratory characteristics of DKA and HHS *

	DKA			HHS
	Mild	Moderate	Severe	
Plasma glucose(mg/dL)	>250	>250	>250	>600
Plasma glucose(mmol/L)	>13.9	>13.9	>13.9	>33.3
Arterial blood pH	7.25-7.30	7.00-7.24	<7.00	>7.30
Serum bicarbonate(mEq/L)	15-18	10-15	<10	>18
Urine ketones	Positive	Positive	Positive	Negative
Serum ketones- Nitroprusside reaction	Positive	Positive	Positive	Normal or weak postive
Serum ketones- Enzymatic assay of Beta hydroxybutyrate (normal range<0.6mmol/L)[#]	3-4 mmol/L	4-8 mmol/L	>8 mmol/L	<0.6 mmol/L
Effective serum osmolality(mOsm/kg) * *	Variable	Variable	Variable	>320
Alteration in sensoria or mental obtundation	Alert	Alert/drowsy	Stupor/coma	Stupor/coma

* There may be considerable diagnostic overlap between DKA and HHS.

Note: Many assays for beta hydroxybutyrate can only report markedly elevated values as>6.0 mmol/L.

* * Calculation: 2[measured Na (mEq/L)] +glucose (mg/dL)/18.

2006 American Diabetes Association. From Diabetes Care Vol 29, Issue 12, 2006.

27.4　Management

(1) Confirm diagnosis (↑ plasma glucose, positive serum ketones, metabolic acidosis).

(2) Admit to hospital; intensive-care setting may be necessary for frequent monitoring if pH<7. 00 or unconscious.

(3) Assess: serum electrolytes, acid-base status and renal function.

(4) Replace fluids: 2-3 L of 0. 9% saline over first 1-3 hours [15-20 mL/(kg · h)]; subsequently, 0. 45% saline at 250-500 mL/h; change to 5% glucose and 0. 45% saline at 150-250 mL/h when plasma glucose reaches 200 mg/dL (11. 2 mmol/L).

(5) Administer short-acting insulin: Ⅳ (0. 1 μ/kg), then 0. 1 μ/(kg · h) by continuous Ⅳ infusion; increase two-threefold if no response by 2-4 hours. If the initial serum potassium is<3. 3 mmol/L, do not administer insulin until the potassium is corrected. If the initial serum potassium is >5. 2 mmol/L, do not supplement K⁺until the potassium is corrected.

(6) Assess patient: What precipitated the episode (non-compliance, infection, trauma, infarction, cocaine)? Initiate appropriate workup for precipitating event.

(7) Measure capillary glucose every 1-2 hours; measure electrolytes and anion gap every 4 hours for first 24 hours.

(8) Monitor blood pressure, pulse, respirations, mental status, fluid intake and output every 1-4 hours.

(9) Replace K⁺:10 meq/h when plasma K⁺<5. 0-5. 2 meq/L (or 20-30 meq/L of infusion fluid), ECG normal, urine flow and normal creatinine documented; administer 40-80 meq/h when plasma K⁺< 3. 5 meq/L or if bicarbonate is given.

(10) Continue above until patient is stable the goal of plasma glucose is 8. 3-13. 9 mmol/L (150-250 mg/dL), and acidosis is resolved. Insulin infusion may be decreased to 0. 05-0. 1 μ/(kg · h).

(11) Administer long-acting insulin as soon as patient could take food orally. Allow for overlap in insulin infusion and SC insulin injection.

Gao Yanxia

Chapter 28

Hyperosmolar Hyperglycemic State

Hyperosmolar hyperglycemic state (HHS, also known as hyperosmotic hyperglycemic nonketotic state, HHNK) is also one of the most serious acute complications of diabetes. Compared to DKA, HHS usually has more severe hyperglycemia but no ketoacidosis. Symptoms of hyperosmolar hyperglycemic state develop more insidiously with polyuria, polydipsia, and weight loss, often persisting for several days before hospital admission. Neurologic symptoms are most common in HHS, such as lethargy, focal signs, obtundation, and even coma. In HHS, fluid losses and dehydration are usually more pronounced than in DKA due to the longer duration of the illness. The patient with HHS is usually older, more likely to have mental status changes, and more likely to have a life-threatening precipitating event with accompanying comorbidities. Even with proper treatment, HHS has a substantially higher mortality rate than DKA.

28.1 Pathophysiology

Relative insulin deficiency and inadequate fluid intake are the underlying causes of HHS. Insulin deficiency increases hepatic glucose production (through glycogenolysis and gluconeogenesis) and impairs glucose utilization in skeletal muscle. Hyperglycemia induces an osmotic diuresis that leads to intravascular volume depletion, which is exacerbated by inadequate fluid replacement. The absence of ketosis in HHS is still not understood. Presumably, the insulin deficiency is only relative and less severe than in DKA.

28.2 Clinical features and laboratory test

The prototypical patient with HHS is an elderly individual with type 2 DM, with a several-week history of polyuria, weight loss, and diminished oral intake that culminates in mental confusion, lethargy, or coma. The physical examination reflects profound dehydration and hyperosmolality and reveals hypotension, tachycardia, and altered mental status. A precipitating event can usually be identified in patients with HHS. The most common events are infection (often pneumonia or urinary tract infection) and discontinuation of or inadequate insulin therapy. Compromised water intake due to underlying medical conditions, particularly in older patients, can promote the development of severe dehydration and HHS. Acute major illnesses such as myocardial infarction, cerebrovascular accident, sepsis can also lead to HHS.

The most notable laboratory features of HHS are the marked hyperglycemia (plasma glucose is usually higher than 33.3 mmol/L), hyperosmolality (more than 350 mOsm/L), and prerenal azotemia. In contrast to DKA, acidosis and ketonemia are absent or mild. Moderate ketonuria, if it presents, is secondary to starvation.

28.3   Diagnosis

In HHS, there is little or no ketoacid accumulation, the serum glucose concentration frequently exceeds 1,000 mg/dL (56 mmol/L), the plasma osmolality may reach 380 mmol/kg, and neurologic abnormalities are frequently presented (including coma in 25% –50% of cases). Most patients with HHS have an admission pH>7.30, a serum bicarbonate>20 mEq/L, a serum glucose>600mg/dL (33.3 mmol/L), and test negative for ketones in serum and urine, although mild ketonemia may present.

The diagnostic criteria proposed by the American Diabetes Association (ADA) for HHS and the differences between HHS and DKA are shown in Table 27–1.

28.4   Management

Fluid supplementation should initially stabilize the hemodynamic status of the patient (1–3 L of 0.9% normal saline over the first 2–3 hours). Because the fluid deficit in HHS is accumulated over a period of days to weeks, the rapidity of reversal of the hyperosmolar state must balance the need for free water repletion with the risk that too rapid reversal may worsen neurologic function. If the serum sodium is>150 mmol/L, 0.45% saline should be used. After hemodynamic stability is achieved, the IV fluid administration is directed at reversing the free water deficit using hypotonic fluids (0.45% saline initially, then 5% dextrose in water). The calculated free water deficit (which averages 9–10 L) should be reversed over the next 1–2 days (infusion rates of 200–300 mL/h of hypotonic solution). Potassium repletion is usually necessary and should be dictated by repeated measurements of the serum potassium. In patients taking diuretics, the potassium deficit could be quite large and may be accompanied by magnesium deficiency.

Rehydration and blood volume expansion lower the plasma glucose initially, but insulin is also required. A reasonable regimen for HHS begins with an IV insulin bolus of 0.1 u/kg followed by IV insulin at a constant infusion rate of 0.1 u/(kg · h). If the serum glucose does not fall, increase the insulin infusion rate by twofold. Glucose should be added to IV fluid when the plasma glucose falls to 13.9–16.7 mmol/L (250–300 mg/dL), and the insulin infusion rate should be decreased to 0.05–0.1 u/(kg · h). The insulin infusion should be continued until the patient has resumed eating and can be transferred to an SC insulin regimen. The patient should be discharged from the hospital on insulin, though some patients can later switch to oral glucose–lowering agents.

Gao Yanxia

Chapter 29

Thyroid Storm

29.1　Introduction

Thyroid storm or thyrotoxic crisis is a rare but severe and potentially life-threatening complication of hyperthyroidism (overactivity of the thyroid gland). It is characterized by a high fever (temperature is often above 40 ℃/104 ℉), fast and often irregular heart beat, vomiting, diarrhea, and agitation.

29.2　Pathophysiology of thyroid storm

Thyroid hormone (TH) is synthesized within the follicular cells of the thyroid gland. Production begins with the uptake of iodine into the follicular lumen. Thyroglobulin, produced within the follicular cell, is bound to iodine and then coupled to produce the thyroid hormones, thyroxine (T4) and triiodothyrinine (T3). Release of thyroid hormone is stimulated by one of the hormones secreted by the pituitary gland, thyroid-stimulating hormone (TSH). In turn, TSH is regulated by thyroid-releasing hormone (TRH) secreted by the hypothalamus. High levels of T4 and T3 act to suppress production of TSH and TRH via a negative feedback loop. TH released from the thyroid gland is in its less active form—T4, which is converted in peripheral organs (kidney and liver) into its 10 times more active derivative—T3. The half life of T3 is significantly shorter, approximately a day, compared with 1 week for T4 In the serum, the majority of TH is bound to thyroid-binding globulin (TBG), making it inactive. The only active forms are free T3 and T4. After TH enters cells, it binds to its nuclear receptor and regulates expression of genes involved in lipid and carbohydrates metabolism and protein synthesis.

29.2.1　Increases in free thyroid hormone

Individuals with thyroid storm tend to have increased levels of free thyroid hormone, although total thyroid hormone levels may not be much higher than in uncomplicated hyperthyroidism. The rise in the availability of free thyroid hormone may be the result of manipulating the thyroid gland. In the setting of an individual receiving radioactive iodine therapy, free thyroid hormone levels may sharply increase due to the release of hormone from ablated thyroid tissue.

29.2.2　Decrease in thyroid hormone binding protein

A decrease in thyroid hormone binding protein in the setting of various stressors or medications may also cause a rise in free thyroid hormone.

29.2.3　Increased sensitivity to thyroid hormone

Along with increases in thyroid hormone availability, it is also suggested that thyroid storm is characterized by enhanced sensitivity to thyroid hormone, which may be related to sympathetic activation.

29.2.4　Sympathetic activation

Sympathetic nervous system activation during times of stress may also play a significant role in thyroid storm. Sympathetic activation increases production of thyroid hormone by the thyroid gland. In the setting of elevated thyroid hormone, the density of thyroid hormone receptors (esp. β-receptors) also increases, which enhances the response to catecholamines. This is likely responsible for several of the cardiovascular symptoms (increased cardiac output, heart rate, stroke volume) seen in thyroid storm.

29.2.5　Thyroid storm as allostatic failure

Usually, in critical illness (e. g. , sepsis, myocardial infarction and other causes of shock) thyroid function is turned down to result in low-T3 syndrome and, occasionally, also low TSH concentrations, low-T4 syndrome and impaired plasma protein binding of thyroid hormones. This endocrine pattern is referred to as euthyroid sick syndrome (ESS), non-thyroidal illness syndrome (NTIS) or thyroid allostasis in critical illness, tumours, uraemia and starvation (TACITUS). Although NTIS is associated with significantly worse prognosis, it is also assumed to represent a beneficial adaptation (type 1 allostasis). In cases, where critical illness is accompanied by thyrotoxicosis, this comorbidity prevents the down-regulation of thyroid function. Therefore, the consumption of energy, oxygen and glutathione remains high, which leads to further increased mortality.

29.3　Clinical presentation

29.3.1　Symptom

Depending on the degree of abnormality, patients will present with varied severity of symptoms. Patients with earlier stages of thyrotoxicosis will report excessive sweating, weight loss, palpitations, anxiety, and heat intolerance. Patients in thyroid storm will present with symptoms of thyrotoxicosis in addition to fever, tachycardia, altered mental status, and often congestive heart failure. In elderly patients, there is a rare form of thyrotoxicosis referred to as apathetic hyperthyroidism, presenting with lethargy, altered mental status, blepharoptosis (drooping of the upper eye lid), weight loss, and atrial fibrillation leading to congestive heart failure.

29.3.2 Signs

Frequent findings in patients with hyperthyroidism owing to Graves disease include goiter, exopthalmos, palmar erythema, and tachy cardia. In thyroid storm, in addition to those findings, patients will have altered mental status, fever, hypertension, and frequently atrial fibrillation.

29.3.3 Auxiliary inspection

As with hyperthyroidism, TSH is suppressed. Both free and serum (or total) T3 and T4 are elevated. An elevation in thyroid hormone levels is suggestive of thyroid storm when accompanied by signs of severe hyperthyroidism but is not diagnostic as it may also correlate with uncomplicated hyperthyroidism. Moreover, serum T3 may be normal in critically ill patients due to decreased conversion of T4 to T3. Other potential abnormalities include the following:

Hyperglycemia likely due to catecholamine-mediated effects on insulin release and metabolism as well as increased glycogenolysis, evolving into hypoglycemia when glycogen stores are depleted.

Elevated aspartate aminotransferase (AST), bilirubin and lactate dehydrogenase (LDH).

Hypercalcemia and elevated alkaline phosphatase due to increased bone resorption.

Elevated white blood cell count.

29.4 Diagnosis

The diagnostic criteria for thyroid storm see Table 29-1.

Table 29-1   The diagnostic criteria for thyroid storm (TS)

Prerequisite for diagnosis
Presence of thyrotoxicosis with elevated levels of free triiodothyronine (FT3) or free thyroxine (FT4)
Symptoms
1. Central nervous system (CNS) manifestations: Restlessness, delirium, mental aberration/psychosis, somnolence/lethargy, coma (≥ 1 on the Japan Coma Scale or ≤ 14 on the Glasgow Coma Scale)
2. Fever: $\geq 38\ ^{\circ}\text{C}$
3. Tachycardia: ≥ 130 beats/min or heart rate ≥ 130 in atrial fibrillation
4. Congestive heart failure (CHF): Pulmonary edema, moist rales over more than half of the lung field, cardiogenic shock, or Class Ⅳ by the New York Heart Assciation or $\geq$ Class Ⅲ in the Killip classification
5. Gastrointestinal (GI)/hepatic manifestations: nausea, vomiting, diarrhea, or a total bilirubin level ≥ 3.0 mg/dL

29.5 Treatment

The main strategies for the management of thyroid storm are reducing production and release of thyroid hormone, reducing the effects of thyroid hormone on tissues, replacing fluid losses, and controlling temperature. Thyroid storm requires prompt treatment and hospitalization. Often, admission to the intensive care unit is needed.

29.5.1 Antithyroid medications

The main action of ATDs(MMI and PTU) is to directly inhibit thyroid peroxidase through the coupling of iodotyrosine in thyroglobulin molecules, resulting in reduced synthesis of new thyroid hormone molecules. The major functional difference between MMI and PTU is that large doses of PTU (at least 400 mg/d) inhibit type I deiodinase activity in the thyroid gland and other peripheral organs, and may therefore acutely decrease triiodothyronine (T3) levels more than MMI. These are the reasons that PTU, rather than MMI, is recommended, however both are commonly used. The median dose of MMI administered was 30 mg (range, 5–120 mg), whereas the median dose of PTU was 450 mg (range, 150–1,500 mg).

29.5.2 Iodine

The administration of inorganic iodide in large doses decreases thyroid hormone synthesis by inhibiting iodide oxidation and organification (the Wolff–Chaikoff effect), and also rapidly inhibits the release of thyroid hormones from the follicular lumen of the thyroid gland. Therefore, inorganic iodide can decrease thyroid hormone levels more rapidly than other agents, including ATDs and corticosteroids. Inorganic iodide be administered at least 1 hour after the administration of ATDs to prevent the organification of iodide. It can be given as strong iodine solution, 1 mL 3 times daily, as potassium iodide, 10 drops of a solution containing 1 g/mL every 4–6 hours, or as sodium iodide, 1 g every 8–12 hours by slow intravenous infusion.

29.5.3 Beta blockers

Beta1-selective AAs[landiolol, esmolol (intravenous), or bisoprolol (oral)] should be selected as the first choice of treatment for tachycardia in thyroid storm. In addition, propanolol at high doses also reduces peripheral conversion of T4 to T3, which is the more active form of thyroid hormone. Although previously unselective beta blockers (e. g. , propranolol) have been suggested to be beneficial due to their inhibitory effects on peripheral deiodinases recent research suggests them to be associated with increased mortality. Therefore, cardioselective beta blockers may be favourable.

29.5.4 Corticosteroids

High levels of thyroid hormone result in a hypermetabolic state, which can result in increased breakdown of cortisol, a hormone produced by the adrenal gland. This results in a state of relative adrenal insufficiency, in which the amount of cortisol is not sufficient. Guidelines recommend that corticosteroids (hydrocortisone and dexamethasone are preferred over prednisolone or methylprednisolone) be administered to all patients with thyroid storm. However, doses should be altered for each individual patient to ensure that the relative adrenal insufficiency is adequately treated while minimizing the risk of side effects.

29.5.5 Supportive measures

In high fever, temperature control is achieved with fever reducers such as paracetamol/acetaminophen, external cooling measures (cool blankets, ice packs) are not recommended. Dehydration, which occurs due to fluid loss from sweating, diarrhea, and vomiting, is treated with frequent fluid replacement. In severe cases, continuous renal replacement therapy may be necessary to reduce plasma thyroid hormone concentration.

Cao Yan

Chapter 30

Rhabdomyolysis

30.1　Introduction

　　Rhabdomyolysis is a condition in which damaged skeletal muscle tissue breaks down rapidly ("rhab-domyo" = skeletal muscle, "lysis" = rapid breakdown). Breakdown products of damaged muscle cells are released into the bloodstream. Some of these, such as the protein myoglobin, are harmful to the kidneys and may lead to kidney failure.

30.2　Common causes

　　Most cases of rhabdomyolysis are considered as part of crush syndrome, a condition that occurs as the result of traumaticskeletal muscle injury. But there are many cases not caused by direct trauma are considered to be the result of several different factors.

　　(1) Prolonged immobilization.

　　(2) Overexertion of muscles.

　　(3) Infections, in particular bacterial and viral infections that cause blood infections.

　　(4) Heatstroke, hyperthermia, electrocution, lightning strikes or a third-degree burn that cause muscle damage.

　　(5) Hypothermia.

　　(6) Status epilepticus, in which the seizure lasts for a prolonged period of time and muscles involuntarily contract.

　　(7) Toxins, such as excessive or long-term alcohol or drug use. This also includes exposure to environmental toxins, including reptile or insect venom, mold, and carbon monoxide.

　　(8) Complications from the venom from snake bites and black widow spider bites.

　　(9) Inherited, caused by genetic conditions such as muscular myopathies.

　　(10) Certain medications (Cholesterol lowering medications, Antidepressant medications) can also lead to rhabdomylosis. For example, the condition is estimated to arise in an estimated 0.3–13.5 cases out

of every 1 million statin prescriptions made. Other medications include anti-psychotic medications and those used to manage muscular conditions such as Parkinson's disease.

(11)Crayfish (though its pathogenesis remains unclear).

30.3   Symptoms and signs

Although mild cases may not cause symptoms, most people with rhabdomyolysis experience a common set of complaints. Most symptoms first appear within hours to days after the condition develops or a cause has occurred.

Common symptoms of rhabdomyolysis mainly include muscle stiffness or aching (often extremely painful aching and throbbing due to muscle necrosis, Figure 30 - 1 and dark -, cola -, or tea-colored urine (which is due to myoglobin being excreted in the urine).

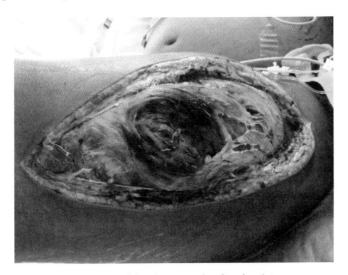

Figure 30-1   **Muscle necrosis after fasciotomy**

In addition to the above symptoms, it is also included symptoms of kidney failure (decreased urine output, shortness of breath as excess fluid builds up in the lungs), symptoms of hyperkalemia (nausea or vomiting, general exhaustion or fatigue, dizziness, or feeling faint, irregular heartbeat, palpitations, ventricular tachycardia and ventricular fibrillation due to heart rhythm disturbances), muscle weakness, muscle swelling or inflammation, confusion or disorientation.

Disseminated intravascular coagulation may present as unexplained bleeding, a condition that occurs when small blood clots begin forming in the body's blood vessels. These clots consume all the clotting factors and platelets in the body, and bleeding begins to occur spontaneously.

30.4   Examinations and laboratory tests

(1)Creatine kinase (CK) level, a product of muscle breakdown.

(2)Serum calcium.

(3)Serum myoglobin.

(4) Serum potassium.

(5) Urinalysis, the dark urine color is due to myoglobin being excreted in the urine. Some affected individuals describe this as blood in the urine, but when it is examined under a microscope, no red blood cells are seen.

(6) Urine myoglobin test, a relative of hemoglobin that is released from damaged muscles.

This disease may also affect the results of the following tests: CK isoenzymes, serum creatinine, and urine creatinine.

Occasionally genetic testing may also be performed in people with suspected cases of rhabdomyolysis, in order to check for the presence of inherited muscle conditions.

30.5 Diagnosis

Most physicians begin by reviewing patient medical history, considering factors including injury, over-exertion, medication use, and other health conditions or symptoms. To make a diagnosis, laboratory confirmation is normally required. This tends to involve detection of elevated CK levels in the blood and the presence of myoglobin in the urine. CK levels>1,000 IU/L and serum myoglobin>150 ng/mL are considered to be evidence of rhabdomyolysis. Activity or physical exertion may raise CK levels temporarily. As a result, tests should be done after avoiding rigorous activity for roughly 7 days. In many instances, muscle biopsies are also carried out to confirm and assess muscle damage.

30.6 Treatment

Early treatment of rhabdomyolysis and its causes are keys to a successful outcome. You can expect full recovery with prompt treatment. Doctors can even reverse kidney damage. However, if compartment syndrome is not treated early enough, it may cause permanent damage. Treatment depends on the severity of the case, symptoms, and presence of additional health complications that may increase the risk of kidney damage.

30.6.1 Fluid therapy

First and most important treatment method is intravenous fluid therapy. Large volumes of fluid (Amounts of 6 to 12 liters over 24 hours are recommended) are often administered intravenously in order to rehydrate the body and flush the myoglobin out of the kidneys. The rate of fluid administration may be altered to achieve a high urine output (200–300 ml/h in adults), unless there are complications, such as heart failure. This fluid should contain bicarbonate, which helps flush. Furosemide, a loop diuretic, is often used to ensure sufficient urine production and keep the kidneys functioning.

30.6.2 Correction of electrolyte disorders

In the initial stages, electrolyte levels are often abnormal and require correction. High potassium levels can be life-threatening, as well as low blood calcium levels (hypocalcemia).

30.6.3 Hemodialysis and hemofiltration

Typically kidney dysfunction develops 1–2 days after the initial muscle damage. If supportive treatment is inadequate to manage this, renal replacement therapy (RRT) may be required. Hemodialysis and hemo-filtration are effective at removing small molecules (such as potassium) and large molecules (such as myo-globin) from the bloodstream.

30.6.4   Symptomatic treatment

If rhabdomyolysis is related to a medical condition, such as diabetes or a thyroid disorder, appropriate treatment for the medical condition will be needed. And if rhabdomyolysis is related to a medication or drug, its use will need to be stopped or replaced with an alternative.

30.6.5   Surgical treatment

30.6.5.1   Fasciotomy

A surgical procedure (fasciotomy) is necessary to relieve tension or pressure and loss of circulation if compartment syndrome is still getting worse and threatens muscle death or nerve damage through the treat-ment above (Figure 30-2). Often, multiple incisions are made and left open until the swelling has re-duced. At that point, the incisions are closed, often requiring debridement (removal of non-viable tissue) and skin grafting in the process.

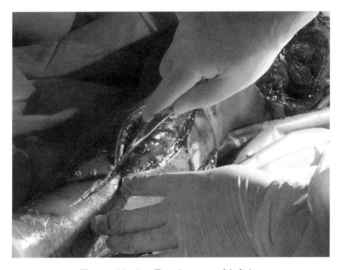

Figure 30-2   **Fasciotomy of left leg**

30.6.5.2   Vacuum sealing drainage

Vacuum sealing drainage (VSD) has been increasingly recognized as a valid treatment approach in the management of various types of tissue injuries. A VSD device facilitates complete wound drainage and elimi-nates dead space decreases wound area, and enhances formation of granulation tissue. It facilitates complete suction (using a sealed wound dressing connected to a vacuum pump) of seepage, necrotic tissues, and pus from the wound area by using a negative-pressure device. Emerging studies have demonstrated that VSD treatment can speed wound healing and reduce incidence of infection. It can also be used in rhabdomyolys-is, especially after fasciotomy and debridement due to compartment syndrome(Figure 30-3).

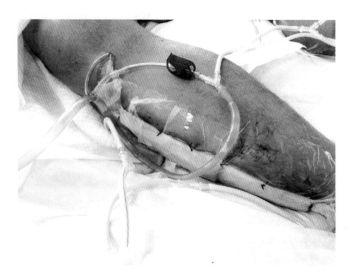

Figure 30 – 3   VSD of right leg after fasciotomy and debridement

Yao Dongqi

Chapter 31

Coma

31.1　Introduction

Coma is a state of unconsciousness in which a person cannot be awakened; fails to respond normally to painful stimuli, light, or sound; lacks a normal wake−sleep cycle; and does not initiate voluntary actions. A person in a state of coma is described as being comatose.

31.2　Epidemiology

31.2.1　Intoxication

Forty percent of comatose states result from drug poisoning. Drugs damage or weaken the synaptic functioning in the ARAS and keep the system from properly functioning to arouse the brain. Secondary effects of drugs, which include abnormal heart rate and blood pressure, as well as abnormal breathing and sweating, may also indirectly harm the functioning of the ARAS and lead to acoma. Seizures and hallucinations also have shown to play a major role in ARAS malfunction.

31.2.2　Lack of oxygen

Generally resulting from cardiac arrest. The Central Nervous System (CNS) requires a great deal of oxygen for its neurons. Oxygen deprivation in the brain, also known as hypoxia, causes neuronal extracellular sodium and calcium to decrease and intracellular calcium to increase, which harms neuron communication. Lack of oxygen in the brain also causes ATP exhaustion and cellular breakdown from cytoskeleton damage and nitric oxideproduction.

31.2.3　Others

Others includes metabolic syndrome, central nervous system diseases, acute neurologic injuries such as strokes or herniations, hypothermia, hypoglycemia, eclampsia or traumatic injuries such as head trauma caused by falls, drowning accidents, or vehicle collisions. It may also be deliberately induced by pharmaceutical agents during major neurosurgery, to preserve higher brain functions following brain trauma, or to save the patient from extreme pain during healing of injuries or diseases.

31.3　Diagnosis

31.3.1　Clinical menifestation

Coma is a severe consciousness disorders characterized by persistent interruption or complete loss of consciousness, which can be divided into the following three stages.

31.3.1.1　Mild coma

Most of the consciousness is lost. There is no independent movement, no response to sound and light stimulation. The patients can show the expression of pain or the shrinking defense reaction to pain stimulation, such as corneal reflex, pupillary light reflex, eye movements, pharyngeal reflex etc.

31.3.1.2　Moderate coma

No reaction to the surroundings and various stimuli, for intense stimulation, patients can appear defensive reflex, along with Hypocorneal reflex, the pupil light reflex slow, the eye could not move.

31.3.1.3　Deep coma

Whole body muscle is relaxation and shows no response to various stimuli, deep and shallow reflection are all disappeared.

31.3.2　Auxiliary examination

(1) Blood tests, urine routines, blood glucose, urea, creatinine, blood gas analysis, blood ammonia, blood electrolytes, and other test items are helpful for diagnosis.

(2) Cerebrospinal fluid examination is very important for understanding changes in intracranial pressure, intracranial infection and bleeding. Normal cerebrospinal fluid is colorless and transparent, uniform bloody cerebrospinal fluid is seen in cerebral hemorrhage or subarachnoid hemorrhage; cerebrospinal fluid turbidity is seen in bacterial meningitis.

(3) Conduct relevant examinations allording to the medical history and condition, related examination include blood biochemical tests such as liver function and renal function, and electroencephalogream, rheo-encephalogram, head CT, magnetic resonance examination. Digital subtraction angiography (DSA) helps in the diagnosis of etiology of subarachnoid hemorrhage and the diagnosis of venous system thrombosis.

31.4　Treatment

31.4.1　General treatment

(1) All patients need to go to the hospital for further treatment as soon as possible.

(2) Keep respiratory tract unobstructed, clear in time the airway foreign bodies, is used for breathing resistance oropharyngeal tube, also can make the patients with stable lateral position, it can control the phar-

ynx jams respiratory tissue, and is helpful for drainage of secretions, prevent the content of the digestive tract reflux aspiration caused by lateral position is therefore a coma patients must be taken prior to admission position.

(3) Support therapy and symptomatic treatment, the establishment of intravenous route, to maintain blood pressure and the balance of water and electricity, for breathing was abnormal breathing support (mask airbag artificial respiration endotracheal intubation doping, etc.), for tic diazepam drugs, such as for patients with high cranial pressure dehydration drugs.

31.4.2   Etiological treatment

According to the primary disease and cause of the coma, targeted treatment measures should be taken, such as anti-infective treatment, oxygen inhalation and mangement of hypoglycemia.

31.4.3   Drug therapy

31.4.3.1   nervous centralis inhibitor

The central nervous inhibition barbiturate drugs could inhibit the brain cell metabolism and make reasonable distribution of cerebral blood flow, relieve cerebral edema, cut the intracranial pressure to reduce calcium internal flow and scaveng free radicals, and so on. The most commonly used pentobarbital, conventional application methods are a high initial close of 10 mg/kg, intravenous for 30 minutes; maintain volume 5 mg/(kg · h) continue to pump note 3 hours, follow-up 1 mg/(kg · h) continue to pump injection, until the outbreak of EEG present sample inhibition or ICP down to target drugs must be monitoring vital signs change during the drug adverse reactions, such as lowering blood pressure and inhibiting respiratory, therefore is not advo cating a routine use

31.4.3.2   Calcium antagonist

Nimodipine can slow down the increase of cytoplasmic free calcium, reduce intracellular calcium overload, reduce ATP depletion, relieve vascular spasm, and reduce intracellular acidosis. The conventional method is 1-2 mg/h, continuous intravenous infusion for 10-20 days.

31.4.3.3   Free radical scavenger (antioxidant)

The commonly used free radical scavenger is idaravone (3-methyl-1-phenyl-2-pyrazoline-5-ketone). The conventional application method is: 30 mg, intravenous infusion, 2 times per day, for 14 consecutive days.

Mu Qiong

Chapter 32

Intracerebral Hemorrhage

Intracerebral hemorrhage (ICH) is a kind of hemorrhage in the cerebral parenchyma and intraventricular hemorrhage caused by rupture of the arteries, veins or capillaries of the brain. Cerebral hemorrhage is a common emergency in emergency room, which is characterized by acute onset, severe illness and high disability rate.

32.1 Clinical manifestation

Intracerebral hemorrhage occurs mostly in patients over 50 years old with history of hypertension. It is more common between the age of 60 and 70. This disease can occur all the year round, the incidence is higher in cold season and times of sudden change in temperature; it usually occurs under agitation, psychentonia, aggravating activities, overexertion, cough and defecation. The disease occur suddenly, and most of the patients do not have prodromal symptoms. The severity of clinical manifestation is related to the following factors: ①the primary bleeding artery; ②direction of hematoma expansion; ③the extent of cerebral parenchymal destruction; ④whether or not to break into the ventricle; ⑤amount of hemorrhage; hematoma enlargement caused by persistent hemorrhage is one of the causes of exacerbation, manifested as sudden or gradual deterioration of consciousness and increased blood pressure.

32.1.1 Prodromal stage

No sign before the onset of the disease. A few patients may have headaches, dizziness, transient vagueness, somnolence, mental symptoms, transient movement and sensation abnormality or unclear speech in a few hours or several days before the bleeding.

32.1.2 Onset stage

The condition is related to the location, the speed and the amount of bleeding. All patients develop rapidly and can develop to peak within minutes or hours, it can also fall into a coma in a few minutes.

(1) The following different clinical manifestations can be found in the course of the disease. ①Headache: It's usually the first symptom, the manifestation is a sudden severe headache, a few patients with supratentorial intracerebral hemorrhage and some elderly patients had mild headache or no headache. ②Dizzi-

ness: may be accompanied by a headache, it can also be the main clinical manifestation, most of them occur in the cerebral hemorrhage of the posterior cranial fossa. ③Nausea and vomiting: it is more obvious. When the headache is intense, it's one of the early symptoms. ④Disorder of consciousness: clouding of consciousness and sleepy can be found in patients with mild conditions, while coma, cerebral ankylosis, high fever in severe patients ; and disorder of consciousness can be absent in patients with very less bleeding. ⑤High blood pressure: The blood presures in most cases are between (170–250)/(100–150) mmHg. ⑥Changes in the pupil: when cerebral hemisphere hemorrhage is small, the pupil size is normal, the light responds well, sometimes the side pupil is relatively small. When brain hernia occurs, the pupil of the affected side is enlarged, and the light reaction is slow or disappearing. If the condition continues to deteriorates, the lateral pupil is also large. When brain stem hemorrhage, pontine hemorrhage and intraventricular hemorrhage enter the subarachnoid space, the pupil tends to be pinpointed. ⑦Else: arteriosclerosis, retinal hemorrhage and papillae edema can be found in fundus examination. Meningeal irritation can occur when hemorrhage enters the subarachnoid space. The occupying effect of hematoma and destruction of the brain tissue by hematoma cause hemiplegia, aphasia, and changes in the eye position.

(2) Certain specific clinical symptoms can be produced according to the location and range of bleeding. The main types of cerebral hemorrhage are described below.

1) Putamen – internal capsule hemorrhage (Figure 32–1) : the most common clinical case, account for about 60% of the cerebral hemorrhage. Hemiplegia, hemiplegia and hemiparesis called three partial syndrome often occur on the contralateral side of the lesion. Both eyes gaze on the focal side of the lesion, predominant hemispheric lesions may lead to aphasia.

2) Thalamus hemorrhage (Figure 32 – 2) : account for about 20% –25% of the cerebral hemorrhage. More common in patients over age of 50 years, and with history of hypertension arteriosclerosis. The most common hemorrhage is thalamic geniculate artery or thalamus perforating artery rupture. The former leads to hemorrhage of lateral thalamic nucleus, the latter leads to hemorrhage of medial thalamic nucleus. Almost all thalamus

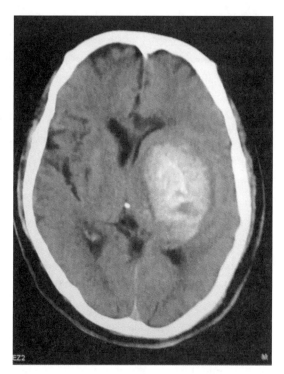

Figure 32–1   Left basal ganglia hemorrhage

hemorrhage has eye movement disorder, for example, inferior optic palsy, pupil reduction, etc. The clinical manifestations include obvious disturbance of consciousness, even coma, contralateral limb complete paralysis, meningeal irritation, etc. The medial or lower thalamic hemorrhage leads to binocular adduction, Inferior optic nasal tip, and upper visual disturbance, which is a typical sign of thalamic hemorrhage.

3) Lobar hemorrhage (Figure 32–3) : also known as subcortical white matter hemorrhage, account for about 13% –18% of the cerebral hemorrhage. the overwhelming majority of the disease is urgent, most patients present with headache, vomiting, convulsion, and urinary incontinence. The disturbance of consciousness is less, and the degree is mild; The incidence of hemiplegia is less than that of basal ganglia hemorrhage, most of the comatose cases are caused by massive hemorrhage and compression of the brainstem.

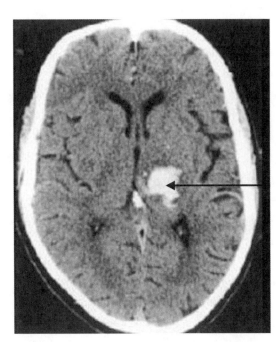
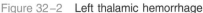

Figure 32-2　Left thalamic hemorrhage

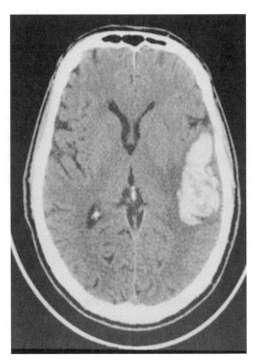

Figure 32-3　Left temporal lobe hemorrhage

4)Cerebellar hemorrhage(Figure 32-4):account for about 10% of the cerebral hemorrhage. The location of the lesion is usually in the dentate nucleus of the cerebellar hemisphere. Most of them are due to rupture of the upper cerebellar artery. Clinically, it can be divided into cerebellar hemorrhage and vermis hemorrhage. Most of them are sudden onset of occipital headache, vertigo, vomiting, limb or trunk ataxia, nystagmus, etc. When hematoma affects the brain stem and circulation of cerebrospinal fluid, brain stem compression and acute obstructive hydrocephalus appear. Small and limited bleeding, mostly cannot be noticed requires CT examination to confirm the diagnosis; patients with severe illness fall into a coma in a short time. Cerebellar tonsil hernia can cause sudden death. Some patients are progressively deteriorating, and gradually fall into a coma, appear signs of brain stem compression. If they can not get timely and correct treatment, they will die within 48 hours.

5)Primary brain stem hemorrhage(Figure 32-5):more than 90% of the primary brain stem hemorrhage caused by hypertension occurs in the pons, and a few occur in the midbrain. ①Hemorrhage in the middle brain:Invasion of one side of the cerebrum foot leads to ipsilateral oculomotor palsy and contralateral limb paralysis (Weber syndrome). ②Pontine hemorrhage:it usually falls into a deep coma, and the pupil is narrowed down to the pin point, but it is present in the light reflex;Four limbs are paralysis, bilateral pyramidal sign is positive. Patients have high fever, irregular breathing, and unstable blood pressure;some patients complicate with gastrointestinal hemorrhage, and the disease progressively deteriorated. Most patients are died within a short time. ③Medulla oblongata hemorrhage:once it happens, patient will die soon.

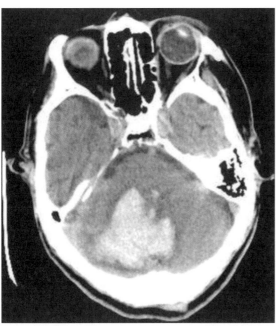

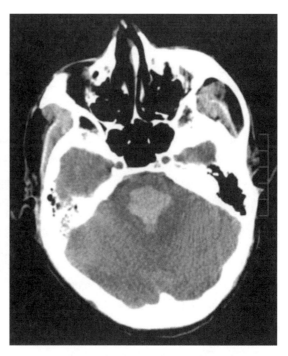

Figure 32-4   **Cerebellar hemorrhage**   Figure 32-5   **Quadriventricular hemorrhage**

6) Intracerebroventricular hemorrhage (Figure 32 – 6) : includes primary intraventricular hemorrhage and secondary intraventricular hemorrhage. The former is characterized by meningeal irritation caused by blood component stimulation and increased intracranial pressure caused by cerebrospinal fluid circulation obstruction. In addition to the above symptoms, the latter is accompanied by neurological dysfunction caused by primary Hemorrhagic focus.

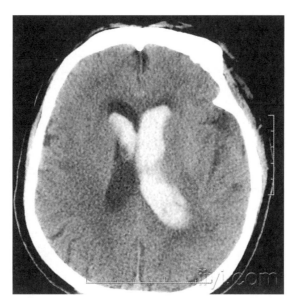

Figure 32-6   **Ventricular hemorrhage**

32.2 Ancillany inspection

32.2.1 Craniocerebral CT scan

On highly clear CT images, the diagnosis of cerebral hemorrhage can reach almost 100%. CT examination is not only an effective diagnostic method, but also an important basis for specifying treatment plan, observing curative effect and judging prognosis. CT Imaging manifestation in different periods of cerebral hemorrhage is not the same.

32.2.2 Craniocerebral MRI scan

MRI characteristics of chronic hematoma: high signal hematoma plus a low signal hemeflavin ring. Although CT is still the first choice for acute intracerebral hemorrhage, MRI is more sensitive than CT in diagnosing subacute and chronic hematoma, especially for the old hematoma, MRI can clearly show the low signal residual cavity containing hemoflavin, which is easy to differentiate from the old cerebral infarction.

32.2.3 Brain angiography

When cerebral arteriovenous malformation or cerebral aneurysm rupture bleeding is suspected clinically, cerebral angiography can identify the cause of disease and has the value that other examinations can not replace.

32.2.4 Lumbar puncture

It has certain value in diagnosing cerebral hemorrhage, but for patients with high intracranial pressure, lumbar puncture has the risk of inducing brain hernia. After extensive application of CT, lumbar puncture has rarely been used to diagnose cerebral hemorrhage.

32.3 Diagnosis and differential diagnosis

32.3.1 Key points of diagnosis

Most diagnoses can be made based on medical history and physical examination: the majority of patients are over 50 years of age having, history of hypertension and arteriosclerosis, most patients develop when they are emotionally excited or physically laboring; sudden onset, headache, nausea and vomiting after the onset of the disease, half of the patients had disturbance of consciousness or convulsion and urinary incontinence. There were obvious signs of localization, such as hemiplegia and meningeal irritation. Blood pressure increases significantly after onset. CT scan and MRI show hemorrhagic focus and cerebrospinal fluid could be bloody.

32.3.2 Differential diagnosis

32.3.2.1 Cerebral infarction

Because cerebral hemorrhage and cerebral infarction are completely different in principle of treatment, it is very important to distinguish them. The use of CT examination can directly determine whether there is bleeding or not(Table 32-1).

Table 32-1　Differential diagnosis of cerebral hemorrhage

Manifestation of disease	Hemorrhagic cerebrovascular disease		Ischemic cerebrovascular disease	
	Cerebral hemorrhage	Subarachnoid hemorrhage	Cerebral thrombosis	Cerebral embolism
Common etiology	Hypertension	Aneurysmor vascular malformation	Atherosclerosis	Cerebral embolism
Age	40-60 years old	Young and middle-aged	Over 65 years of age	35-45 years old
Onset	Emergent	Emergent	Slower	The most emergent
Cause	Emotional excitement, Force	Emotional excitement, Force	Rest, sleep	Atrial fibrillation
Headache	Common	Severe	No	No
Vomiting	More common	More common	No	Probably
Hemiplegia	Yes	No	Yes	Yes
Meningeal irritation sign	Yes	Obvious	No	No
Cerebrospinal fluid pressure	Increase	Increase	Normal	Probably increase
Bloody cerebrospinal fluid	Yes	Yes	No	No

32.3.2.2　Subarachnoid hemorrhage

Sudden onset, accompanied by severe headache, vomiting, transient disturbance of consciousness. There are obvious signs of meningeal irritation, few signs of focal neurological signs, and general identification is not difficult. Clinically, hemiplegia usually occurs in cerebral hemorrhage, and meningeal irritation occurs only when blood breaks into the ventricular system and subarachnoid space. The rupture and bleeding of aneurysms and arteriovenous malformations can enter the subarachnoid space directly, so there is a meningeal irritation sign and then a hemiplegia. Cerebral angiography can help clear diagnosis.

32.3.2.3　Intracranial tumor hemorrhage

Long course of disease, the original symptoms usually have an acute exacerbation, it can also be the first symptom. Enhanced CT and MRI have diagnostic value for tumor hemorrhage.

32.4　Treatment

The treatment of acute stage of cerebral hemorrhage mainly includes on-site emergency treatment, medical treatment and surgical treatment.

32.4.1　Emergency treatment

For patients with coma, the secretion of oral cavity and respiratory tract should be removed in time to maintain airway open. For patients with respiratory failure, tracheal intubation is necessary for artificial ventilation. The doctor should ask for a brief medical history and do a comprehensive physical examination. Patients with high blood pressure, cerebral hernia crisis and convulsions should be treated in time to minimize unnecessary movements. It is also necessary to establish venous access and monitor life signs.

32.4.2 Medical treatment

In the acute period of the disease, the principle of medical treatment is to maintain vital signs, stop bleeding and prevent rebleeding, reduce and control brain edema, and prevent and treat various complications; The main purpose is to save patients' lives, reduce disability rate and prevent recurrence(Figure 32-7).

32.4.2.1 General treatment

①Absolute bed rest and monitoring of vital signs. If the patient is dysphoria, use diazepam and prohibit morphine. ②Maintain airway open, oxygen inhalation, tracheal intubation or tracheostomy if necessary. Catheterization should be retained in patients with urinary retention; comatose patients need to be turned over regularly to prevent pressure sore. ③Maintaining water and electrolyte balance and nutritional support, 24- 48 hours in the acute period should be fasted. Appropriate rehydration should be given and the total amount should be controlled at 1 500-2 000 ml/days. If the patient has a better consciousness and no swallowing disorder, after 48 hours he/she can try to get into the diet with a small amount of meal, otherwise the patient should be given tube feeding to maintain nutrition. Keep the functional position and prevent the deformity of the limbs.

32.4.2.2 Special treatment

①Treatment of hypertension in the acute period: When systolic blood pressure is greater than 200 mmHg, antihypertensive drugs should be given, which is also the key to prevent further bleeding. Keep blood pressure around 160/100 mmHg. ②Control cerebral edema and reduce intracranial pressure: Dehydrating agent should be used immediately. The effect of mannitol is the most accurate and the most effective. The common use is 20% mannitol solution 125-250 ml, intravenous drip, once every 4-6 hours, mannitol should be used for patients with brain hernia immediately. Patients of relatively stable can use glycerin fructose, 250-500 ml, intravenous drip, 2 times/day. ③The application of hemostatic drugs: In addition to patients with bleeding tendency and those with concurrent gastrointestinal bleeding, the majority of patients need does not routinely. ④Brain protective agent and hypothermia therapy: Commonly used drugs are nimodipine, vitamin E, vitamin C. Mannitol also has the effect of scavenging free radicals. Hypothermia can reduce cellular metabolism, inhibit the synthesis and release of monoamine and excitatory amino acid transmitters, and have a definite protective effect on damaged brain tissue. Commonly used measures are pillow ice bag and ice caps, which can play a certain role. Hibernation therapy combined with ice blanket and ice cap can lower the temperature to 35 centigrade and play a protective role in the brain.

32.4.3 Emergency operation

There is no uniform standard for indication of emergency surgical treatment. According to the amount of bleeding, when putamen hemorrhage more than 30 ml, thalamic hemorrhage more than 14 ml, cerebellar hemorrhage more than 15 ml, surgical treatment should be given. It should be determined according to the amount of bleeding, the location of bleeding, the time between operation and bleeding, the patient's age and general condition, and the experience of the surgeon.

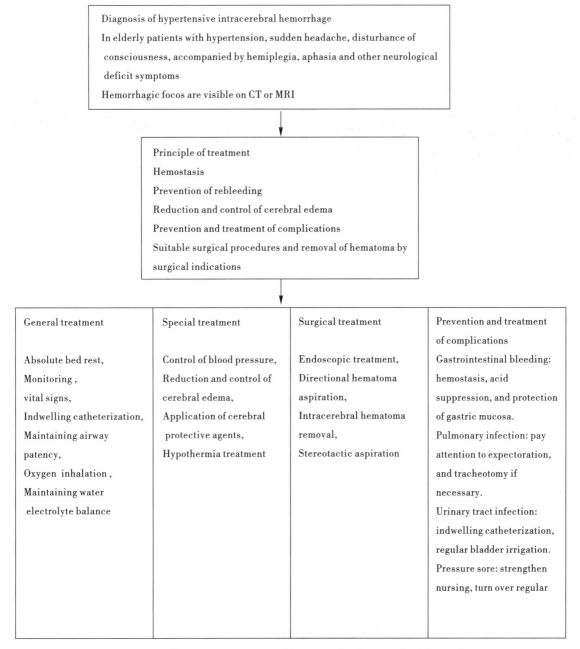

Figure 32-7   The rescue process of hypertensive intracerebral hemorrhage

32.4.4   Prevention and treatment of complications

Common complications of cerebral hemorrhage include gastrointestinal bleeding, pulmonary infection, urinary tract infection, pressure ulcer, and renal failure. The basic principle of treatment is to reduce intracranial pressure, control brain edema, reduce the damage to the hypothalamus and brain stem, and deal with it according to the patient's condition.

Shi Jinhe

Chapter 33

Meningitis

33.1 Introduction

Meningitis is an acute inflammation of the protective membranes covering the brain and spinal cord, known collectively as the meninges. The most common symptoms are fever, headache, and neck stiffness. Other symptoms include confusion or altered consciousness, vomiting, and an inability to tolerate light or loud noises. Young children often exhibit only nonspecific symptoms, such as irritability, drowsiness, or poor feeding. If a rash is presented, it may indicate a particular cause of meningitis; for instance, meningitis caused by meningococcal bacteria may be accompanied by a characteristic rash (Table 33-1).

Table 33-1　Meningitis

Meningitis

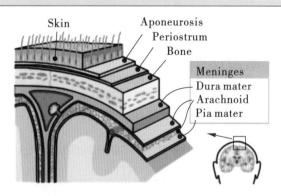

Meninges of the central nervous system: dura mater, arachnoid mater, and pia mater.

Specialty	Infectious disease, neurology
Symptoms	Fever, headache, neck stiffness

Continue to Table 33-1

Meningitis	
Complications	Deafness, epilepsy, hydrocephalus, cognitive deficits
Causes	Viral, bacterial, other
Diagnostic method	Lumbar puncture
Differential diagnosis	Brain tumor, lupus, Lyme disease, seizures, neuroleptic malignant syndrome, naegleriasis
Prevention	Vaccination
Medication	Antibiotics, antivirals, steroids

33.2   Signs and symptoms

Clinical features: in adults, the most common symptom of meningitis is a severe headache, occurring in almost 90% of cases of bacterial meningitis, followed by nuchal rigidity (the inability to flex the neck forward passively due to increased neck muscle tone and stiffness). The classic triad of diagnostic signs consists of nuchal rigidity, sudden high fever, and altered mental status; however, all three features are presented in only 44% –46% of bacterial meningitis cases. If none of the three signs are presented, acute meningitis is extremely unlikely. Other signs commonly associated with meningitis include photophobia (intolerance to bright light) and phonophobia (intolerance to loud noises). Young children often do not exhibit the aforementioned symptoms, and may only be irritable and look unwell. The fontanelle (the soft spot on the top of a baby's head) can bulge in infants aged up to 6 months. Other features that distinguish meningitis from less severe illnesses in young children are leg pain, cold extremities, and an abnormal skin color.

Nuchal rigidity occurs in 70% of bacterial meningitis in adults. Other signs include the presence of positive Kernig's sign or Brudziński sign. Kernig's sign is assessed with the person lying supine, with the hip and knee flexed to 90 degrees. In a person with a positive Kernig's sign, pain limits passive extension of the knee. A positive Brudzinski's sign occurs when flexion of the neck causes involuntary flexion of the knee and hip. Although Kernig's sign and Brudzinski's sign are both commonly used to screen for meningitis, the sensitivity of these tests is limited. They do, however, have very good specificity for meningitis: the signs rarely occur in other diseases. Another test, known as the "jolt accentuation maneuver" helps determine whether meningitis is presented in those reporting fever and headache. A person is asked to rapidly rotate the head horizontally; if this does not make the headache worse, meningitis is unlikely.

33.3   Etiology

Meningitis is typically caused by microbial infection. Most infections are due to viruses, with bacteria, fungi, and protozoa being the next most common causes. It may also result from various non-infectious causes. The term *aseptic meningitis* refers to cases of meningitis in which no bacterial infection can be demonstrated. This type of meningitis is usually caused by viruses but it may be due to bacterial infection that has already been partially treated, when bacteria disappear from the meninges, or pathogens infect a space adjacent to the meninges (e. g. ,sinusitis). Endocarditis (an infection of the heart valves which spreads small clusters of bacteria through the bloodstream) may cause aseptic meningitis. Aseptic meningitis may also result from infection with spirochetes, a group of bacteria that includes *Treponema pallidum* (the cause of syphilis) and *Borrelia burgdorferi* (known for causing Lyme disease). Meningitis may be encountered in cerebral malaria (malaria infecting the brain) or amoebic meningitis, meningitis due to infection with amoebae such as *Naegleria fowleri*, contracted from freshwater sources.

33.3.1 Bacterial

In adults, *Neisseria meningitidis* and *Streptococcus pneumoniae* together cause 80% of bacterial meningitis cases. Risk of infection with *Listeria monocytogenes* is increased in persons over 50 years old. The introduction of pneumococcal vaccine has lowered rates of pneumococcal meningitis in both children and adults.

Recent skulltrauma potentially allows nasal cavity bacteria to enter the meningeal space. Similarly, devices in the brain and meninges, such as cerebral shunts, extraventricular drains or Ommaya reservoirs, carry an increased risk of meningitis. In these cases, the persons are more likely to be infected with Staphylococci, Pseudomonas, and other Gram-negative bacteria. These pathogens are also associated with meningitis in people with an impaired immune system. An infection in the head and neck area, such as otitis mediaor mastoiditis, can lead to meningitis in a small proportion of people. Recipients of cochlear implants for hearing loss are more at risk for pneumococcal meningitis.

Tuberculous meningitis, which is meningitis caused by *Mycobacterium tuberculosis*, is more common in people from countries in which tuberculosis is endemic, but is also encountered in persons with immune problems, such as AIDS.

33.3.2 Viral

Viruses that cause meningitis include enteroviruses, herpes simplex virus (generally type 2, which produces most genital sores; less commonly type 1), varicella zoster virus (known for causing chickenpox and shingles), mumps virus, HIV, and LCMV.

33.3.3 Fungal

There are a number of risk factors forfungal meningitis, including the use of immunosuppressants (such as after organ transplantation), HIV/AIDS, and the loss of immunity associated with aging. It is uncommon in those with a normal immune system but has occurred with medication contamination. Symptom onset is typically more gradual, with headaches and fever being presented for at least a couple of weeks before diagnosis. The most common fungal meningitis is cryptococcal meningitis due to *Cryptococcus neoformans*.

33.3.4 Parasitic

A parasitic cause is often assumed when there is a predominance of eosinophils (a type of white blood cell) in the CSF. The most common parasites implicated are *Angiostrongylus cantonensis*, *Gnathostoma spinigerum*, *Schistosoma*, as well as the conditions cysticercosis, toxocariasis, baylisascariasis, paragonimiasis, and a number of rarer infections and noninfective conditions.

33.3.5 Non-infectious

Meningitis may occur as the result of several non-infectious causes: spread of cancer to the meninges (*malignant or neoplastic meningitis*) and certain drugs (mainly non-steroidal anti-inflammatory drugs, antibiotics and intravenous immunoglobulins). It may also be caused by several inflammatory conditions, such as sarcoidosis (which is then called neurosarcoidosis), connective tissue disorders such as systemic lupus erythematosus, and certain forms of vasculitis (inflammatory conditions of the blood vessel wall), such as Behcet's disease. Epidermoid cysts and dermoid cysts may cause meningitis by releasing irritant matter into the subarachnoid space.

33.3.6 Mechanism

In bacterial meningitis, bacteria reach the meninges by one of two main routes: through the bloodstream or through direct contact between the meninges and either the nasal cavity or the skin. In most cases, meningitis follows invasion of the bloodstream by organisms that live upon mucous surfaces such as the nasal cavity. This is often in turn preceded by viral infections, which break down the normal barrier provided by the mucous surfaces. Once bacteria have entered the bloodstream, they enter the subarachnoid space in places where the blood-brain barrier is vulnerable—such as the choroid plexus. Meningitis occurs in 25% of newborns with bloodstream infections due to group B streptococci; this phenomenon is less common in adults. Direct contamination of the cerebrospinal fluid may arise from indwelling devices, skull fractures, or infections of the nasopharynx or the nasal sinuses that have formed a tract with the subarachnoid space (see above); occasionally, congenital defects of the duramater can be identified.

The large-scale inflammation that occurs in the subarachnoid space during meningitis is not a direct result of bacterial infection but can rather largely be attributed to the response of the immune system to the entry of bacteria into the central nervous system. When components of the bacterial cell membrane are identified by the immune cells of the brain (astrocytes and microglia), they respond by releasing large amounts of cytokines, hormone-like mediators that recruit other immune cells and stimulate other tissues to participate in an immune response. The blood-brain barrier becomes more permeable, leading to "vasogenic" cerebral edema (swelling of the brain due to fluid leakage from blood vessels). Large numbers of white blood cells enter the CSF, causing inflammation of the meninges and leading to "interstitial" edema (swelling due to fluid between the cells). In addition, the walls of the blood vessels themselves become inflamed (cerebral vasculitis), which leads to decreased blood flow and a third type of edema, "cytotoxic" edema. The three forms of cerebral edema all lead to increased intracranial pressure; together with the lowered blood pressure often encountered in acute infection, this means that it is harder for blood to enter the brain, consequently brain cells are deprived of oxygen and undergo apoptosis (programmed cell death).

33.4 Diagnosis

33.4.1 Blood tests and imaging

The most important test in identifying or ruling out meningitis is analysis of the cerebrospinal fluid through lumbar puncture (LP, spinal tap). However, lumbar puncture is contraindicated if there is a mass in the brain (tumor or abscess) or the intracranial pressure (ICP) is elevated, as it may lead to brain herniation. If someone is at risk for either a mass or raised ICP (recent head injury, a known immune system problem, localizing neurological signs, or evidence on examination of a raised ICP), a CT or MRI scan is recommended prior to the lumbar puncture. This applies in 45% of all adult cases. If a CT or MRI is required before LP, or if LP proves difficult, professional guidelines suggest that antibiotics should be administered first to prevent delayed treatment, especially if this may be longer than 30 minutes. Often, CT or MRI scans are performed at a later stage to assess for complications of meningitis.

In severe forms of meningitis, monitoring of blood electrolytes may be important; for example, hyponatremia is common in bacterial meningitis. The cause of hyponatremia, however, is controversial and may include dehydration, the inappropriate secretion of the antidiuretic hormone (SIADH), or overly aggressive intravenous fluid administration.

33.4.2　Lumbar puncture

A lumbar puncture is done by positioning the person, usually lying on the side, applying local anesthetic, and inserting a needle into the dural sac (a sac around the spinal cord) to collect cerebrospinal fluid (CSF). When this has been achieved, the "opening pressure" of the CSF is measured using a manometer. The pressure is normally between 6 and 18 cm water (cmH_2O); in bacterial meningitis the pressure is usually elevated. In cryptococcal meningitis, intracranial pressure is markedly elevated. The initial appearance of the fluid may prove an indication of the nature of the infection: cloudy CSF indicates higher levels of protein, white and red blood cells and/or bacteria, and therefore may suggest bacterial meningitis.

The CSF sample is examined for presence and types of white blood cells, red blood cells, protein content and glucose level. Gram staining of the sample may demonstrate bacteria in bacterial meningitis, but absence of bacteria does not exclude bacterial meningitis as they are only seen in 60% of cases; this figure is reduced by a further 20% if antibiotics were administered before the sample is taken. Gram staining is also less reliable in particular infections such as listeriosis. Microbiological culture of the sample is more sensitive (it identifies the organism in 70% –85% of cases) but results can take up to 48 hours to become available. The type of white blood cell predominantly present (Table 33-2) indicates whether meningitis is bacterial (usually neutrophil–predominant) or viral (usually lymphocyte–predominant), although at the beginning of the disease this is not always a reliable indicator. Less commonly, eosinophils predominate, suggesting parasitic or fungal etiology, among others.

Table 33-2　CSF findings in different forms of meningitis

Type of meningitis	Glucose	Protein	Cells
Acute bacterial	Low	High	PMNs, often>300/mm^3
Acute viral	Normal	Normal or high	Mononuclear, < 300/mm^3
Tuberculous	Low	High	Mononuclear and PMNs, < 300/mm^3
Fungal	Low	High	<300/mm^3
Malignant	Low	High	Usually mononuclear

The concentration of glucose in CSF is normally above 40% of that in blood. In bacterial meningitis, it is typically lower; the CSF glucose level is therefore divided by the blood glucose (CSF glucose to serum glucose ratio). A ratio ≤ 0.4 is indicative of bacterial meningitis; in the newborn, glucose levels in CSF are normally higher, and a ratio below 0.6 (60%) is therefore considered abnormal. High levels of lactate in CSF indicate a higher likelihood of bacterial meningitis, as does a higher white blood cell count. If lactate levels are less than 35 mg/dl and the person has not previously received antibiotics, then this may rule out bacterial meningitis.

33.4.3　Postmortem

Meningitis can be diagnosed after death has occurred. The findings from a post mortem are usually a widespread inflammation of the piamater and arachnoid layers of the meninges. Neutrophil granulocytes tend to have migrated to the cerebrospinal fluid and the base of the brain, along with cranial nerves and the spinal cord, may be surrounded with pus—as may the meningeal vessels.

33.4.4　Prevention

For some causes of meningitis, protection can be provided in the long term through vaccination, or in the short term with antibiotics. Some behavioral measures may also be effective.

33.4.5　Behavioral

Bacterial and viral meningitis are contagious, but neither is as contagious as the common cold or flu. Both can be transmitted through droplets of respiratory secretions during close contact such as kissing, sneezing or coughing on someone, but cannot be spread by only breathing the air where a person with meningitis has been. Viral meningitis is typically caused by enteroviruses, and is most commonly spread through fecal contamination. The risk of infection can be decreased by changing the behavior that led to transmission.

33.4.6　Vaccination

Meningococcus vaccines are avaiable against groups A, B, C, W135 and Y. In countries where the vaccine for meningococcus group C was introduced, cases caused by this pathogen have decreased substantially.

Routine vaccination against *Streptococcus pneumoniae* with the pneumococcal conjugate vaccine (PCV), which is active against seven common serotypes of this pathogen, significantly reduces the incidence of pneumococcal meningitis. The pneumococcal polysaccharide vaccine, which covers 23 strains, is only administered to certain groups (e. g. , those who have had a splenectomy, the surgical removal of the spleen); it does not elicit a significant immune response in all recipients, e. g. , young children. Childhood vaccination with Bacillus Calmette—Guérin has been reported to significantly reduce the rate of tuberculous meningitis, but its waning effectiveness in adulthood has prompted a search for a better vaccine.

33.4.7　Antibiotics

Short—term antibiotic prophylaxis is another method of prevention, particularly of meningococcal meningitis. In cases of meningococcal meningitis, preventative treatment in close contacts with antibiotics (e. g. , rifampicin, ciprofloxacin or ceftriaxone) can reduce their risk of contracting the condition, but does not protect against future infections.

33.5　Treatment

Meningitis is potentially life—threatening and has a high mortality rate if untreated, delayed treatment has been associated with a poorer outcome. Thus, treatment with wide—spectrum antibiotics should not be delayed while confirmatory tests are being conducted. If meningococcal disease is suspected in primary care, guidelines recommend that benzylpenicillin be administered before transfering to hospital. Intravenous fluids should be administered if hypotension (low blood pressure) or shock are present. It is not clear whether intravenous fluid should be given routinely or whether this should be restricted. Given that meningitis can cause a number of early severe complications, regular medical review is recommended to identify these complications early and to admit the person to an intensive care unit if deemed necessary.

33.5.1 Bacterial meningitis

33.5.1.1 Antibiotics

Empiric antibiotics (treatment without exact diagnosis) should be started immediately, even before the results of the lumbar puncture and CSF analysis are known. The choice of initial treatment depends largely on the kind of bacteria that cause meningitis in a particular place and population.

Empirical therapy may be chosen on the basis of the person's age, whether the infection was preceded by a head injury, whether the person has undergone recent neurosurgery and whether or not a cerebral shunt is present.

33.5.1.2 Steroids

Additional treatment with corticosteroids (usually dexamethasone) has shown some benefits, such as a reduction of hearing loss, and better short term neurological outcomes in adolescents and adults from high–income countries with low rates of HIV.

Professional guidelines therefore recommend the commencement of dexamethasone or a similar cortico-steroid just before the first dose of antibiotics is given, and continued for four days. Given that most of the benefit of the treatment is confined to those with pneumococcal meningitis, some guidelines suggest that dex-amethasone should be discontinued if another cause for meningitis is identified.

33.5.2 Viral meningitis

Viral meningitis typically only requires supportive therapy; most viruses causing meningitis are not a-menable to specific treatment. Viral meningitis tends to run a more benign course than bacterial meningitis. Herpes simplex virus and varicella zoster virus may respond to treatment with antiviral drugs such as aciclo-vir, but there are no clinical trials that have specifically addressed whether this treatment is effective. Mild cases of viral meningitis can be treated at home with conservative measures such as fluid supplement, bed-rest, and analgesics.

33.5.3 Fungal meningitis

Fungal meningitis, such ascryptococcal meningitis, is treated with long courses of high dose antifun-gals, such as amphotericin B and flucytosine. Raised intracranial pressure is common in fungal meningitis, and frequent (ideally daily) lumbar punctures to relieve the pressure are recommended, or alternatively a lumbar draining.

33.6 Prognosis

Untreated, bacterial meningitis is almost always fatal. Viral meningitis, in contrast, tends to resolve spontaneously and is rarely fatal. With treatment, mortality from bacterial meningitis depends on the age of the person and the underlying cause.

Shi Junxia

Chapter 34

Disorders of Hemostasis

34.1 Introduction

The disorder of the coagulation system in severe patients is very common and can range from only abnormal laboratory examination to severe DIC, unless very alert, often until severe bleeding tendency occurs. Symptoms of shock or organ failure will attract clinical attention. At present, the acquired disorder of coagulation secondary to severe diseases is generally referred to as "acquired coagulation disease", its incidence rate is as high as 10% –40%. The mechanism of its pathogenesis is very complicated. If it is not well understood or improperly handled, it can lead to disastrous consequences. Therefore, it is very important to recognize and deal with the problem of coagulation disorder in the treatment of severe patients.

34.2 Pathophysiology

34.2.1 Definition

Coagulation dysfunction is a hemorrhagic disease caused by lack of coagulation factors or abnormal function.

34.2.2 Coagulation functional basis

34.2.2.1 Vessel Wall

After the blood vessel is damaged or stimulated, there are many smooth muscle vessels (such as arterioles, arterioles, etc.), first of all, autonomic nerve reflex contraction which makes blood flow slow or blocked, which is beneficial to hemostasis. Vascular Willebrand factor(vWF), which is synthesized and released by endothelial cells (EC), participates in platelet adhesion and aggregation, activated platelets release thromboxane A_2 (TXA_2), 5–Hydroxytryptamine (5–HT), Endothelin–1 (ET–1), Angiotensin and other vasoactive substance to strengthen the vasoconstriction, make the injured vessel wound more narrow. At the same time, the activation of factor XII (F XII) and the release of tissue factor(TF), which activates respectively to produce Thrombin and fibrin Fibrin(Fb) to reinforce the hemostatic effect. If fibrinolytic activity is reduced, so that the formed blood clot is difficult to dissolve, to consolidate the effect of hemostasis.

34.2.2.2　Blood cells

Platelet has the function of maintaining the integrity of vascular wall, capillary permeability and so on. When the blood vessel wall is not damaged, the platelet is in a static state. If the blood vessel is damaged, the aggregation of the platelet adhesion factor and glycoprotein II b/III aforms the white thrombus; activated platelet—releasing active substances (such as ADPP—ATPase PF4) promote platelet aggregation, vasoconstriction, blood clot contraction (thromboplastin), and provide membrane phospholipid surface and coagulation reaction medium.

34.2.2.3　Blood coagulation system

There are 12 classical coagulation factors, namely F I —XIII (in which factor VI has been abolished), and two factors in the kallikrein system, namely, prekallikrein PK, and high molecular weight kallikrein Kininogen (HMWK). With the exception of F IV (Ca^{2+}) as metal ions, all other proteins, except for tissue factor(TF), are present in plasma.

34.2.3　Normal coagulation process

Blood coagulation can be roughly divided into three stages.

In the first stage, the formation of prothrombin activator was divided into endogenous coagulation system and exogenous coagulation system according to its formation pathway(Figure 34–1). Exogenous coagulation system, also known as tissue coagulation, is the release of coagulation factor III from injured tissues, which enters the plasma and forms a complex with factor VII and Ca. It can catalyze the conversion of factor X into the activating factor Xa. Xa, Va, Ca and platelet phospholipid to form prothrombin activator. Endogenous coagulation system, also known as blood coagulation, refers to all the substances involved in coagulation exist in the blood. In pathological conditions such as atherosclerosis and vasculitis, vascular intima is injuried, blood does not flow out. Factors in plasma are activated by exposure to collagen fibers exposed to injured blood vessels. With the participation of platelet—released platelet factor and Ca, some coagulation factors (X,IX,VIII) have been activated successively, X, V, together form prothrombin activator. From this point, there is no difference between exogenous and endogenous coagulation processes. The bleeding after tissue injury is bound to be accompanied by vascular injury, so the blood flow out of the blood coagulation process in vitro, both exogenous coagulation system and endogenous coagulation system involved. In the second stage, prothrombin activator catalyzes the transformation of prothrombin (factor II) into an active thrombin (II a) with the participation of Ca. In the third stage, the soluble fibrinogen in plasma was transformed into insoluble fibrinogen under the catalysis of thrombin Ca and factor XIII. Fibrin is filamentous, crisscross, meshes a large number of blood cells and forms gel—like blood clots. From the time of blood flowing out of the body to the appearance of filamentous fibrin, the normal time of coagulation is 2–8 minutes (glass plate method).

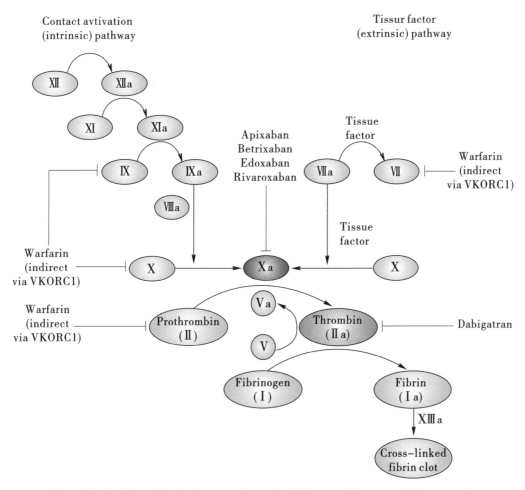

Figure 34-1　Interaction between anticoagulant drugs and the coagulation cascade

34.2.4　Anticoagulant mechanism

At the same time, the anticoagulant mechanism starts quickly, and almost every step of the coagulation process is involved. In human body, the most important anticoagulants are antithrombin (AT3), formerly called AT-Ⅲ (protein) and tissue factor pathway inhibitor (TFPI).

34.2.4.1　Antithrombin

A glycoprotein, mainly synthesized in liver and endothelial cells, inhibits the activation of serine proteases, so it inhibits the activation of most of the coagulation factors such as Ⅱ, Ⅶ, Ⅸ. However, the inhibitory activity of AT alone is very low, and the inhibitory rate of AT combined with heparin sulfate (HSH) or heparin could be increased by more than a thousand times.

34.2.4.2　Protein C

Synthesized in liver, activated by thrombin or thrombin/thrombomodontin complex, Ⅴa and Ⅷa. PC is inactivated by protein S. It also inhibits platelet binding and inactivates plasminogen activator inhibitor (plasminogen activator), promotes plasminogen activator release.

34.2.4.3　Tissue factor pathway inhibitor

A glycoprotein synthesized and released by endothelial cells exists in plasma in the forms of free type and lipoprotein binding type, but the anticoagulant effect is free type. It binds with Ⅶa-TF complex to form Xa-TFPI-Ⅶa-TF tetrachloride, which makes Ⅶa-TF inactive.

34.2.4.4 Fibrinolytic mechanism

The function of fibrinolysis system is to break fibrin so that it can be cleared in time after completing its mission. Plasminogen is synthesized in liver and bone marrow and activated by endogenous and exogenous pathways.

34.2.4.5 Therole of endothelial cells

The anticoagulant effect of endothelial cells is dominant in normal state, and it has anti-platelet effect (PGI2NO-ADPN), anticoagulant effect (tissue factor pathway inhibitor, thrombomodulin, antithrombin, heparin-like molecule), and fibrinolysis (tissue plasminogen activator). Endothelial cells secrete TFF, coagulation factors V and VIII, von Willebrand factor VWfN and plasminogen activator inhibitor.

34.3　Classification of coagulation

There are two main types of coagulation substances in patients with severe coagulation: low coagulation and high coagulation. Low coagulation is lack of coagulation substance or functional damage; high coagulation is hypercoagulant mechanism or insufficient anticoagulant mechanism; hypercoagulability is only a stage of the course of the disease and will eventually fall into low coagulation due to severe consumption of coagulation substances.

According to its pathophysiological mechanism, severe coagulation can be divided into three types: dilute coagulation, functional coagulation and consumptive coagulation.

34.3.1　Dilute coagulation

Through fluid resuscitation in patients with severe blood loss caused by dilute coagulation disease, insufficient clotting substances are not provided, which resultes in severe dilution and lack of platelet and coagulation factors, which is especially prominent today when blood component transfusion is widely used. The degree of hemodilution has obvious influence on coagulation function. This clotting disease is called dilute clotting.

34.3.2　Functional coagulation

Hypothermia ($< 35 ℃$) is also a major cause of coagulation dysfunction. For example, severe trauma or shock, mild hypothermia therapy, continuous blood purification or massive hypothermia fluid resuscitation can lead to hypothermia in severe patients. During hypothermia, lipid oxidase and cyclooxygenase pathway of arachidonic acid metabolism are interfered, which resulte in the reduction of thromboembolization and vasoconstriction, hypothermia also decreases the activity of protein kinase C, which affects platelet aggregation and adhesion. These changes damage the "preliminary coagulation". In addition, hypothermia can also reduce the activity of serine enzyme, inhibit the cascade of coagulation factors, and eventually "secondary coagulation" is also affected. The coagulation process is an enzymatic reaction which requires an appropriate acid-base environment, so severe acidosis can affect the coagulation of severe patients. Because red blood cells can produce lactic acid, and the longer the time is, the higher the acidity is, and a large amount of transfusion of stored blood can affect the coagulation function of patients to a certain extent. Coagulation dysfunction caused by hypothermia and acidosis is called functional coagulation disease.

34.3.3 Consumptive coagulation diffuse intravascular

Disseminated intravascular coagulation(DIC) is a pathophysiological process characterized by hyperco-agulation-thromboplasmosis and hyperfibrinolysis caused by severe infection,craniocerebral injury,obstetric emergencies,etc. It is characterized by the injury of microvascular system by pathogenic factors,the activation of blood coagulation,the formation of systemic microvascular thrombosis,the massive consumption of coagulation factors and secondary hyperfibrinolysis,which can lead to hemorrhage and microcirculation failure,and eventually to the occurrence of multiple organ dysfunction.

34.4 Clinical symptoms of coagulation dysfunction

34.4.1 Thrombosis and ischemic necrosis arteriole

Capillary thrombosis or venous thrombosis can cause various organ microthrombus obstruction,leading to organ perfusion insufficiency and dysfunction,or even failure. Hemorrhagic plaque in the end of the skin caused by obstruction of the arterioles. The outbreak is characterized by gangrene of the fingers or toes. Renal cortical necrosis causes hematuria,oliguria or even anuria,secondary tubular necrosis and further impairment of renal function. Pulmonary interstitial haemorrhage affects respiratory function with different degrees of hypoxemia. Gastric and duodenal submucosal necrosis can produce superficial ulcers,leading to gastrointestinal bleeding. Hepatocytic jaundice may occur in patients with chronic infection and hypotension often exacerbating liver damage. Acute adrenocortical failure caused by adrenocortical hemorrhage and necrosis is called Waterhouse-Friderichsen syndrome. Pituitary hemorrhage caused by pituitary microthrombus leads to pituitary failure.

34.4.2 Bleeding symptom

Hemorrhage was the first and most common clinical manifestation of DIC. The most common bleeding site is skin,followed by kidney,mucosa,gastrointestinal tract,which present as skin ecchymosis,purpura, hemoptysis,hemoptysis gastrointestinal bleeding,etc. Only local bleeding (such as needle injection) occurs in the mild cases,and multiple bleeding occurs in the heavy cases.

34.4.3 Microvascular hemolytic anemia

Patients with microvascular hemolytic anemia may be associated with microvascular hemolytic anemia due to hemorrhage and erythrocyte destruction. Unstable,loose fibrin filaments are deposited in small blood vessels,and when circulating red blood cells flow through the reticulum made of fibrin filaments,they often stick or hang on fibrin filaments,and with the constant impact on blood flow,red blood cells are ruptured. Red blood cell fragments are found in peripheral blood smears. The clinical manifestations are anemia,hemoglobinemia and hemoglobinuria.

34.4.4 Shock

Extensive microthrombus formation in shock resulted in a significant decrease in the volume of blood returned to the heart,combined with a decrease in blood volume caused by extensive bleeding,resulting in a decrease in cardiac output. A variety of vasoactive substances (kinin,complement C3a and C5a) are produced during the formation of shock. DIC by aggravating the disturbance of microcirculation, results in the relaxation of microvascular smooth muscle, vascular dilatation, increase in permeability and decrease in the volume of blood returned to the heart.

Liu Liping

Section 4

Surgical Emergencies

Chapter 35

The Principle of Trauma Treatment

Trauma refers to a variety of physical, chemical, and biological factors that act on the body, resulting in structural integrity damage or dysfunction. The occurrence rate is high and the harm is great. If the treatment is not timely, it will lead to serious consequences. Each year, about 3.5 million people died from various kinds of accidental injuries around the world. The number of injured and disabled people is about 100 – 500 times the number of deaths. Trauma has become the first public hazard in modern society.

The trauma emergency is an important part of emergency medicine. It reflects the inevitable needs of modern medical advancement and economic development, and is also widely concerned and highly valued by the society. At the same time, it is also the first link to improve the quality of medical care, increase the survival rate of the wounded, and reduce the disability rate.

35.1 Principles of emergency organization management

35.1.1 The staffs

Trauma emergency organizations must have a team of well-trained and skilled professionals.

35.1.2 Rescue focused

After the emergency personnel arrive at the emergency scene, they must immediately carry out the necessary emergency treatment for the injury that threatens the life of the patient, and send the patient to a nearby, better-conditioned treatment unit.

35.1.3 Prompt CPR

For the injured people who need CPR, resuscitation is performed immediately, and the injured person is fully judged at the same time of recovery. When necessary, it can be handed over to another group of staff for treatment.

35.1.4 Equipment of emergency center

Trauma emergency centers should have a variety of emergency equipments in particular, various laboratories and relevant equipment, radiology facilities and blood banks.

35.2　First aid for mass casualty

When first-aid at the scene of a trauma, especially the treatment of a group of wounded people, should be focused on, and targeted to take a different approach.

35.2.1　Hidden dangers elimiration

Paying attention to site safety and immediately eliminating hidden dangers at the scene of the accident, such as cutting off the power and preventing the explosion from happening.

35.2.2　Counting the number of the wounded

The designated person is responsible for the immediate inventory of the number of the wounded, looking for potentially wounded casualties, such as being crushed by ruined or destroyed vehicles.

35.2.3　Initial evaluation

The initial assessment of the wounded is conducted by experienced physicians (according to A-B-C and mental situation), the on-site casualty is divided into light, heavy and critically ill and wounded casualties. ①Critical injuries are applied to those who are in danger of immediate medical care and are marked in red. Immediate traumatic basic life support (BTIS) is needed and transshipment of the relevant hospital as soon as possible. ②Severe injury is not immediately life-threatening, but the wounded who must undergo surgery can be marked in yellow. ③All minor injuries, marked in green. ④Rescuing the dead and wounded is a time-consuming and difficult operation. The critically ill wounded, who have poor treatment and survival opportunities, are marked in black.

35.2.4　Seeking help

For the lack of the rescue participants and equipment, you can timely ask for help from the relevant department near the medical units to add personnel.

35.2.5　Proper transport

According to the regulations for the transport of various types of wounded, the wounded shall be transported properly and the relevant hospital should be informed to make appropriate first aid preparations.

35.3　Trauma basic life support

35.3.1　CPR

For patients with airway obstruction and/or cardiac arrest, timely removal of airway obstructions and maintenance of airway patency are performed simultaneously with cardio-pulmonary resuscitation measures such as external cardiac compression and synchronized artificial respiration.

35.3.2   Effective hemostasis

For obvious external hemorrhage, finger pressure, pressure dressing, gauze packing, and hemostasis should be used to stop bleeding. Pay attention to monitor and redress hypovolemia.

35.3.3   Fracture fixation

Temporary and effective fixation of the fracture is needed before transporting the wounded.

35.3.4   Timely delivery

Hospitals or emergency units that are closest to the site and have better conditions should be selected to transport the sick or wounded to rescue timely as soon as possible.

35.4   Observation and monitoring

35.4.1   Paying attention to the changes in vital signs

Severely injured patients in the brain or other parts should be observed for the changes of consciousness and barrier holes on a regular basis; The changes in vital signs include respiration, blood pressure, pulse, and heart rate.

35.4.2   Observe after recovery

The consciousness, heartbeat, and respiration of the patient after resuscitation should be observed and monitored closely so that remedial measures can be taken in time to maintain respiration and circulation.

35.4.3   External bleeding

It should be paid attention on effectiveness of hemostasis and existed active bleading.

35.4.4   The cantent of care

For the coma patient, close attention should be paid to the position of body and head, making sure to keep airway open and prevent suffocation.

Zhu Changju

Chapter 36

Multiple Injuries

36.1　Introduction

Broadly speaking, the body that has suffered more than two anatomic lesions at the same time is called multiple trauma. At present, most scholars define multiple injuries as referring to the same serious mechanical damage (direct, indirect violence, mixed violence). The body suffers from more or more serious damage to two or more anatomical sites or organs at the same time, or at least one injury. Life-threatening or concomitant traumatic shock is called multiple trauma. The high mortality rate of multiple injuries poses a threat to the patient's life and requires emergency treatment.

36.2　The characteristics of multiple injuries

The multiple traumatic injuries are serious and can cause a series of circulatory and oxygen metabolic disorders that affect the function of the tissue cells in a short period of time, such as physiological imbalances, microcirculatory disturbances, and severe hypoxia. Improper handling may rapidly endanger the lives of the wounded.

36.2.1　Complexity of damage mechanisrm

The injury caused by different mechanisms of the same patient may exist at the same time.

36.2.2　Heavy injury and quickly changes

Multiple injuries have aggravating effect, and the total injury is more serious than the total injuries of all organ. The injury progresses rapidly, requires timely and accurate judgment and processing.

36.2.3　Severe physiological disorders

The complexity of multiple injuries, often involving multiple important organs, can cause direct tissue damage and function. Due to the pathophysiological changes, such as acute hypovolemia, hypoperfusion and hypoxia, a series of complex systemic stress reactions are often associated. As well as sepsis and other secondary damage caused by tissues and organs, prone to shock, hypoxemia, metabolic acidosis, increased intracranial pressure, if these pathological changes can not be effectively controlled, can lead to the synthesis of multiple organ dysfunction sign (MODS).

36.2.4　Diagnostic difficulties

Due to the large number of injuries, complicated injuries, severe injuries, and difficulty in collecting medical history, missed diagnoses are easily caused in patients with multiple injuries.

36.2.5　Processing sequence and principles

The treatment of multiple injuries should adhere to the principle of saving life first. Then estimate the iniury in a timely, accurate and comprehensive manner, and quickly deal with the most life-threatening injuries such as hemorrhagic shock, acute respiratory dysfunction and cerebral hernia. Under the premise of full resuscitation, the injured organs should be repaired with the simplest operation and the fastest speed, so as to reduce the burden of the wounded, reduce the risk of operation and save the lives of the wounded.

36.2.6　Complication

Due to the extensive damage and destruction of tissues and organs in patients with multiple injuries, as well as the great loss of blood and serious systemic physiologic disorders, various complications are prone to occur. Serious infections and sepsis are common due to the reduced defensive system after immune system impairing.

36.3　Diagnosis

A person who has suffered more than two anatomical lesions and meets one of the following injuries may be diagnosed with multiple injuries.

(1) Skull fractures are associated with disturbances of consciousness in intracranial hematoma, brain contusion, and maxillofacial fractures.

(2) Neck trauma with large blood vessel damage, hematoma, cervical spine injury.

(3) Multiple rib fractures, pneumothorax, pulmonary contusion, injury of mediastinum, heart, large vessels, and rupture of the trachea.

(4) Intra-abdominal bleeding, ruptured intra-abdominal organs, large retroperitoneal hematoma.

(5) Kidney rupture, bladder rupture, uterine rupture, urethral rupture, vaginal rupture.

(6) Complex pelvic fracture.

(7) Vertebral fracture, dislocation with spinal cord injury, or multiple vertebral fractures.

(8) Upper limb scapula, long bone fracture, upper limb off.

(9) Lower long bone fracture, lower limb off.

(10) Extensive skin avulsion.

36.4 The principle of treatment

36.4.1 Life support

First-aid life support for multiple wounded in emergency room.

36.4.1.1 Respiratory management

In the first aid, various factors that block the airway should be quickly removed to keep the airway open. For coma patients, tracheal intubation is needed, cricothyroid membrane puncture and tracheotomy can be performed in emergency. Among the methods to establish artificial airway, the most common used is tracheal intubation, which can completely control the airway, prevent aspiration, maintain oxygen supply and facilitate administration.

36.4.1.2 Cardiopulmonary resuscitation(CPR)

CPR is a life-saving technique for patients with sudden cardiac and respiratory arrest. The aim of CPR is to restore the spontaneous respiration and circulation of the patients. Cardiac arrest in patients with multiple injuries will lead to the termination of effective cardiac pump and circulatory function, resulting in severe ischemia, hypoxia and metabolic disorders of cells in the whole body. Once cardiac arrest occurs, if cardiopulmonary resuscitation is not performed in time (within 4-6 minutes), it will cause irreversible damage to the patients' brain and other organs.

36.4.1.3 Anti-shock treatment

Most patients with multiple injuries are associated with hypovolemic shock. For patients with obvious trauma, traumatic bleeding should be controlled immediatelly. The severity of shock is assessed by closely monitoring blood pressure, pulse and skin temperature. Mare than two intravenous access should be quickly established or central venous catheterization should be performed to facilitate the expansion and monitoring of blood volume.

36.4.2 Thorough evaluation

Medical staff should first observe the consciousness, breathing, blood pressure, pulse and bleeding of the injured, as well as the presence or absence of respiratory tract obstruction, shock, massive hemorrhage and other life-threatening signs. To avoid missing major injuries, examinations can be performed in the following order: criculation, respiratory, abdomen, spine, head, pelvis, limbs, arteries and veins, and nerves. If life-threatening injuries are found, effecive emergency measures should be taken.

36.4.3 Improvement of inspection

For patients with multiple injuries, routine examinations should be performed, such as blood routine, blood type and cross matching, electrolytes, liver and kidney function, arterial blood gas analysis, thoracic and abdominal puncture and so on. If the whole condition of the wounded permits, and can be moued, the X-ray examination, ultrasound exmaination, CT examination and MRI examination should be carried out; if the condition is critical, blood pressure and breathing are unstable, and it is not suitable to move, bedside photography and ultrasound examination should be done.

Multiple injuries are changeable dynamic injuries, and the early signs of some concealed injuries are not obvious. There fore, the conclusion of the initial inspection is not comprehensive and dunamic observation must be carried out.

36.4.4   Damage control

Multiple surgical procedures for the treatment of multiple injuries and one-stage surgical treatment for multiple trauma patients with more than two sites requiring surgery, the order of choice is the key to successful rescue. The principle of multi-injury resuscitation is to repair the injured organs with the simplest surgical method, the fastest speed, to reduce the burden on the wounded, reduce the risk of surgery, and save the lives of the wounded.

36.4.5   Nutritional support

The body is in a state of high metabolism after trauma, energy consumption increases, a large number of protein break down and cause, negative nitrogen balance, if not promptly corrected, the patient is prone to malnutrition, infection and multiple organ failure. Therefore, post-traumatic nutritional support is particularly important.

36.4.6   Infection control

There are many ways to prevent infection from multiple infections. They can originate from open wounds, from nosocomial infections caused by improper use of various catheters, from bacterial translocation in the intestine, and long-term use of broad-spectrum antibiotics. Double infection, infection triggers SIRS to develop into MODS and MOF, which is the most important cause of post-traumatic death. Therefore, the prevention and treatment of infection is an important part of reducing the mortality of multiple injuries.

Zhu Changju

Chapter 37

Abdominal Trauma

37.1 Overview

37.1.1 Definition

Abdominal trauma refers to a variety of physical, chemical, and biological exogenous factors that act on the body, resulting in damage to the structural integrity of the internal organs of the abdominal wall and/or abdominal cavity and a series of dysfunctions that occur at the same time or in succession.

37.1.2 Epidemiology

Abdominal trauma is common in both peacetime and wartime. It is an important part of the spectrum of traumatic diseases. Its incidence usually accounts for 0.4% –1.8% of various injuries; it accounts for about 5% –8% in wartime. Usually more common in traffic accidents, work injuries, crashes, fighting, disasters and so on.

37.1.3 Classification

Generally, it can be divided into two types: open injury and closed injury. Among them, the open injury is divided into two types according to whether the peritoneum is intact: penetrating wounds in the peritoneal membrane, most of which are associated with internal organ damage, and nonpenetrating wounds in the absence of peritoneal membrane damage. Damage to internal organs: among them, the projectile has an exit, the entrance is a penetrating wound, and the entranceless one is a blind tube injury. The penetrating injury can be further divided into a stab wound and a gunshot wound. Closed injury may be limited to the abdominal wall, but it may also be associated with abdominal visceral injury. In addition, a variety of puncture, endoscopy, enema, curettage, abdominal surgery and other diagnostic and treatment measures can even cause some iatrogenic injuries.

37.1.4 Combined injury

For abdominal wounds, both open and closed injuries can cause damage to the internal organs of the abdominal cavity. Commonly damaged internal organs are liver, small intestine, stomach, colon, and large blood vessels in open lesions, followed by spleen, kidney, small intestine, liver, and mesentery in closed lesions. Other organs, such as the pancreas, duodenum, hernia, rectum, etc., have a lower incidence of injury due to the deeper anatomy.

37.2   Clinical manifestations

Simple abdominal wall injuries can manifest as pain at the injury site, swelling of the abdominal wall, subcutaneous bruising, and tenderness. The characteristic is that the degree and scope do not increase or expand over time. Abdominal wall injury usually does not show nausea, vomiting or shock.

With intra-abdominal organ damage, its clinical manifestations depend on the nature and extent of damage to the damaged organs. Injury to the parenchyma or large vessels of the liver, spleen, pancreas, kidney, etc. is mainly manifested as intra-abdominal (or retroperitoneal) hemorrhage. More than 1,500 mL of bleeding or 30% bleeding rate can cause hypovolemic shock. The wounded is irritability, pale, clammy skin, pulse is breakdown, pulse pressure becomes smaller, blood pressure decreases; abdominal symptoms are persistent abdominal pain, mild to moderate tenderness, rebound tenderness, and muscular tension. Mobile dullness is the late presentation of intra-abdominal hemorrhage.

Intra-abdominal cavity organ damage (stomach, gallbladder, bladder, etc.) ruptured, mainly manifested as diffuse peritonitis. When the upper gastrointestinal tract is ruptured, it immediately cause severe abdominal pain, tenderness, rebound tenderness, and abdominal muscle tension; when the lower gastrointestinal tract is ruptured, peritonitis shows progressiveness, but the bacterial pollution caused is far more severe than that of the upper gastrointestinal tract. With the progress of peritonitis, fever, obdominal distension and other symptoms gradually aggravate, while bowels sounds may weaken or disappear. After the rupture of the stomach, duodenum, or colon, there may be a reduction or disappearance of the hepatic dullness, and rupture of the retroperitoneal duodenum may sometimes manifest as testicular pain, scrotal hematoma, and abnormal penile erection.

37.3   Diagnosis

37.3.1   History of trauma and symptom

Trauma history collection and physical examination are still the most basic diagnostic methods for abdominal trauma. The doctors should ask detailed questions about conscious patients and witnesses at the scene include the time of injury, passing, type of injury, the site of action, direction, etc., as well as changes in the condition and handling measures.

Abdominal open injuries, due to the presence of wounds, and mostly penetrating injuries, can generally be diagnosed and treated in a timely manner. However, careful inspection should be conducted to avoid omissions.

The diagnosis of blunt trauma is relatively difficult. Abdominal muscle tension and tenderness are important signs of abdominal organ injuries, but should be differentiated from simple abdominal wall bruises. Abdominal wall contusion patients with pain relief when resting quietly, when the contraction of the abdominal muscles is significantly aggravated, the disease gradually reduces the trend. and the abdominal wall injury is generally not gastrointestinal symptoms; The relationship is not serious and the condition is progressively worse. Abdominal organ injuries should be considered in the following cases:①early shock;②persistent abdominal pain with symptoms such as nausea and vomiting, and aggravating trends;③fixed abdominal tenderness and muscle tension;④hematemesis, hematochezia or hematuria;⑤the abdomen shows shifting dullness.

37.3.2 Auxiliary inspection

37.3.2.1 Lab tests

The decreased values of red blood cells, hemoglobin, and hematocrit suggest bleeding. The increase in the total number of white blood cells and neutrophils can be seen in the abdominal organ injury, but also a stress response to the body. Elevated blood or urine amylase indicates pancreatic injury or perforation of the gastrointestinal tract. Hematuria is an important sign of urinary system damage, but the degree may not be directly proportional to the injury.

37.3.2.2 X-ray

When there is more than 50 mL of free gas in the abdominal cavity, it can be shown on the X-ray film, which is the clear evidence of rupture of the gastrointestinal tract. Retroperitoneal gas accumulation suggests a retroperitoneal duodenal or knot, rectal rupture. In teh case of retroperitoneal hematoma, the shadow of the psoas is disappeared. When the left side of the sacrum is more than enough to see the stomach bubble or bowel into the chest.

37.3.2.3 Diagnostic abdominal puncture

The operation is relatively simple, safe and reliable, the positive rate of up to 90%. Suspected liver, spleen, gastrointestinal tract and other organ injuries, in particular, the history of trauma is unknown, post-injury coma and shock is difficult to use other parts of the interpretation of the injury, peritoneal puncture could be applied. The positive rate of abdominal puncture is higher, positive results have diagnostic value, but negative results can not completely rule out visceral injury, if it is necessary, repeated puncture or peritoneal lavage could be conducted.

37.3.2.4 Diagnostic peritoneal lavage

It is applicable to patients with blunt trauma who are suspected of having intra-abdominal lesions that are not clearly identified by abdominal puncture. Diagnostic peritoneal lavage is a very sensitive examination with few false-negative results, but more than 10% of those who are positive have undergone laparotomy to prove that they do not need this surgery. Therefore, it is not appropriate to use lavage positivity as an absolute indication for exploratory laparotomy. For retroperitoneal injury (pancreatic head, duodenal retroperitoneal part and kidney), peritoneal lavage has no diagnostic significance.

37.3.2.5 Ultrasonography

Ultrasonography is an effective method to evaluate substantial abdominal organ damage (liver, spleen, pancreas, and kidney, etc.). The majority of lesions can be clearly identified by their location and extent, and dynamic observation.

37.3.2.6 CT

It is the preferred method for diagnosing substantial organ injuries such as liver, spleen, and kidney. It is simple, rapid, safe, painless, with high resolution, clear anatomy, and less dependent on the examiner's skills and experience than ultrasound.

37.3.2.7 MRI

It is only considered when the injury is allowed and the diagnosis is difficult. It can be used for the examination of liver, pancreas, spleen, kidney and biliary tract injury, abdominal aortic dissection, and rupture of abdominal aortic aneurysm. However, it should be emphasized that the abdominal MRI examination time is relatively long, so it should be closely observed when critical patients are examined to prevent accidents.

37.4 Treatment

37.4.1 Initial treatment

37.4.1.1 Pre-hospital treatment

Pre-hospital care for patients with severe abdominal trauma includes airway management, respiratory support, and circulatory support. A smooth infusion channel is quickly established in the upper limbs, rapid expansion, application of anti-shock pants, and chest cardiac compression. Penetrating wounds should be promptly bandaged; when the intestine is exposed out of the abdominal wall, the intestine should not be returned to the abdominal cavity to avoid increased abdominal contamination. The prolapsed bowel can be covered with a large sterile dressing, and the rice bowl is buckled for protective dressing. If the abdominal wall defect leads to a large number of prolapse of the bowel, excessive bowel escaping to pull the mesenteric blood vessels to affect blood pressure, or out of the intestinal incarceration, etc., the intestine can be sent back to the abdominal cavity, dressing the abdominal wound.

37.4.1.2 Emergency department treatment

After arriving at the emergency department, the doctors should first deal with the greatest threats to life, such as maintaining airway patency, controlling significant external bleeding, managing open pneumothorax or tension pneumothorax, restoring circulating blood volume as soon as possible, controlling shock, and managing rapid epidural hematoma and other brain injury. In addition, the treatment of abdominal trauma should be given priority, because intra-abdominal hemorrhage can cause shock, gastrointestinal rupture can cause severe consequences such as abdominal infection.

37.4.2 Non-surgical treatment

For the diagnosis of a clear, mild and simple substantial organ injury, vital signs and hemodynamically stable wounded people are feasible non-surgical treatment. After detailed physical examination and auxiliary examination, if it is difficult to determine whether there is injury to the abdominal organs, and temporary non-surgical treatment is suitable.

While performing non-surgical treatment, we must closely observe the condition of the wounded, including: ①monitoring of vital signs (body temperature, pulse rate, respiration, blood pressure); ②checking abdominal signs every half hour, paying attention to changes; ③every other one hour ordering the blood routine, paying attention to changes of red blood cells, hemoglobin, hematocrit and white blood cell.

During the treatment period, it is forbidden to move casualties casually; use of painkillers should be with caution. Fasting, decompression of the gastrointestinal tract, giving fluids and broad-spectrum antibiotics are suggested. If the condition is aggravated, a laparotomy may be considered.

37.4.3　Laparotomy

37.4.3.1　Surgical indication

Correct selection and definitive treatment as soon as possible is the key to reducing the mortality and complication rate after abdominal trauma. The following conditions should be followed by laparotomy: ①there is a clear peritoneal irritation sign. ②Continuous hypotension and difficult to explain with reasons other than the abdomen. ③Wound bleeding a lot, or with gastrointestinal contents, bile, urine. ④Intestinal bleeding through the abdominal wall. ⑤Abdominal X-ray film with free gas, intraperitoneal metallic foreign body retention, abdominal puncture or lavage positive, gastrointestinal bleeding, hematuria, etc. suggesting abdominal organ injury. ⑥Abdominal wall penetration injured person, or abdominal or lower chest or waist and abdomen high-speed projectile penetration or blind wound.

37.4.3.2　Preoperative preparation

After the completion of the establishment of infusion channel rehydration, laboratory tests, auxiliary examinations, preparation of blood, gastrointestinal decompression, catheterization, broad-spectrum antibiotics should be given to prevent infection. Traumatic or colorectal injuries should be injected with tetanus antitoxin. Patients with intra-abdominal hemorrhage should be quickly taken to the operating room.

37.4.3.3　Anesthesia

Because abdominal trauma patients often face the threat of shock, and can not move, doctors should choose endotracheal intubation anesthesia.

37.4.3.4　Principle of surgery

For the abdominal road traffic injury, the exploratory laparotomy is mainly based on the principle of "rescuing life first and organ preservation second" and should follow the principle of system and order. Intraoperative procedures include: ①control of bleeding. After the removal of hemoperitoneum, hemorrhage should be controlled first. Temporary measures include clamps, tamponade, or compression. Certain measures include vascular ligation, substantial organ bleeding, etc. ②Exploration. All organs in the abdominal cavity should be inspected in an orderly manner to identify the site of injury and to control abdominal contamination. ③The principle of damage control should be followed for serious injuries. ④Definitive treatment. According to the abdominal injury and the general condition of the patient, the treatment and reconstruction of the injured organs should be completed.

37.4.3.5　Close the incision

After the organ injury is repaired completely, foreign bodies, tissue fragments, food residues and feces in the abdominal cavity should be completely removed. The abdominal cavity should be washed with a large amount of isotonic saline, and the heavily polluted site should be flushed repeatedly. If it is necessary, the drainage tube should be indwelt to prevent the accumulation of fluid under the armpit and in the pelvic cavity.

Zhu Changju

Chapter 38

Fracture of Femur and Hip

38.1 Introduction

38.1.1 Basics

Hip fractures are cracks or breaks in the top of the thigh bone (femur) close to the hip joint. They're usually caused by a fall or an injury to the side of the hip, but may occasionally be caused by a condition, such as cancer, weakening the hip bone. Falls are very common in older people, who may have reduced vision or mobility and balance problems. Hip fractures are also more common in women, who are more susceptible to osteoporosis (weak and fragile bones).

38.1.2 Symptoms

Symptoms of a hip fracture after a fall may include: ①pain; ②not being able to lift, move or rotate (turn) the leg; ③being unable to stand or put weight on the leg; ④bruising and swelling around the hip area; ⑤a shorter leg on the injured side; ⑥the leg turning outwards more on the injured side. A hip fracture won't necessarily cause bruising or prevent one from standing or walking.

38.1.3 Seeking medical help

For patients with fractrue, call 120 for an ambulance. Before the ambulance arrives at the scene, open fracture with bleeding can be oppressed with clean sterilized gauze. When the compression cannot stop the bleeding, a tourniquet rins can be used to tie the upper part of the wound (near the heart) to stop bleeding. If the bleeding is dark red and the bleeding rate is relatively slow, bandage the distal end of the wound to stop venous bleeding. If the bleeding is bright red and shows a rapid gush, which suggest arterial bleeding, then the artery should be bandaged near the heart of the wound. If the facture is exposed out, do not try to put the fracture end back to the original place, so as not to bring bacteria into the deep part of the wound to cause deep infection.

The fractured limb should be fixed with a splint, which is longer than the upper and lower joint of the fracture site, a soft object should be padded between the splint and the limb, and then fixed with a bandage, so as to reduce the pain of the patient, avoid secondary injury and faciliate bandling and transport.

38.2 Diagnosis

38.2.1 Hospital assessment

After arriving at hospital with a suspected hip fracture, the overall condition of the patient will be assessed. The doctor carrying out the assessment may: ①ask how the patient were injured and whether had a fall; ②ask if this is the first time the patient has fallen (if the patient did fall); ③ask about any other medical conditions the patient have; ④ask whether the patient is taking any medication; ⑤assess how much pain the patient is in; ⑥assess the mental state of the patient (if the patient fell and hit his/her head); ⑦take the temperature of the patient; ⑧make sure the patient is not dehydrated. After a while, the patient may be moved from the emergency department to a ward, such as an orthopaedic ward.

38.2.2 Imaging diagnostic

To confirm whether the patient's hip has been fractured, many imaging tests may be needed, such as: an X-ray, a magnetic resonance imaging (MRI) scan, a computerised tomography (CT) scan.

38.3 Treatment

38.3.1 Primary treatment

38.3.1.1 Relieve pain

Hip fractures can be very painful. During diagnosis and treatment, patient should be given medication to relieve pain.

Depending on the outcome of assessment, patient may be given: ①painkilling medication; ②a local anaesthetic injection near the hip; ③intravenous fluid; ④the health care professionals treat the patient to make sure he/she is warm and amfortable.

38.3.1.2 Preventing infection

Antibiotics should be used before operation, which is to reduce the risk of wound infected after surgery.

38.3.1.3 Prevention of thrombosis

Long-term bed rest may be required after operation, which increases the risk of thrombosis, so it is necessary to monitor thrombosis regulaxly and take preven tive measures. For example, get out of bed as early as possible after surgery, or use anticoagulants such as heparin.

38.3.2 Conservative treatment

Conservative treatment is the alternative to surgery. It involves a long period of bed rest and isn't often used because it can: ①make people more unwell in the long-term; ②involve a longer stay in hospital; ③slow down recovery. However, conservative treatment may be necessary if surgery isn't possible—for example, if someone is too fragile to cope with surgery, or if the fracture occurred a few weeks earlier and has already started to heal.

38.3.3   Surgical treatment

38.3.3.1   Surgical time

Hip fractures are usually treated in hospital with surgery.

Most people will need surgery to fix the fracture or replace all or part of their hip, ideally on the day they're admitted to hospital or the day after.

The National Institute for Health and Care Excellence (NICE) recommends that someone with a hip fracture should have surgery within 48 hours of admission to hospital. However, surgery may sometimes be delayed if the person is unwell with another condition and treatment would significantly improve the outcome of the operation.

38.3.3.2   Influential factors of surgical treatment

There are a number of different operations, which are described below. The type of surgery will depend on: ①the type of fracture (where in the femur the fracture is); ②the age of the patient; ③how physically mobile he/she was before the hip fracture; ④the mental ability of the patient to take part in the post−surgery rehabilitation programme; ⑤the condition of the bone and joint−for example, whether or not the patient has arthritis.

38.3.3.3   Surgical methods

(1) Internal fixation

Internal fixation means using pins, screws, rods or plates to hold the bone in place while it heals. It tends to be used for either: ①extracapsular fractures (outside the socket of the hip joint); ②intracapsular fractures (inside the socket of the hip joint) −if they're stable and haven't moved significantly (undisplaced). If internal fixation is used for an intracapsular fracture, the patient will need follow−up appointments over several months with X−rays to check healing.

(2) Hemiarthroplasty

Hemiarthroplasty means replacing the femoral head with a prosthesis (false part). The femoral head is the rounded top part of the femur (upper thigh bone) that sits in the hip socket. The procedure is often the preferred option for intracapsular fractures (inside the socket of the hip joint), which occur in people who already had reduced mobility before the fracture. In this type of fracture, a replacement is the preferred option, as the fracture is unlikely to heal well.

(3) Complete hip replacement

A complete hip replacement is an operation to replace both the natural socket in the hip and the femoral head with prostheses (false parts). This is a more major operation than hemiarthroplasty and isn't necessary in most patients, but may be considered if the patient already has a condition that affects his/her joints, such as arthritis, or he/she is very active.

38.3.3.4   Complications of hip surgery

Complications can arise from surgery, including: ①infection−the risk is reduced by using antibiotics at the time of surgery and careful sterile techniques. Infection occurs in about 1%−3% of cases and requires further treatment and often further surgery. ②Blood clots−can form in the deep veins of the leg (deep vein thrombosis, or DVT) as a result of reduced movement. DVT can be prevented using special stockings, exercise and medication. ③Pressure ulcers (bedsores)−can occur on areas of skin under constant pressure from being in a chair or bed for long periods.

38.4 Recovery

How long the patient will need to stay in hospital will depend on his/her condition and mobility. It may be possible to be discharged in three to five days.

Evidence suggests that prompt surgery and a tailored rehabilitation programme that starts as soon as possible after surgery can significantly improve a person's life, reduce the length of the hospital stay and help him/her recover his/her mobility faster.

Wang Nan ,Zhu Changju

Chapter 39

Limb Trauma

39.1 Introduction

39.1.1 The concept of fracture

Fracture refers to the interruption of the integrity and continuity of the bone.

39.1.2 The causes of fractures

Fractures can be caused by trauma and skeletal diseases, such as bone destruction caused by osteomyelitis and bone tumors, and fractures that occur when minor external forces are called pathological fractures.

(1) Direct violence: the direct effect of violence causes fractures in the injured area, often accompanied by varying degrees of soft tissue injury.

(2) Indirect violence: violence causes fractures in the far limbs through conduction, leverage, rotation, and muscle contractions.

(3) Accumulated strains: long-term, repeated, and minor direct or indirect injuries can cause fractures in a specific part of the limb.

39.1.3 The classification of fractures

(1) Classification according to the integrity of the skin and mucous membranes at the fracture site

Closed fracture: the skin or mucous membrane is intact at the fracture site, and the fractured end is not exposed out.

Open fractures: the skin or mucous membrane of fracture site is ruptured, fractures site is exposed out.

(2) Classification according to degree and shape of fracture

• Incomplete fracture can be divided into fissured fracture and greendstick fracture.

• Complete fracture: the integrity and continuity of bone are completely interrupted and can be divided according to the direction of the fracture line and its morphology.

Transverse fracture: the fracture line is approximately perpendicular to the longitudinal axis of the bone shaft.

Oblique fracture: the fracture line is at an angle to the longitudinal axis of the backbone.

Spiral fracture: the fracture line is spiral.

Comminuted fractures: bone fragmentation into three or more.

Intercalated fractures: the fractures intercalated with each other and are more common in metaphyseal fractures.

Compression fractures: bone masses are deformed by compression and are more common in cancellous bones such as vertebrae and calcaneus.

Depressed fractures: the fracture sites are partially depressed and are more common in the skull.

(3) Classification based on the stability of fractures

Stable fractures: fractures are not easily displaced or displaced after reduction, such as fissured fracture, greendstick fracture, transverse fractures, compression fractures, and intercalated fractures.

Instability fracture: easy to shift the fracture end or easy to reposition after reduction, such as oblique fractures, spiral fractures, comminuted fractures.

39.1.4   Clinical manifestations

Most fractures usually cause only local symptoms. Severe fractures and multiple fractures can lead to systemic reactions.

(1) Systemic performance

Shock: the main cause of shock caused by fractures is bleeding, especially pelvic fractures, femoral fractures, and multiple fractures.

Fever: the body temperature is generally normal after fracture. Fractures with large amount of blood loss may have low fever, and high fever may occur after open fracture infection.

(2) Local symptoms

• General manifestations of fractures: local pain, swelling, and dysfunction.

• Specific signs of fracture.

Malformation: mainly manifested as shortening, angulation or rotational malformation.

Abnormal activity: abnormal activities after fracture.

Friction or bone rubbing: after the fracture, the two fractured ends rub against each other to produce a bone fricative or bruise.

39.2   Diagnosis

With one of the three specific signs above, a fracture can be diagnosed. X-ray examination is of great value in the diagnosis of fractures. The X-ray examination of a fracture should generally be taken to include the front and side views adjacent to one joint. If necessary, an X-ray film at a specific location should be taken.

39.3   Complications of fractures

Fractures are often caused by severe trauma. In some complicated injuries, sometimes the fracture itself is not important. It is important that the fracture is accompanied by or caused by damage to important tissues or vital organs, which often causes severe systemic reactions and even endangers the patient's life.

(1) Early complications

Severe shock caused by major bleeding or damage to vital organs.

Fat embolism syndrome: occurs in adults because the tension in the intramedullary hematoma at the fracture is too large, the bone marrow is destroyed, and fat droplets enter the ruptured venous sinus, which can cause lung and brain fat embolism. Clinically, respiratory insufficiency, cyanosis, and widespread lung consolidation occur. Arterial hypoxemia can cause irritability, drowsiness, and even coma and death.

Important internal-organ damage: rupturing of liver and spleen; lung injury; damage of bladder and urethra; rectal injury.

Important surrounding tissue damage: vital vascular injury; peripheral nerve injury; spinal cord injury.

Osteofascial compartment syndrome: a series of early syndromes caused by acute ischaemia in the muscles and nerves of the fascia compartments formed by the osteoporotic membrane, intermuscular space, and deep fascia.

(2) Late complications

Hypostatic pneumonia: mainly occurs in patients who are bedridden for a long time due to fractures, especially in the elderly, infirm, and patients with chronic diseases.

Pressure sores: patients with severe traumatic fractures, long-term bedridden, body bone protrusion at the pressure, local blood circulation disorders are easy to form pressure sores. Common parts include the patella, hip, and heel.

Deep venous thrombus of lower extremity: it is more common in pelvic fractures or lower extremity fractures. Patients who have a long braking of the lower extremities, slow venous return, companing with hypercoagulable states of the wounds, are easy to form thrombosis.

Infection: open fractures, especially those with heavier pollution or severe soft tissue injuries. If debridement is not complete, poor tissue or soft tissue coverage may result in infection.

Traumatic ossification: also known as myositis ossificans. Due to the fracture of the subperiosteal hematoma and the extensive ossification in the soft tissue near the joints, serious joint motion dysfunction is caused.

Traumatic arthritis: intra-articular fractures, destruction of the articular surface, and can not be accurately reset, after the bone healing, the joint surface is not smooth, long-term wear and tear can easily lead to traumatic arthritis, resulting in pain when the joint is in motion.

Stiffness of joint: the injured limbs are immobilized for a long time, and venous and lymphatic drainage are not smooth. Fibrous exudation and fibrin deposition in the tissues around the joints result in fibrous adhesion. It also has joint capsule and peripheral muscle contracture, resulting in joint motion disorders.

Acute bone atrophy (Sudeck's atrophy): a painful osteoporosis near the joint is also known as reflex sympathetic dystrophy.

Ischemic necrosis of bone: fractures cause the blood supply to a fractured segment to be destroyed and the ischaemic necrosis occurs.

Ischemic contracture: it is a serious consequence of improper handling of compartment syndrome. It can be caused directly by fractures and soft tissue injuries, and is more common in external fixation.

39.4 The process of fracture healing

Fracture healing is a complex and continuous process. From histological and cytological changes, it is usually divided into three stages:

(1) Hematoma and inflammation formative period: fractures cause hemorrhage and rupture of bone marrow cavity, periosteal and surrounding tissues, and form hematoma at the ends of fracture.

(2) Primary callus formation period: periosteum, neovascularization and osteoblasts proliferate, synthesize and secrete bone matrix and form new bone.

(3) Bone plate forming period: the new bone of trabecular bone in the original callus gradually thickens, and the arrangement is gradually regular and dense. The necrotic bone at the fracture end is invaded by osteoclasts and osteoblasts, completing the crawling replacement process of sequestration and new bone formation.

39.5 Treatment

39.5.1 First aid for fractures

The purpose of first aid for fracture is to use the simplest and most effective method to save lives, protect limbs, and quickly transfer. So that it can be properly handled as soon as possible.

(1) Rescue shock: the first thing is to check the general condition of the patient. Those with the shock should be kept warm, reduce the moving, and immediately infusion, blood transfusion. Patients with craniocerebral injury coma should maintain airway patency.

(2) Bind up the wound: patients with open fractures, the vast majority of wound bleeding should be dressed around properly.

(3) Proper fixation: fixation is an important measure of first aid for fractures. The purpose of fixation: ①to avoid the surrounding tissues damage during the transportation; ②to reduce the activities of the fracture end to reduce patient pain; ③to facilitate the delivery.

(4) Rapid transfer: after initial treatment and proper fixation, the patient should be transferred to the nearest hospital for treatment as soon as possible.

39.5.2 Treatment of fracture

The treatment of fractures has three principles, namely, reduction, fixation, and rehabilitation.

(1) Reduction of fracture

Anatomic reduction: the fracture segment is restored to a normal anatomical relationship by repositioning, and the anatomical reduction is described when the alignment (the contact surface of the two fracture ends) and the alignment (the relationship between the two fracture segments on the vertical axis) is completely satisfactory.

Functional reduction: after the reduction, although the two fracture segments do not return to the normal anatomical relationship, there is no significant effect on the limb function after the fracture healing, and the function is reset.

(2) Fixation of fracture

There are two types of fixation of fractures, namely, external fixation (fixation the outside of the body), and internal fixation(fixation inside the body).

External fixation: external flxation is mainly used for patients with fractures after manual reduction, and some fractures are treated with open reduction and internal fixation. Currently used external fixation methods include small splints, plaster bandages, outriggers, continuous traction and external fixation.

Internal fixation: internal fixation is mainly used for open reduction, the use of metal internal fixation, such as bone plates, screws, absorbable screws, intramedullary nails or interlocking intramedullary nails and compression plate, etc. , to fix the fracture segment to the position of anatomical reduction.

(3) Rehabilitation therapy for fracture

Early stage: within 1−2 weeks after the fracture, the goal of rehabilitation in this period is to promote blood circulation of the affected limb, eliminate swelling, and prevent muscle atrophy.

Middle stage: after 2 weeks of fracture, the swelling of the affected limb has subsided, the local pain is relieved, and the fracture site has been connected with fiber and becomes stable.

Late stage: fractures have reached the standard of clinical healing, external fixation has been removed.

Zhang Junqiang

Chapter 40

General Approach to Poisoning

40.1　Introduction

Most poisoned patients seen in the emergency department are adults with acute oral drug overdoses. Other common clinical scenarios include accidental poisoning in children; drug abuse through smoking, snorting, or injection; chronic poisoning from drug abuse or from environmental, industrial, and agricultural chemical exposure; medication reactions or interactions; and envenomation. Poisoning is very common in our daily life, every doctor must learn to treat poisoning.

40.2　The general approach to the poisoning

40.2.1　Emergency management

(1) Resuscitation with airway establishment, adequate ventilation and perfusion, and maintaining all vital signs must first be accomplished.

(2) Continuous cardiac and pulse monitoring is essential at the same time.

(3) Rapid-sequence intubation may be indicated.

(4) Inserting an intravenous (IV) line and drawing appropriate blood samples.

(5) Naloxone 2 mg (IV), thiamine 100 mg (IV), and 50% glucose 50 mL (IV) (if the patient is hypoglycemic) are given to all patients in coma.

(6) Maintaining blood pressure and tissue perfusion may require adequate volume replacement, correcting acid-base disturbance, antidotal therapy, and pressor agents.

(7) Cardiac arrhythmias and seizures should be treated appropriately if possible.

40.2.2　Clinical evaluation

Use all your senses, search for the clues. Such as look, track marks, pupil size, feel, temperature, sweating, smell, and so on. Take alcohol poisoning as an example, patient presenting with multisystem involvement should be suspected of poisoning until proved otherwise. A thorough history and physical examination are essential.

40.2.3   Eliminating poison from the gastrointestinal tract, skin, and eyes or removal from the site of exposure in inhalation poisoning

40.2.3.1   Inhaled poisons

Objective：move the patient to fresh air；optimize ventilation and protect personnel from exposure.

40.2.3.2   Absorbed poisons

Objective：remove poison from skin.

Liquid：wash with copious amounts of water.

Powder：brush off as much as possible, then wash with copious amounts of water.

Protect personnel from exposure.

40.2.3.3   Dilute/irrigate/wash

Use soap, shampoo for hydrocarbons.

No need for chemical neutralization—heat produced by reaction could be harmful.

40.2.3.4   Eye irrigation

Wash for 15 minutes.

Use only water or balanced salt solutions.

Remove contact lenses.

Wash from medial to lateral.

40.2.3.5   Ingested poisons

Objective：remove the poisons from GI tract before absorption occurs. The majority of poisoning occurs via the gastrointestinal tract. Gastric decontamination is indicated to reduce absorption of the poisonous substance. Principal modalities in historical order include induced vomiting, gastric lavage, activated charcoal, and whole—bowel irrigation. Firstly we should do induced vomiting. This is may be recommended if the time since ingestion of the poison is less than 30 minutes. We can use digital stimulation or use syrup of ipecac.

Ipecac is rarely used anymore. If used, has to be initiated within 30 minutes after ingestion. Vomiting in 20—30 minutes. This way only removes about 32% of contaminate. There are many contraindications. For example alcohol and corrosive.

Ipecass dose：15 cc if the patient is 12 months to 12 years old, 30 cc if the patient is more than 12 years old, and follow with 2—3 glasses of water.

Keep patient ambulatory if possible, and repeat it if no vomiting after 20 minutes, repeat. When emesis occurs, keep head down. And we should collect, save vomitus for analysis.

The contraindications of Ipecac is following：

Comatose or no gag reflex；Seizing or has seized；caustic（such as acid or alkali）ingestion；late term pregnancy；severe hypertension and cardiovascular insufficiency, possible AMI（Acute myocardial infarction）.

Gastric lavage is also used in elimination of poison. Gastric lavage is contraindicated in patients who have ingested corrosives or petroleum distillate hydrocarbons because of the risk of aspiration—induced hydrocarbon pneumonitis and gastroesophageal perforation. It is commonly used in emergency departments. It can removes about 31% of substance. It helps get activated charcoal in patient, especially if patient is unconscious. It is not helpful for sustained release tablets.

Activated charcoal is another way in elimination of poison. Activated charcoal, as a suspension in water either alone or with a cathartic, is given orally via a nippled bottle(for infants), or via a cup, straw, or small –bore nasogastric tube. The recommended dose is 1 – 2 g/kg body weight.

Activated charcoal adsorbs compounds, prevents movement from GI(gastrointestinal) tract. It is very effective at adsorbing substances. It can binds about 62% of toxin. We use activated charcoal when inactivates Ipecac. Do not give it until vomiting stops.

Whole–bowel irrigation is performed by administering a bowel–cleansing solution containing electrolytes and polyethylene glycol orally or by gastric tube.

40.2.4   Administering an antidote

The 4th phase of poisoning treatment is antidotes. For example:

(1)Naloxone for all morphine–like drugs.

(2)Atropine sulphate and pralidoxime, for anticholinesterase poisoning.

(3)Desferrioxamine for iron poisoning Methionine or N–acetyl cysteine in severe paracetamol poisoning.

(4)Nikethamide for alcohol or barbiturate.

40.2.5   Elimination of absorbed substance

The 5th phase of poisoning treatment is elimination of absorbed substance.

(1)We use diuresis and forced diuresis;for such as phenobarbital;salicylate poisoning.

(2)We use alkalinization of urine for such as salicylate;barbiturates poisoning.

(3)We use hemoperfusion for such as Lithium;methanol;ethylene glycol;salicylate poisoning.

(4)We use hemodialysis for theophyline;barbiturates poisoning.

Criteria for hemodialysis/hemoperfusion(HD/Hp) include:

The presence of complications.

Renal failure.

Severe and probably fatal poisoning with grade IV coma.

High ingested dose and blood levels.

Progressive deterioration with apnea.

Circulatory failure.

Hypothermia.

Conscious level include:

Grade I :drowsy, confused, responds to command, reflexes brisk.

Grade II :unconscious, does not respond to command, responds to minimal painful stimulus.

Grade III :deeper, responds only to severe stimulus, respiration depressed.

Grade IV :coma, no responses, hypotension severe respiratory depression or apnea.

40.2.6   Supportive therapy

The 6th phase of poisoning treatment is supportive therapy.

(1)Indiscriminately using drugs, antidotes, and gastric lavage should be avoided.

(2)Hospitalization in an intensive care unit is often indicated for the serious poisoning.

40.2.7   Observation and disposition

The 7th phase of poisoning treatment is observation and disposition.

Gao Yanxia

Chapter 41

Organophosphorus Poisoning

41.1 Introduction

The first organophosphate insecticide, triethyl pyrophosphate, was synthesized in 1859, but did not replace nicotine as a pesticide until World War II. After World War II, these compounds were used as chemical warfare agents, as organophosphorus and carbamate insecticides, and as medicinal agents. Organophosphates are widely used because of their great etfficacy and unstable structure; the latter militate against long-term environmental contamination. Organophosphate insecticides account for nearly 80% of all hospitalizations for pesticide poisoning. Although all organophosphates should be considered toxic, individual differences in toxicity are significant; the most toxic of this group are generally used for agricultural purposes (ethyl parathion, mevinphos) and the least are available for household use(malathion, dichlorvos). An intermediate group exists(ronnel, trichlorfon) and is most often used as animal poisons.

41.2 Principles of organophosphorus poisoning

Organophosphorus pesticides work by persistently inhibiting the enzyme acetylcholinesterase, the enzymatic deactivator of the ubiquitous neurotransmitter acetylcholine. Because of the global penetration of organophosphorus compounds, inhibition occurs at tissue sites [true acetylcholinesterase and represented by erythrocyte or red blood cell (RBC) cholinesterase] and in plasma(circulating pseudocholinesterase). Inhibition of cholinesterase results in the accumulation and subsequent prolonged effect of acetylcholine at a variety of neurotransmitter receptors, including sympathetic and parasympathetic ganglionic nicotinic sites, postganglionic cholinergic sympathetic and parasympathetic muscarinic sites, skeletal muscle nicotinic sites, and central nervous system sites.

41.3　Clinical presentation

The first signs and symptoms of organophosphate poisoning are caused by stimulation of muscarinic, parasympathetic receptors and include nausea, vomiting, abdominal cramping, chest pain, dyspnea, wheezing, miosis, bradycardia, diaphoresis, blurred vision, bronchorrhea, and the SLUD response (salivation, lacrimation, urination, diarrhea). As toxicity increases, stimulation of nicotinic sites and central muscarinic receptors becomes manifest; nicotinic or peripheral sympathetic stimulation results in tremors, twitching, weakness, fasciculations, paralysis, tachycardia, hypertension, mydriasis, and pallor. CNS effects include anxiety, restlessness, insomnia, confusion, delirium, giddiness, emotional lability, headache, weakness, ataxia, tremors, seizures, slurred speech, decreased respirations, hypotension, and coma.

41.4　Laboratory tests

Laboratory tests should include routine admission tests and measurement of arterial blood gases. Confirmation of organophosphate poisoning is based on depression of red blood cell acetylcholinesterase activity; depressions greater than 25% are diagnostic of exposure, greater than 50% associated with the expectation of symptoms, and greater than 80% –90% is indicative of severe poisoning. Serum cholinesterase levels may be measured and the urine analyzed to determine the specific pesticide involved.

41.5　Treatment

Treatment must be promptly initiated before laboratory confirmation of pesticide toxicity; the clinical diagnosis is based on a history compatible with exposure and the expected symptoms. Ingested organophosphates should be removed by the usual gastrointestinal tract decontamination procedures; gastric lavage is followed by the administration of charcoal and cathartics. Victims of skin contamination or inhalation of organophosphates obviously do not benefit from gastrointestinal tract decontamination, but removal of the material from the skin surface is indicated. The patient's clothing must be removed and placed into plastic bags. The patient's skin and hair are then thoroughly washed with mild soap, followed by copious irrigation; asymptomatic patients may take shower. The medical staff must be protected from secondary contamination using waterproof gowns or aprons, gloves, and goggles. At an alkaline pH, both organophosphates and carbamates are hydrolyzed, and irrigation of the skin with diluted 0.5% sodium hypochlorite (1 part household bleach with 10 parts water) may increase the effectiveness of skin irrigation. The eyes are then irrigated with normal saline.

To patients with moderate poisoning, atropine is given to reverse the peripheral muscarinic parasympathetic effects as well as many of the CNS effects. Importantly, atropine will not reverse nicotinic neuromuscular paralysis or other neurologic dysfunction associated with severe poisoning. This is because atropine does not separate the organophosphate from the cholinesterase enzyme. Atropine, 1–2 mg intravenous (0.05 mg/kg intravenous for children) is given slowly as required; patients with severe symptoms will require 2–4 mg up to every 2-3 minutes as needed to reverse symptomatic bradycardia, excessive bronchial secretions, and so on. Massive doses, of up to 50 mg/d or more, have occasionally been required. In addition, pralidoxime (2-PAM) is a specific antidote that acts to cleave the organophosphate from the cholinesterase enzyme; it thereby frees the enzyme to hydrolyze excess acetylcholine. Pralidoxime must be given before irreversible phosphorylation has occurred; this agent has the greatest affinity for the phosphorylated enzyme at the nicotinic neuromuscular junction and in this context is used to reverse skeletal muscle paralysis. It does not, however, readily cross the blood-brain barrier and has poor affinity for peripheral muscarinic sites so that coadministration of atropine is always required. Pralidoxime is given intravenously, 1 g in 100 mL of normal saline at a rate not to exceed 500 mg/min. Children should be given 25-50 mg/kg (a maximum of 1 g) over 15-30 minutes. This dose may be repeated in 20 minutes. If muscle strength has not returned and then as needed to maintain strength; up to 0.5 g/h has been required in critically ill patients. Pralidoxime may also be administered as a deep intramuscular injection.

Gao Yanxia

Chapter 42

Paraquat

42.1 Introduction

Paraquat and diquat are representative of the dipyridyl compounds. Paraquat is the more toxic, with more than 600 lethal cases of poisoning to date, of which nearly 60% were suicides. The toxic effects of dipyridyl compounds are thought to be caused by superoxide radial formation, its caustic nature, and its aliphatic petroleum solvent. Dermal and inhalational toxicity is low, but ingestion is potentially lethal.

42.2 Principles of paraquat poisoning

Paraquat is the most significant in terms of number of cases and toxic effects. Paraquat use is tightly regulated in China, but is widespread throughout the world. Paraquat is absorbed through the skin, gastrointestinal tract, and respiratory tract. Almost all fatal exposures have resulted from the ingestion of paraquat, although a few case reports have involved extensive skin contamination. Toxicity has occurred, but no fatal cases have been reported from inhalation of paraquat vapor or aerosols.

Paraquat's toxic effect is from the production of superoxides created during cyclic oxidation−reduction reactions of the compound in tissues. Lipid peroxidation of cellular membranes seems to be one significant pathway of cellular injury.

Paraquat selectively concentrates in the lungs because of an amine uptake mechanism in alveolar cells. In addition, high concentrations of oxygen significantly increase the extent of paraquat−induced injury so that the lungs are the major target organs. The pathophysiologic lesions include direct injury to the alveolar-capillary membrane followed by surfactant loss, adult respiratory distress syndrome, progressive pulmonary fibrosis, and respiratory failure. Paraquat damages other major organ systems by the same cellular membrane effects, including the liver, kidneys, heart, and central nervous system.

42.3   Clinical presentation

Paraquat is extremely corrosive and cause nausea, vomiting, and severe chemical burns of the oropharynx soon after ingestion. Patients with dermal paraquat exposures show significant skin irritation, and ocular exposures may produce severe corneal burns. Acute toxicity is marked by causticulcerations of buccal, oral, and esophageal epithelium; corneal ulceration is seen when either compound is splashed into the eyes. Ingestions of greater than 30 mg/kg are associated with multiple organ failure, including hepatic, pulmonary, cardiac, renal, and the CNS. Death typically occurs within hours to days. Paraquat ingestion of more than 4 mg/kg produces reversible renal failure within 24 hours and irreversible pulmonary fibrosis. The paraquat–induced pulmonary injury usually progresses during 1–3 weeks, although the clinical course varies considerably with severity of poisoning, involvement of other organ systems, and underlying medical problems. Myocarditis, epicardial hemorrhage, and adrenal gland injury are also reported.

42.4   Laboratory tests

Laboratory studies should be performed to provide baseline values for all major systems; paraquat is measurable in the blood. As long as the time of acute exposure is known, the level serves as an accurate prognostic marker. serial chest roentgenograms and measurement of arterial blood gases to follow pulmonary function are indicated. Paraquat can be detected by gas and high–pressure liquid chromatography.

42.5   Treatment

There are no studies comparing various treatment strategies, but the key to successful treatment of an acute paraquat exposure probably depends on early decontamination measures to limit absorption. There are no effective treatments once clinical effects are seen. Thorough skin cleansing is obvious and straight forward in dermal exposures. Careful gastric lavage and administration of activated charcoal may be lifesaving and should be undertaken in consultation with a poison center or a medical toxicologist. These treatments may be hazardous in the context of a corrosive ingestion. Early endoscopy and surgical intervention may be necessary if there is evidence of esophageal perforation and mediastinitis. Although fuller's earth and bentonite are recommended as adsorbents in paraquat ingestions, activated charcoal is much more readily available in China and has equal if not greater efficacy.

Oxygen treatment can theoretically exacerbate paraquat toxicity by the production of superoxides. Therefore, oxygen should be used only as minimally necessary in these cases.

Although it is controversial, many experts recommend rapid initiation of charcoal hemoperfusion to rapidly lower plasma paraquat levels and to limit pulmonary and other organ system uptake of paraquat. Many also recommend serial and combined hemoperfusion and hemodialysis, particularly during the first 24 hours after exposure.

Cyclophosphamides in combination with corticosteroids have also been investigated as a means to attenuate paraquat toxicity. Whereas the results have been mixed, this therapy has been recommended by some experts in the setting of significant paraquat toxicity.

Early application of glucocorticoid hormone may be beneficial in patients with moderately severe acute paraquat poisoning, recommended for early treatment in patients with severe paraquat poisoning, a prednisolone 15 mg/(kg · d) or equivalent dose of hydrogenated pine. The specific dose, treatment time, side effects, remains to be further discussed.

There are other suggested treatment adjuncts, such as N-acetylcysteine, nitric oxide, deferoxamine, and cytoprotective agents such as amifostine, but no single therapy has been proved consistently successful.

Gao Yanxia

Chapter 43

Sedative–hypnotic Poisoning

43.1 Toxicological characteristics

Sedative hypnotics have inhibitory effect on the central nervous system, and the large dosage can suppress the whole nervous system, including the medullary center. Taking an overdose at a time can cause acute poisoning, showing coma, respiratory depression, shock, etc. , and even life–threatening, known as acute sedative–hypnotic poisoning. Sedative–hypnotic drugs are generally classified into Barbiturates, Benzodiazepines(BDZ), –Nonbenzodiazepine–nonbarbiturates and Phenothiazines.

The commonly used sedative–hypnotic drugs before 1950 were barbiturates. In 1960, benzodiazepines began to be used, which have both sedative and anti–anxiety effects. Currently, these drugs have almost replaced most other sedative–hypnotic drugs in hypnosis and anti–anxiety.

The sedative–hypnotic drugs are all fat–soluble and can be easily passed through the blood–brain barrier, acting on the central nervous system. Its absorption, distribution, protein binding, metabolism, excretion and onset time and effect duration are all related to the lipid soluble strength of the drug. The central nervous inhibitory effect of benzodiazepines is associated with the enhancement of the neurologic function of GABA. Barbiturates have a similar effect on GABA neurons with benzodiazepines. Benzodiazepines act selectively on the limbic system and the diencephalon, affecting mood and memory. Barbiturates are widely distributed, but they mainly act on the ascending activation system of the reticular structure to produce diffuse inhibition in the whole cerebral cortex, and the toxic amount can cause the disturbance of consciousness. The inhibitory effect of barbiturates on the central nervous system is dose–effect. With the increase of dose, its inhibitory effect gradually enhances from sedative and hypnotic to anesthesia, and even cause the respiratory center paralysis of medulla oblongata, which leads to respiratory failure, with further blood vessel central motor paralysis, blocking α–adrenergic receptor, drop in blood pressure and leads to shock. In addition, hepatic and renal function damage can be complicated. The mechanism of nonbenzodiazepine–nonbarbiturates poisoning is similar to that of barbiturates. The pharmacological action of phenothiazine is complex and diverse, involving cortex and subcortical center, which mainly acts on the whole brain stem reticular structure, and works by suppressing the dopamine receptors in the synapses.

43.2 Diagnosis

43.2.1 History

The patient has a history of oral or intravenous drug overdose. The vomitus, stomach contents, blood and urine specimens of the victim should be retained for identification and toxicological analysis.

43.2.2 Clinical manifestations

43.2.2.1 Barbiturate poisoning

The poisoning symptom is positively correlated with the dose. In the case of severe poisoning, the inhibition of the central nervous system gradually aggravates, the disturbance of consciousness and the inhibition of respiratory and cardiovascular functions are deeper, the coma lasts longer, and there are more complications. The clinical manifestations are from narcolepsy to deep coma, from shallow breathing to cessation of breathing, from hypotension to shock; hypothermia is common; the muscle tension decreases and the tendon reflexes disappear; gastrointestinal peristalsis slows down. Long-term comatose patients can be complicated with pneumonia, pulmonary edema, cerebral edema, renal failure and life - threatening. Liver damage or jaundice can occur in survivors.

43.2.2.2 Benzodiazepine poisoning

It is characterized by inhibition of the central nervous system, but no extrapyramidal system and plant antagonistic system symptoms. If there is no other sedative-hypnotic drug poisoning, severe poisoning is rare, and there are few serious symptoms such as prolonged deep coma, and no obvious inhibition of respiration and circulation. If it occurs, taking with other sedative-hypnotic drugs or alcohol should be considered at the same time.

43.2.2.3 Nonbenzodiazepine-nonbarbiturates poisoning

Chloral hydrate poisoning, in addition to its inhibitory effect on the central nervous system, has great damage to the heart, liver and kidney. Mental disorders of Glutethimide poisoning has cyclical fluctuations; because its directly action in vasomotor centers, cardiovascular suppression is more serious; it also has anticholinergic nerve function, showing dilated pupils, dry mouth, constipation, and urinary retention. In addition to lethargy, Meprobamate poisoning often shows red complexion, dilated pupils and decreased blood pressure. In the rescue of the severe poisoning patient, they can still die even the symptoms significantly improved, because of the low water solubility and slow absorption of this drug.

43.2.2.4 Phenothiazine poisoning

In addition to narcolepsy and coma, the extrapyramidal reaction is obvious, which is manifested as muscle tone enhancement, tremor, and lockjaw. There is also an antagonistic effect of alpha adrenergic nerve, which shows hypothermia, hypotension, shock, arrhythmia, and even cardiac arrest. The anticholinergic symptoms can be seen with dilated pupils, dry mouth, urinary retention, tachycardia, and reduced intestinal peristalsis, etc. Liver damage or jaundice often occurs in survivors.

43.2.3 Laboratory Examination

(1) Qualitative and quantitative determination of drugs in blood, urine and gastric juice; it is useful for

diagnosis.

(2) Arterial blood gas analysis and blood oxygen saturation monitoring: it can assess the respiratory depression.

(3) Blood biochemical examination, such as blood glucose, transaminase, urea nitrogen, creatinine, electrolyte, and ECG monitoring, which can evaluate the extent of body damage.

43.3　Differential diagnosis

43.3.1　Cerebrovascular accident

There are many local positioning signs, and brain CT scanner can help make a definitive diagnosis.

43.3.2　Epilepsy

There is a history of seizures in the past, and EEG examination is helpful for diagnosis.

43.3.3　Diabetic ketoacidosis coma and hyperosmolar nonketotic coma

Blood sugar, urine sugar, blood ketone, and serum electrolyte determination can help diagnose.

43.3.4　Uremia coma

First there is fidget, delirium, and finally into coma. Others like increased blood urea nitrogen, decreased blood carbon dioxide binding force and metabolic acidosis.

43.3.5　Hysteria

Clinically it is not uncommon. According to the accompanying symptoms, signs, exposure history of toxins, and the mental and emotional state of the patient before the onset of the disease, the final diagnosis can be assisted by toxicological analysis if necessary.

43.4　Treatment

Treatment principle: clear poison, close monitoring, timely application of specific antidote, maintain the basic physiological functions of several suppressed organs, until all toxins metabolized and excreted in many ways.

43.4.1　Clear poison

43.4.1.1　Gastric lavage

The general preference is 1 : 5,000 potassium permanganate solution, also can be washed with lukewarm water, each time the liquid is about 250 mL, rinse repeatedly until the solution is completely clarified.

43.4.1.2　Adsorption and catharsis

After the gastric lavage, activated carbon suspension can be perfused by gastric tube, which is effective for the adsorption of various sedative and hypnotic drugs; At the same time, 50% sodium sulfate solution

40-60 mL can be injected. It should be noted that since magnesium sulfate can be absorbed by a small a-mount, which can aggravate the central nervous system inhibition, so it is not suitable for the catharsis of this disease.

43.4.1.3   Fluid infusion, diuresis, alkalization of urine

Generally, furosemide and sodium bicarbonate can be used to promote the excretion of poisons from the kidney, which is good for barbiturates, and is not effective for phenothiazines.

43.4.1.4   Blood purification treatment

One of the following indications can be carried out: ①The amount of ingested medicine has reached le-thal levels and is estimated to have been absorbed. ②The symptoms of poisoning are severe and the symp-toms of central inhibition gradually deepen. ③With severe water, electrolyte and acid-base balance disor-der. ④Heart and kidney failure. Hemodialysis is preferred.

43.4.2   Specific antidote

Barbiturates, nonbenzodiazepine-nonbarbiturates and phenothiazines poisoning have no specific anti-dote. Flumazenil is a benzodiazepine antagonist, which can block the inhibitory function in central nervous system of benzodiazepine, through competitive binding to the benzodiazepine receptors. Dosage: 0.5 mg each time, slow intravenous injection, repeated injection when needed, total amount can reach up to 2 mg.

43.4.3   Maintain organic physiological functions of comatose patients

43.4.3.1   Keep the airway open

The deep comatose patients require tracheal intubation or tracheotomy and, if necessary, mechanical ventilation to ensure adequate oxygen intake and carbon dioxide removal.

43.4.3.2   Maintain respiratory center excitation

In the case of deep coma or respiratory depression, moderate use of central stimulants is appropriate. The first choice is Bemegride, which can promote the recovery of consciousness. Drug usage: Dilute 50 mg Bemegride with 10 mL 5% glucose solution, intravenous injection, every 5-10 min. Or Dilute 200-300 mg drugs with 500 mL 5% -10% glucose solution, slow intravenous drip. Lobeline and Nikethamide also can be used.

43.4.3.3   Maintain the blood pressure

Low blood pressure in acute poisoning is caused by blood vessel dilation, and the blood volume should be supplemented with fluid infusion. If it is not effective, vasoactive drugs can be considered.

43.4.3.4   Promote the recovery of consciousness

Naloxone has certain curative effect, each time 0.4-0.8 mg, intravenous injection, and can be repeated every 15 minutes to half an hour according to the condition.

43.4.3.5   Supportive and symptomatic treatment

Maintain the water-electrolyte balance, control the arrhythmia, correct acidosis, prevent infection, pul-monary edema, cerebral edema, renal failure, etc. If the extrapyramidal reaction of Phenothiazine poisoning is obvious, Benzhexol and Scopolamine can be used to treat the muscle tremor. Muscle spasm and tension disorder can be treated by giving diphenhydramine 25-50 mg orally or 20-40 mg intramuscularly.

Jian Xiangdong, Zeng Mei

Chapter 44

Opioids Poisoning

44.1   Summary

Drugs refer to opium, heroin, morphine, marijuana, cocaine, and other narcotic drugs and psychotropic substances regulated by the State Council make people addicted. The world health organization (WHO) divides drugs into eight categories: morphine, barbiturate, alcohol, cocaine, Indian hemp, Benzedrine, Khat, and hallucinogens. At present, there are more than 200 kinds of drugs. The United Nations commission on narcotic drugs classifies drugs into six categories: ①Morphine-type drugs, including opium, morphine, codeine, heroin and poppy, which are the most dangerous drugs; ②Cocaine and Cocaleaf; ③Marijuana; ④Amphetamine and other synthetic stimulants; ⑤Narcotic sedatives, including barbiturates and methaqualone; ⑥psychotropic drug, like diazepam.

The main methods of drug use include: smoke inhalation, ironing, nasalodor, oral administration, and injection. ①Smoke inhalation: mix the drug into the tobacco and inhaling through smoking. ②Ironing: the heroin is placed on aluminum foil or metal spoons, which are heated by fire, and the drug is sublimated into smoke. ③Nasal odor: use the tube to align ones nostrils and inhale the drug through the mucous membrane. ④Oral administration: Take drugs orally, such as oral meth tablets, ecstasy tablets, etc. ⑤Injection: subcutaneous injection, intramuscular injection and intravenous injection. In addition, hiding drugs in the body can also lead to the death due to drug absorption.

44.2   Opioids poisoning

44.2.1   Morphine poisoning

44.2.1.1   Pharmacological characteristics

The main pharmacological characteristics of morphine include:

(1) The central nervous system

It mainly includes: ① strong analgesic and sedative effect; ② respiratory depression; ③ antitussive effect; ④others: such as myosis, nausea, vomiting, etc.

(2) The digestive system

It has an exciting effect on the smooth muscle and sphincter of the gastrointestinal tract, which increases the tension of the gastrointestinal tract and weakens the peristalsis. Therefore, it has the effect that stops diarrhea and causes constipation, also can induce the biliary colic.

(3) The cardiovascular system

It has hypotensive effect, and can cause postural hypotension and bradycardia.

(4) Other

It can enhance the bladder sphincter tension, resulting in urinary retention and so on.

44.2.1.2　Diagnosis

(1) History

The patient has a clear history of morphine abuse.

(2) Clinical manifestations

Acute morphine poisoning is initially characterized by euphoria and excitement, followed by panic, dizziness, sweating, thirst, nausea, vomiting, pallor, delirium, coma, and respiratory depression. In the later stage, the pupil shrinks like pinpoint, and the light reflex disappears. The pulse is weak, blood pressure drops, shock, and finally death from respiratory and circulatory failure.

Withdrawal symptoms of morphine mainly include: excitement, insomnia, tears, runny nose, sweating, tremor, vomiting, diarrhea, fever, elevated blood pressure, muscle pain, spasm, loss of consciousness, etc.

(3) Laboratory examination

①Blood routine, urine routine, stool routine, liver and kidney function tests, creatinase, arterial blood gas analysis, electrocardiogram examination, etc. ②Serological examination of related diseases, such as viral hepatitis and AIDS. ③Toxicological analysis.

44.2.1.3　Differential diagnosis

It should be identified with other drug poisoning and organophosphorus poisoning.

44.2.1.4　Treatment

First aid measures mainly include:

(1) Gastric lavage and emetic: 1 : 2,000 potassium permanganate.

(2) Catharsis: injecting through stomach tube or feeding of sodium sulfate 15-30 g to promote the expulsion of toxic substances.

(3) Inhibit the absorption of drugs: if the subcutaneous injection is applied, the rubber belt or cloth belt should be used to tighten the upper part of the injection site and cold compresses at the same time, to delay the absorption of poison. The ligation area should be relaxed for 1-2 minutes every 20-30 minutes and can not be ligated continuously.

(4) Oxygen therapy and keep airway open: mechanical ventilation is administered during respiratory failure.

(5) Naloxone: using it as early as possible.

44.2.2　Pethidine poisoning

44.2.2.1　Pharmacological characteristics

Pethidine is a synthetic narcotic drug, and its function and mechanism are similar to morphine. It is commonly used in clinical, and has weak analgesic and anesthetic effects, with only amount to 1/10-1/8 of morphine.

44.2.2.2   Diagnosis

(1) History

There is a clear history of pethidine abuse.

(2) Clinical manifestations

Pethidine abuse is one of the current drug problems faced by our country. Its side effects are relatively smaller, nausea, vomiting, constipation and other symptoms are mild, and the respiratory inhibition is weak, generally without dyspnea. However, excessive doses can also inhibit respiration, and can cause tremor, muscle contracture, hyperreflexia and even convulsions.

Withdrawal symptoms mainly include lethargy, general malaise, tears, runny nose, vomiting, diarrhea, insomnia, and even collapse in severe cases.

(3) Laboratory examination

It's the same as morphine poisoning.

44.2.2.3   Differential diagnosis

It should be identified mainly with other drug intoxications.

44.2.2.4   Treatment

Refer to the treatment of morphine poisoning, barbiturates should be given as anticonvulsants.

44.2.3   Heroin poisoning

44.2.3.1   Pharmacological characteristics

Heroin, or diacetylmorphine, is the purest and most virulent substance in the opiate series, which was once known as the "king of world drugs". It is one of the main drugs used by drug users in China. Studies have reported that 90% of the deaths from drug use are attributed to heroin abuse. Heroin is more water−soluble and fat−soluble than morphine, so it is absorbed quickly by the body, and can easily enter the central nervous system through the blood brain barrier, and produce a strong reaction. It has a stronger inhibitory effect than morphine, and its analgesic effect is also 4−8 times that of morphine. It also has a stronger drug dependence than morphine, commonly used dosage for two weeks or less can lead to addiction, resulting in severe drug dependence.

44.2.3.2   Diagnosis

(1) History

There is a clear history of heroin abuse, and there may be many needle marks on the body.

(2) Clinical manifestations

Heroin can be used for nose, inhalation, subcutaneous injection and intravenous injection. The latter two methods are more common.

Acute poisoning: non−cardiogenic pulmonary edema and arrhythmias are more common, which may lead to sudden death. ①Breathing very slowly, 4−6 times per minute, respiratory central paralysis, respiratory failure; ②The pupil is narrowed like a pinhole; ③Deep coma with no orbital reaction; ④A cyanosis of limbs and lips; ⑤The heart rate slows down; ⑥Skin clamminess; ⑦Skeletal muscle weakness. ⑧Others: heroin addicts are vulnerable to infection such as abscesses, septicemia, tetanus, viral hepatitis, AIDS, etc.

Withdrawal symptoms: ①Symptoms of flu−like symptoms, such as runny nose, tears, yawning, chills, headache, and muscle and joint pain. ②Symptoms of sympathetic hyperfunction, such as hyperthermia, increased blood pressure and pulse rate, shallow breathing, abdominal pain, diarrhea or spermatorrhea. ③The symptoms of anxiety, including sitting restlessness, attack, self-injury and automutiation. ④Sleep disorders. ⑤There is a persistent craving for drug use in order to repeat the pleasure of taking drugs.

(3) Laboratory examination

Qualitative detection of morphine in urine is helpful for diagnosis. Other tests are the same as morphine poisoning.

44.2.3.3 Differential diagnosis

It should be identified with other drug poisoning and organophosphorus insecticides poisoning. Patients with heroin poisoning are usually characterized by coma, pinpoint pupil and severe respiratory depression, but cholinesterase activity is not reduced. Doctors should be alert to the possibility of pesticide suicide by drug users.

44.2.3.4 Treatment

(1) Clear poison: gastric lavage, enema and catharsis can be used if administered orally; A tourniquet should be used quickly if administered intravenously. Tighten the upper part of the injection site and delay the absorption.

(2) Oxygen therapy: high flow oxygen therapy, keep the airway open, use the respiratory stimulant properly, intubation and mechanical ventilation if necessary.

(3) Fluid infusion, diuretic: rapid fluid infusion, correct water-electrolyte disturbance and maintain the acid-base balance, use diuretics to accelerate the excretion of the drug and their metabolites.

(4) Rational use of glucocorticoids.

(5) Prevention of cerebral edema.

(6) Specific antidote: Naloxone treatment should be early, rapid and sufficient. Immediately intravenous injection of 0.4-0.8 mg, if there is no improvement in breathing, repeat after 3-5 min until consciousness recovery and respiratory improvement.

(7) Withdrawal syndrome: in the case of comatose patients with history of drug addiction, severe heroin withdrawal syndrome should be highly suspected if they have shallow breathing, and 5-10 mg of morphine can be injected intravenously, which often results in rapid remission.

Jian Xiangdong, Zeng Mei

Chapter 45

Ethanol Intoxication

Ethanol (C_2H_5OH) is also known as alcohol. It's colorless flammable volatile liquid. It has a fragrant smell. The molecular weight is 46.07.

45.1　Toxicological characteristics

Ethanol is absorbed mainly through the gastrointestinal tract and respiratory tract. About 80% of oral ethanol is absorbed by the duodenum and jejunum, and the rest is absorbed by the stomach. Gastric contents, the activity capacity of gastrointestinal tract and the type of alcohol and alcohol content can affect the absorption rate of gastrointestinal tract. The absorption can reach 80%–90% within 30–60 minutes after oral administration of healthy adults, but the food in the stomach can delay the total absorption time to 4–6 hours. When the human body takes ethanol at the concentration of 11–20 g/m^3, the average absorption rate is 62%. The absorbed ethanol is distributed to the body's water–bearing tissues and is easily accessible through the blood–brain barrier and placenta. Alcohol in the body is mainly metabolized in the liver. There are three main metabolic pathways of ethanol in hepatocytes, which are most important in the ethanol dehydrogenase pathway of cytoplasm. Ethanol dehydrogenase first oxidizes ethanol to acetaldehyde. Then the acetaldehyde is oxidized to acetic acid ester by aldehyde dehydrogenase, and finally converted into acetyl–coA, which is oxidized to carbon dioxide and water through the tricarboxylic acid cycle. When the concentration of ethanol in the body increases, the microsomal ethanol–oxidation system of hepatocyte endoplasmic reticulum will play an important role. In addition, peroxidases in the peroxisome, and the catalase system also participates in the metabolism of ethanol. Most of the absorbed ethanol is metabolized into carbon dioxide and water, and then eliminated from the body, and only 5%–10% are excreted in the original form exhalation and urine.

45.2　Diagnosis

45.2.1　History

Alcohol is used as industrial solvent, antifreeze and fuel; it is also used in chemical, pharmaceutical, synthetic rubber, plastic, resin, synthetic fiber, adhesives, cosmetics, ink and other industries. And it is used in medical treatment for disinfection. Daily alcoholic beverages contain different amounts of ethanol as well.

45.2.2　Clinical manifestations

45.2.2.1　Acute poisoning

It is mainly seen in heavy drinkers and is rare in occupational poisoning. Mild poisoning and early poisoning shows excitement, euphoria, speech, facial blushing or pale, gait instability, mild action uncoordinated, impaired judgment, incoherent, nystagmus, and even coma. Severe poisoning can show deep coma, shallow breathing or tidal breathing. And patients may die from respiratory paralysis or circulatory failure. A small number of patients with reduced swallowing reflex, vomiting after eating, can show aspiration pneumonia or suffocation death. The pupils of severe patients often shrink, body temperature and blood pressure drop, the pulse rate slows, and the concentration of ethanol in the blood is more than 65.1 mmol/L(3,000 mg/L). Inhalation of high concentration of ethanol vapor can appear drunk feeling, dizziness, fatigue, irritability and mild eyes, upper respiratory tract mucosal irritation and other symptoms, but generally do not cause severe poisoning.

45.2.2.2　Diagnostic criteria for acute poisoning

(1) There is a recent history of excessive alcohol consumption.

(2) Maladjustment behaviors, such as sexual misconduct or aggressive impulsion, mood instability, impaired judgment, social or occupational impairment.

(3) At least one of the following signs：①enunciation unclear；②ataxia；③instability of gait；④nystagmus；⑤facial flushing or pallor.

(4) Exclude any physical illness or other mental illness.

45.2.2.3　Chronic poisoning

Long-term alcoholic can show facial telangiectasia, skin nutrition disorder, chronic gastritis, stomach ulcer, hepatitis, cirrhosis, liver failure, myocardial damage, myopathy, multiple neuropathy, and Wernicke-Korsakoff syndrome. etc.

The skin, which repeatedly exposed to ethanol fluid, can show local dry, desquamate, chapped and dermatitis.

45.2.3　Laboratory examination

The smell of ethanol in breath and vomit us can help diagnose acute poisoning. An increase in the concentration of ethanol in the blood can show as evidence of the cause. The arterial blood gas analysis in acute alcoholic intoxication showed mild metabolic acidosis. Acute, chronic alcohol intoxication can be seen low blood potassium, low blood magnesium, and low blood calcium. Hypoglycemia can be seen in acute alcoholism. Acute and chronic alcoholic liver disease can have abnormal liver function. Alcoholic cardiomyopathy can show arrhythmia and myocardial damage.

45.3　Differential diagnosis

Acute ethanol poisoning needs to be identified with methanol, isopropyl alcohol and other chemicals poisoning, drug poisoning, meningitis and head injury.

45.4   Treatment

Acute ethanol poisoning: inhalation victims should be removed immediately from the scene. Mild cases of acute alcoholism need no special treatment. Keep the patient in bed, keep warm, drink strong tea or coffee, and then they will gradually recover. Pay attention to keep warm and prevent aspiration pneumonia. However, the following measures should be taken promptly for severe patients.

45.4.1   Clean poison

Because of the fast absorption of alcohol, it is of little significance to give gastric lavage. If a large amount of ethanol is ingested within 2 hours, it may be considered to use 1% sodium bicarbonate or 0.5% activated carbon suspension and physiological saline for gastric lavage, but disable apomorphine, lest accentuate the inhibitory effect of alcohol. A person with severe vomiting may be spared from the gastric lavage. For severe cases of prolonged coma, respiratory depression and shock, dialysis should be performed as soon as possible to save the patient's life.

45.4.2   The application of naloxone

Symptoms of alcoholism are caused by increased endorphins. Naloxone is a central morphine receptor antagonist. Severe alcoholism patients with coma, hypotension, shock, and respiratory depression can be applied with the Naloxone 0.4-0.8 mg intravenous infusion, which can be repeated for 20min if necessary; or add 1.2-2 mg to the liquid for continuous drip. .

45.4.3   Promote alcohol oxidative metabolism

Patients can be given 100 mL 50% glucose solution intravenously and 100 mg vitamin B_1, B_6 and niacin intramuscularly, in order to accelerate the metabolism of alcohol in the body.

45.4.4   Symptomatic and supportive therapy

(1) Maintain respiration function and oxygen therapy. Those with respiratory failure can be given a moderate amount of respiratory stimulants such as coramine and lobelia, etc.

(2) Correct shock and replenish blood volume. Correct lactic acidosis at the early stage. The initial dose is 150 mL 5% sodium bicarbonate solution, followed by alkali supplementation according to the results of blood gas analysis. Vasoactive drugs such as dopamine can be given when necessary.

(3) Prevention of cerebral edema: 20% mannitol liquid 250 mL, or 50% glucose solution 60 mL, or dexamethasone 5-10 mg intravenous drip. It can be reused after 4-6 hours according to the condition of the patient and blood pressure.

(4) Rapidly correct the hypoglycemia: some cases can show hypoglycemic coma, and should be identified with the direct effects of alcohol.

(5) The application of sedatives: they should be used with caution. For patients with restlessness and hyperexcitability, we can use Diazepam 5-10 mg muscle injection or intravenous injection, or chlorpromazine 25-50 mg intrmuscular injection, or hydrated chloral 0.5-1.0 g orally or retention enema. Morphine and barbiturates are prohibited.

(6) Infection prevention: comatose patients can be treated with prophylactic antibiotics.

45.4.5 Others

There are also literature reports on the application of glutathione, ginseng and salvia miltiorrhiza, and obtain certain curative effect.

Complete abstinence, pay attention to liver protection, treat multiple neuropathy and give other symptomatic treatment.

Jian Xiangdong, Zeng Mei

Chapter 46

Carbon Monoxide Poisoning

Carbon monoxide is a widely distributed asphyxiating gas. Acute carbon monoxide poisoning is an acute cerebral hypoxia disease caused by inhalation of high concentration of carbon monoxide (CO). A few patients may have delayed neuropsychiatric symptoms. Some of the patients may also have hypoxic changes in other organs. Whether carbon monoxide can cause "chronic carbon monoxide poisoning" is still in debating.

46.1 Toxicological characteristics

Carbon monoxide(CO) with molecular weight 28.01, freezing point −207 ℃, boiling point 190 ℃, is colorless and odorless gas. Carbon monoxide poisoning mainly causes tissue hypoxia. The affinity of carbon monoxide to hemoglobin is 240 times greater than oxygen, 85% of the carbon monoxide is combined with hemoglobin to form stable carboxyhemoglobin, after it enters the body. Carboxyhemoglobin cannot carry oxygen and difficult to separate, whose dissociation rate is 1/3,600 of oxyhemoglobin. The presence of carboxyhemoglobin also makes the oxyhemoglobin dissociation curve move to the left, and the blood oxygen is not easily released to the tissues, resulting in cell hypoxia. When carbon monoxide poisoning occurs, the brain and heart are most vulnerable due to high metabolism and less vascular anastomosis.

46.2 Diagnosis

Acute carbon monoxide poisoning can be diagnosed according to the exposure history of inhaled high concentrations of carbon monoxide and the signs and symptoms of acute central nerve damage, combined with blood carbonyl hemoglobin (HbCO) measurement, the scene of hygiene investigation and measurement data of carbon monoxide concentration in the air, and ruling out other causes.

46.2.1 History

Carbon monoxide poisoning can be divided into living contact poisoning and productive contact poisoning. Living poisoning mostly occurs in winter in the north of China. Acute carbon monoxide poisoning can be caused by poor indoor ventilation when burning coal for heating, blocking air leakage by chimney, downdraft and improper use of gas water heater. There are also reports of poisoning from a broken gas pipeline. In addition, excessive concentration of carbon monoxide at the site of fire can also cause acute poisoning. Productive poisoning is common in steelmaking, coking, kilns, indoor test vehicles, mine drilling and shooting, coal mine gas explosion, etc.

46.2.2　Clinical manifestations

46.2.2.1　Acute carbon monoxide poisoning

The symptoms of acute carbon monoxide poisoning are closely related to the proportion of carboxyhemoglobin in the blood and the time of poisoning. Poisoning patients present unique cherry red skin and mucosa. The main clinical manifestation of this disease is the central nervous system damage caused by acute cerebral hypoxia. Therefore, different levels of consciousness are the important basis for clinical diagnosis and classification.

(1) Contact reaction

It shows headache, dizziness, heart palpitations, nausea and other symptoms, symptoms can disappear after inhalation of fresh air.

(2) Mild poisoning

It has either of the followings: ①severe headache, dizziness, weakness, nausea and vomiting; ②mild to moderate conscious disturbance, but no coma. The blood carboxyhemoglobin concentration can be higher than 10%.

(3) Moderate poisoning

In addition to the above symptoms, the disturbance of consciousness presents as superficial to moderate coma, and can recover without obvious complications after rescue. The blood carboxyhemoglobin concentration can be higher than 30%.

(4) Severe poisoning

It has one of the following: ①the disturbance of consciousness is deep coma or decerebrate state. ②the patient had a conscious disturbance and is accompanied by any of the followings: cerebral edema; shock or severe myocardial damage; pulmonary edema; respiratory failure; upper gastrointestinal bleeding; focal lesion of the brain, such as cone system or extrapyramidal damage signs. The concentration of carboxyhemoglobin can be higher than 50%. In addition to the above, this period also can appear other serious complications, such as cerebral infarction, myocardial infarction, rhabdomyolysis and acute renal failure, pulmonary infection, bullous skin, liver and kidney dysfunction, mononeuropathy or auditory vestibular organ damage, cortical blindness, etc.

46.2.2.2　Delayed encephalopathy in acute carbon monoxide poisoning

After the consciousness disturbance of acute carbon monoxide poisoning recovers, after about 2 – 60 days of "fake heal" period, and one of the following clinical symptoms occurs: ①the spirit and consciousness disturbance, including dementia, delirium or decerebrate state; ②extrapyramidal nervous disorders: the appearance of Parkinson's syndrome; ③the neurological damage of the pyramidal system: such as hemiplegia, pathological reflex or incontinence of urine and stool; ④focal dysfunction in the cerebral cortex: shows loss of speech, blindness, or secondary epilepsy.

46.2.3   Laboratory examination

46.2.3.1   Brain CT or MRI examination

In cerebral edema, the brain CT/MRI appears pathological low density areas. Delayed encephalopathy usually shows demyelination.

46.2.3.2   Blood carboxyhemoglobin test

The concentration of carboxyhemoglobin in mildly intoxicated blood can be higher than 10%, moderate poisoning can be higher than 30%, and heavy toxicity can be more than 50%. However, after away from the poisoning environment, the concentration of HbCO in blood can decrease and sometimes dose not parallel with the clinical manifestations. The HbCO concentration in patients who have stopped contact with carbon monoxide for more than 8 hours is generally less than 10%, and carboxyhemoglobin examination is not necessary.

46.2.3.3   Electroencephalography examination

Electroencephalogram (EEG) examination can reveal moderate and highly abnormal conditions.

46.2.3.4   Blood biochemical examination

There can be electrolyte changes.

46.3   Differential diagnosis

Mild acute carbon monoxide poisoning needs to be identified with colds, high blood pressure, food poisoning, Meniere syndrome, etc. For patients with moderate and severe cases, we should pay attention to the coma identification caused by other causes (such as diabetes, stroke, sleeping pills); for patients with delayed encephalopathy, the differential diagnosis should be made with other psychiatric, Parkinson's and cerebrovascular diseases. Delayed encephalopathy in acute carbon monoxide poisoning and sequela are different, the latter directly by the symptoms of acute phase continuation, and delayed encephalopathy refers to the acute carbon monoxide poisoning coma after waking up, after a period of 2–60 days off the stage, suddenly appeared with consciousness disorder, extrapyramidal system of cone or damage of encephalopathy, therefore, patients with moderate and severe acute carbon monoxide poisoning coma after waking, should be observed for 2 months.

46.4   Treatment

Quickly remove the patient from the toxic site, loosen the collar, keep warm and observe the state of consciousness closely.

46.4.1   Correct the hypoxia

High flow oxygen therapy, hyperbaric oxygen therapy as soon as possible.

46.4.2   The treatment of cerebral edema

Dehydration, diuresis and glucocorticoid. Furosemide 20 mg intravenous injection, 20% mannitol

125 mL intravenous drip, alternate between the two, q 6h or q 8 h. Methylprednisolone 120 mg is added into the fluid by intravenous infusion, once a day, and then stopped after improvement.

46.4.3 Control convulsions and hyperthermia

Treat patients with sedative agents such as diazepam and phenobarbital. Patients with high fever can be given physical cooling. Diazepam 10 mg intravenous injection, which can be reused according to the condition; or Phenobarbital 100 mg muscle injection, q 8 h.

46.4.4 Anti-infection treatment

Infected patients can be treated with broad-spectrum antibiotics. If necessary, bacterial culture and drug susceptibility test can be made.

46.4.5 Promote the metabolism of brain cells

To give energy mixture and other drugs. Also nerve growth factor, ganglioside ester and others can be given.

46.4.6 Active treatment of complications and postoperative complications

Keep the airway open and tracheotomy if necessary. Pay attention to nursing during coma, prevent bedsore and aspiration pneumonia, strengthen nutrition support.

46.4.7 For patients with delayed encephalopathy

Hyperbaric oxygen, glucocorticoids, vasodilators or antiparkinsonian drugs and other symptomatic and supportive treatments can be given to patients with delayed encephalopathy.

Jian Xiangdong, Zeng Mei

Chapter 47

Venomous Snakebite/Snake Envenoming

47.1　Perspective

Venomous snakebite is a common disease in rural, mountainous or coastal areas in China, especially in Guangdong, Guangxi, Fujian and Yunnan province. With the increase of green landscape area, the number of snake bite injuries of citizens also grows. After a venomous snake bites, potential symptoms, such as muscle paralysis, coagulation dysfunction, acute kidney injury and other multiple organ damage may occur. In extreme cases, respiratory or circulatory failure could also happen.

47.2　Epidemiology

There are nearly 3,000 snakes species in the world, among which 650 species of them are venomous snakes, and 195 highly virulent ones. According to taxonomy, the snakes are classified into 14 families and the venomous snakes takes up 5 of them. There are 61 identified species of snakes in China, belonging to 4 families:Polygonidae, Crotalidae (Viperidae), Elapidae and Hydrophiidae. Compared to other three species, Elapidae is the most virulent species. The classification and distribution of venomous snake are shown in the Table 47-1.

Snakes live in all provinces in China, but they are seen mostly in the south of the Yangtze River and the southwestern regions. The snake species varies among regions and provinces. Guangdong is dominated by Naja, Deinagkistrodon (five-step snake), Bungarus multicinctus, and Trimeresurus stejnegeri (green bamboo snake). Guangxi is dominated by Bungarus multicinctus. Zhejiang province is dominated by Agkistrodon halys. Western part of Hunan is dominated by Deinagkistrodon(five-step snake).

Table 47−1　The classification and distribution of venomous snake

Family	Common species	Distribution in the world	Distribution in China
Viperidae	Viper, "iron head snake"	Worldwide except America	Guangdong, Guangxi, Fujian, Taiwan
Crotalidae	Rattlesnake, sistrurus, trimeresurus (green bamboo snake), agkistrodon acutus (five − step snake), adder (copperhead snake)	America, Asia	Yangtze River region, southeastern and southwestern regions. (Adder can be found across the country except Tibetan Plateau)
Elapidae	Cobra, king cobra, Krait, coral snake,	Worldwide except Europe	South of the Yangtze River
Hydrophiidae	Pelamis platurus	The Indian Ocean & the Pacific Ocean	Coastal areas, especially the southeastern coastal areas
Colubridae	Dispholidus, occamy	Africa	(Not found yet)

Venomous snakebite happens closely related to climate and time of a day. Snakes are poikilotherm, or cold−blooded animals, thus the injuries are frequent in summer and fall, whilst fewer cases are recorded because of their hibernation in winter. In the daytime, the most active species are cobra, king cobra and viper. At night, it is mainly a krait, a coral snake, or a "iron head snake". During the sun rises and sets, Trimeresurus (green bamboo snake), Agkistrodon, Deinagkistrodon (five−step snake), or viper are mostly seen.

The victims of venomous snakebite are mostly young adults, mostly men than women, and rural than urban. The body parts where most of the bites take place are limbs, which accounts for 70% from the lower limbs.

47.3　Pathophysiology

The venom apparatus of the snake is inside their head, which consists of venom gland, the duct and the fangs. The morphology of fangs can help identify the species. When the venomous snake bites, its palatal muscles contract, squeezing the venom gland, and the venom is delivered through the ducts to the fangs, injected into the bite wound, spreading along lymphatic and blood circulation systems, causing local and systemic poisoning symptoms. The absorption of venom happens fast at early stage and slows down overtime. It is distributed across the body, but it's seen mostly in kidneys and the least in the brain. The metabolic decomposition of venom mainly happens in the liver, and it is excreted by the kidneys and partly by the liver.

47.3.1　Local effect

The venoms of Viperidae, Crotalidae, Colubridae mainly cause local effect, inducing the vascular wall injury, necrosis, edema and hemorrhage in the wound, with the proteolytic enzymes and small molecular peptides.

47.3.2　Systemic effect

According to the toxicological effects, snake venom can be divided into three categories.

47.3.2.1　Neurotoxin

Neurotoxin is found in the venom of Elapidae and Hydrophiidae, as well as some certain Viperidae. Neurotoxin could block nerve conduction before and/or after synapse, especially in the neuromuscular transmission, causing the whole body striated muscle relaxative paralysis. This will appear in sequence of head, chest, diaphragm and lower limb, and recover in reverse order. The cause of death is respiratory failure caused by paralysis of the respiratory muscles (intercostal muscle and diaphragm), which make neurotoxin the most venomous. However, neurotoxin has no obvious venomous effects on internal organs.

47.3.2.2　Hemotoxin

Hemotoxinis mainly found in the venom of viper, agkistrodon acutus(five-step snake), trimeresurus (green bamboo snake), iron head snake. Cobra and adder can also contain hemotoxin. There are many types of hemotoxin, such as hemorrhagin, haemorrhagin, anticoagulant, fibrinolytic toxin, cardiotoxin, etc. , which could produce a variety of toxic effects, mainly in the circulatory and hematologic system. In the hematologic system, coagulation dysfunction may occur, as well as bleeding, fibrinolysis, and disseminated intravascular coagulation (DIC). In the circulatory system, hemotoxin could reduce vascular resistance and weaken myocardial contractility with arrhythmia, leading to hemodynamic instability, blood pressure decrease and distributed shock.

47.3.2.3　Snake venom enzyme

The snake venom enzymes contain proteolytic enzyme, phospholipase A_2(PLA_2), hyaluronidase, collagenase etc, which can be found in various species. Proteolytic enzyme could injure vessel endothelial cells, causing the increasing vessel permeability and plasma exudation. Furthermore, it produces the edema, hemorrhage and necrosis, which triggers the body to release histamine and vasoactive substances, causing pain and blood pressure drop, actuating the formation of distributed shock. PLA_2 could hydrolyze the lecithin of cell membrane, causing red blood cells lysis, platelets disintegration, and nerve tissues injury, or assist neurotoxins and cardiotoxins being transferred into nervous system and present neurological symptoms. Hyaluronidase and collagenase could hydrolyze connective tissue, resulting in the spread and aggravation of snake venom.

47.4　Diagnostic apporach

47.4.1　History

History of poisonous snake bites. It can be diagnosed of snakebite if there are 1-2 (or 3-4) large and deep tooth marks left on the wound with local and systemic symptoms. Snakebite wounds often have a pair of large and deep tooth marks or two rows of small tooth marks with a pair of large tooth marks on the surface of the wound. Some big tooth marks even have broken teeth. In addition, there is significant swelling and pain around the wound or there is feeling of numbness in the area, and there are spots, blisters, or blood stasis in the area. Systemic symptoms are also more obvious. Non-venomous snake bites have no tooth marks or two symmetrical small tooth marks. If a snake bite does not show the serpentine shape at night, or if it is impossible to tell if it was a snake, it must be treated as a poisonous snake bite.

47.4.2　Distinguish the type of viper

It is more difficult to accurately determine which viper is causing the wound. It is best to catch the snakes and bring them to the hospital for identifing the species of viper reference books, or to ask the patient or the person in attendance about the serpent morphology. It also can be differentiated according to the snake shape, tooth marks, local symptoms, and systemic symptoms, etc. Identification of poisonous snakes and non-venomous snakes is shown in the Table 47-2.

Table 47-2　Identification of poisonous snakes and non-venomous snakes

	Venomous snake	Non-venomous snake
Snake profile	Venomious snake's head is mostly triangular in shape with brightly colored patterns. And its tail is short and thin, and the upper jaw has pairs of fangs, which can be distinguished from non-venomous snakes	The non-venomous snake 's head is oval in shape, with a monotonous color and a thin, long tail
Tooth mark		Only zigzag tooth marks
Local symptoms	Burns, pain, and rapid expansion (except nerve venomous snake bites). Rapid expansion of redness and swelling(except Bungarus multicinctus or Bungarus fasciatus bites). Hemotoxin can lead to persist bleeding, bruises or blisters on the wound. And mixed poison can cause local skin purpura, ulcers, and necrosis	No obvious redness and swelling, less bleeding and, stop bleeding quickly, no ecchymosis or blood stasis
Systemic symptoms	Dizziness, vertigo, chest tightness, palpitations, chills, even coma, shock, heart and kidney failure, respiratory muscle paralysis, etc.	Prostraion may occur because of patient's mental tension, and there is no other symptoms of systemic poisoning

47.5　Physical examination

Two (or three to four) large and deep tooth marks can be seen on the wound. Severe snake bite poisoning can cause fever, hypotension, tachycardia or bradycardia, which are manifestations of shock or cardiovascular involvement. Neurotoxin can cause ptosis, unclear pronunciation, salivation, ataxia, trismu and reduced nerve reflex. Respiratory failure caused by respiratory muscle paralysis can lead to shortness of breath, hypopnea and even respiratory arrest. Hemotoxin can cause marked redness, fever, tenderness, bleeding, and subcutaneous bleeding. Swelling and subcutaneous bleeding can quickly spread to the entire limb with swelling and pain in nearby lymph nodes. The whole body skin may have blemishes and ecchymosis, jaundice may be seen if hemolysis occurs. Cobra bites cause local tissue necrosis, and local skin becomes dark and loses its sensation, and even forms ulcers. Snake venom sprayed into the eyes can lead to conjunctival and corneal congestion and swelling.

47.6   Ancillary inspection

47.6.1   Basic inspection

47.6.1.1   Blood tests

Almost all viper bites can cause a rise in the total number of white blood cells and in the number of myelocytes, and the degree of increase is related to the degree of poisoning, so blood tests can help identify venomous snake bites and non-venomous snake bites. Those with blood system involvement may have thrombocytopenia, anemia.

47.6.1.2   Urine examination

It helps to understand the damage of the kidneys. Red blood cells in the urine suggest bleeding. Red blood cell negative and protein positive may indicate myoglobinuria.

47.6.1.3   Blood biochemical examination

Routine examination of aspartate aminotransferase (AST), lactate dehydrogenase (LDH), creatine phosphokinase (CK), help to determine the degree of poisoning and the damage to the body. These three enzymes can be significantly elevated account for tissue necrosis caused by cobra bites, and CK can often increases by several hundred times. The renal function is examined to determine the acute renal injury. Elevated blood urea nitrogen (BUN) and creatinine (Cr) suggest acute kidney injury. Blood glucose and electrolytes are also routine examination items which can help to evaluate the volume of the patients. Special attention should be paid to the level of serum potassium. Those with significantly elevated CK should also checked the CK-MB, LDH and troponin.

47.6.2   Special inspection

Laboratory identification examination of snake species can be performed on wound venom, blood or urine by immunological methods such as counter immunoelectrophoresis, ELISA double antibody sandwich, latex agglutination inhibition test and radioimmunoassay. However, most of them are currently in the laboratory research stage and are not commonly used clinically.

47.6.3   Alternative inspection

47.6.3.1   Coagulation function

Person with snake bite of hemotoxin should be examined of prothrombin time (PT), activated partial prothrombin time (APTT). Patients with bleeding tendencies must be checked for complete blood counts, platelet counts, PT, APPT, international normalized ratio (INR), and other coagulation parameters.

47.6.3.2   Blood gas analysis

Patients with respiratory failure should be performed.

47.6.3.3   Electrocardiogram

Patients with cardiac involvement or hyperkalemia may have ectopic rhythm, ST-T changes, QT prolongation and cardiac conduction block, etc.

47.7 Diagnositc table

The diagnosis and treatment of snake bite includes two parts, out-of-hospital and in-hospital rescue. As an adjunct doctor, the primary task is to assess the patient's basic vital signs. Under the premise of maintaining the basic vital signs, the doctor should rapidly identify the severity and type of snake bite, as well as assess the degree of damage to the whole body organs, and fully protect important organ functions. The process of diagnosis and treatment is shown in Figure 47-1.

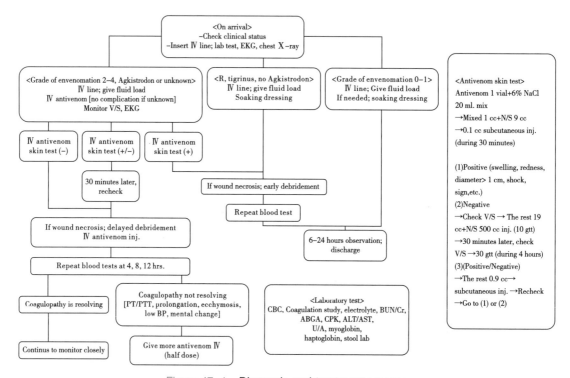

Figure 47-1　Diagnosis and treatment process

47.8 Disposition and management

47.8.1 On-site first aid

To calm the patient first. If it is not clear whether it is a bite by a venomous snake temporarily, it should be initially treated as a snake bite and closely observed. The bite time is recorded, and the size of the bite wound and the surrounding upper and lower ranges are measured to assist in comparing changes in the degree of swelling in the future.

47.8.2 Initial treatment

(1) Using soapy water, distilled water to wash the wound.

(2)Bleeding of the injured limbs: the injured limb can be temporarily braked and then placed in a low position to slow down the spread of venom to the body. At the same time, the limbs and joints should be kept in functional positions to prevent swelling or joints from moving and be promptly taken to the hospital.

(3)If necessary, giving appropriate sedatives to keep the patient quiet. Traditional methods of tying and ice are not recommended, because there is currently no evidence that it can improve the prognosis of snake bite patients.

(4)It is necessary to remove jewelry and tight clothing due to the risk of local swelling.

47.9　Emergency treatment

47.9.1　Rapid stabilization and assessment

Assessing of airway, breathing, circulation rapidly, giving basic life support at the same time. Monitoring of ECG, blood pressure and oxygen status, as well as racing against time to rescue life-threatening toxic effects and protect organ function. According to the clinical symptoms of the patient and the length of symptoms, the clinical grading is performed, as shown in Table 47–3.

Table 47–3　Snake bite severity rating

Severity scale		Manifestations
Grade 0	No envenomation	Local or systemic signs or symptoms absent No symptom development during first 12 hours
Grade I	Minimal	Local swelling<15 cm Absence of systemic signs, normal laboratory findings No systemic involvement after 12 hours
Grade II	Moderate	Swelling extending past bite sites (15–30 cm) One or more systemic sign or symptom Abnormal laboratory findings
Grade III	Severe	Marked (>30 cm) swelling, tissue loss Immediate, multiple, or severe systemic signs, rapid progression of symptoms
Grade IV	Very severe	Sudden pain, rapid development of local reaction, ecchymosis, necrosis, blebs, blisters, swelling severe enough to obstruct venous or arterial flow, swelling may involve ipsilateral trunk Systemic manifestations within 15 minutes*

* Systemic manifestations: nausea & vomiting, dyspnea, dizziness, visual disturbance, hematuria

47.9.2　Wound treatment

Washing wounds can destroy, neutralize, and reduce venom. We can choose 1 : 5,000 potassium permanganate solution, 3% hydrogen peroxide, physiological saline, soapy water, or 1 : 5,000 nitrofurazone solution to wash the wounds. The wounds can be warmed after flushing the them. When flushing, suction can be used. It is not recommended to expand wounds or cut wounds, which may increase tissue damage and local irritation, and there are no proven benefits. It is also not recommended to remove the venom by oral or mechanical suction because there is no evidence that this method is effective. In addition, oral suction can introduce bacteria into the wound and increase the possibility of superinfection or abscess formation. Poisonous fluids may be absorbed through the oral mucosa and may pose a risk to care givers.

47.9.3　Local detoxification

The same or corresponding anti-venom serumcan can block the continued absorption of snake by its ability to neutralize the principle of snake venom. Lidocaine, methylprednisolone, and the same kind of anti-venom serum can be used to add saline to the joints at the proximal end of the wound. In addition, using a 20% magnesium sulfate solution to wet dress the swelling wound can relieve pain, reduce inflammation, reduce tissue allergic reaction to venom and neutralize the effects of snake venom.

47.9.4　Using anti-venom serum as early as possible

The anti-venom serum is an internationally recognized special drug for the treatment of snake wounds. The main component is the horse venom immunoglobulin after digestion by stomach enzymes. Anti-venom serum is rapidly neutralizing and destroying snake venom through antigen-antibody neutralization reactions. The early use of anti-venom serum can make the patient away from poisoning symptoms, and it can control the development of the disease. The anti-venom serum has no direct protective effect on organ damage caused by snake venom.

47.9.4.1　Principle of use

Using the corresponding anti-venom serum according to the type of snake bite. If unknown snake species, drugs can be selected according to the propensity of diagnosis, and even combination therapy can be used.

47.9.4.2　Application timing

The sooner the better, strive to use the best effect within 2 hours after injury. Anti-venom serum should be listed as a regular drug within 24 hours after injury.

47.9.4.3　Dosage of application

In clinical, anti-venom serum application dose, should be based on clinical symptoms, combined with the snake bite time to determine the degree of poisoning.

47.9.4.4　Usage

Opening two intravenous channels to have anti-allergy and anti-venom serum therapy at the same time. The treatment response should be closely observed during anti-venom serum treatment.

47.9.5　Treatment of severe adverse reactions with anti-venom serum

Symptoms include sudden dejection or irritability, pale or flushing, chest tightness or wheezing, cold sweats, nausea or abdominal pain, rapid pulse, low blood pressure, severe coma. Treatment: to stop using anti-venom serum, retain intravenous access, inhale oxygen, inject epinephrine subcutaneously, and to use anti-allergic drugs and adrenocortical hormones. If necessary, add vasopressors.

47.9.6　Strengthen monitoring to prevent possible complications

The monitoring content of different types of snake injury can be focused. Nerve poisonous snake poisoning monitoring focuses on respiratory function including respiratory frequency, rhythm, blood oxygen saturation and blood gas analysis; blood circulation poisonous snake poisoning focuses on monitoring blood routine, urine routine, hourly urine volume; monitoring coagulation function, early prevention and treatment DIC, if necessary, platelets, fibrinogen, etc. Patients with severe anaemia may be given blood transfusions, trying to give fresh blood to supplement clotting factors. Monitor electrocardiogram, myocardial enzymes, detect fatal arrhythmia, and pump failure should be promptly given corresponding treatment, and use of myocardial nutrient. Liver function, serum creatinine, blood urea nitrogen, etc.

47.9.7   The rest of the treatment

(1) Choosing a reasonable antibiotic to control infection.

(2) Short-term use of glucocorticoids can improve the body's venom stress, which also has a certain therapeutic effect on hemorrhage, hemolysis and cell necrosis.

(3) Injecting tetanus antitoxin to prevent tetanus.

(4) Infusion therapy to maintain water and electrolyte balance, maintaining the energy support as well. Critically ill patients with more than 3 days of illness should be given nutritional support.

(5) Chinese herbal medicine treatment. Literature reported that such as Guangdong snake medicine, Nantong snake medicine, etc. can help improve the snake bite symptoms, The doctors flexible to use of local medicine sources.

(6) Surgical treatment. Swelling of snakebite wounds on limbs may consider incision and drainage for decompression, necrotic tissue must be cleared early, so as not to increase the absorption of toxins, promote multiple organ failure. For wound ulceration (mainly found in cobras), it can be treated with plastic surgery.

Wang Lin

Chapter 48

Heat Illness

Heat illness is a heat damage disease caused by the excessive loss of water and electrolyte and the dysfunction of heat dissipation in the human body. It is a life-threatening emergency, which can cause death and permanent brain damage and renal failure due to the central nervous system and circulatory dysfunction. According to the severity of clinical manifestations, it can be divided into: premonitory heat illness, mild heat illness and severe heat illness. Severe heat illness is often divided into heat cramps, heat exhaustion and heatstroke according to its main pathogenesis and clinical manifestations. The three types can develop sequentially or overlapped.

48.1 Etiology and pathogenesis

Heatillness occurs when the rise of temperature is not controlled and beyond the ability of self cooling, while the thermal set point of hypothalamus is often unchanged. Inadequate adaptation to high temperature is the main cause of heat illness. When following factors existed, such as rising atmospheric temperature (above 32 ℃), humidity (above 60%) and wind free environment, long time work or strong manual labor, lack of heat illness prevention, and those who can not adapt to high temperature environment, people are very easy to suffer from heat illness. In addition, in the environment with high temperature and poor ventilation, old and weak and obese people are also prone to heat illness. Generally, the environment with high temperature and humidity is more prone to heat illness than dry heat (high temperature and strong radiation). In the summer heat season, factors such as aging, body weakness, fatigue, obesity, alcohol consumption, hunger, water loss, loss of salt, and wearing tight or impermeable pants and fever, hyperthyroidism, diabetes, cardiovascular diseases, extensive damage of skin, congenital absence of sweat glands, and the use of atropine or other anticholinergic drugs to influence the secretion of sweat glands, are often the cause of the onset of heat illness.

The damage of heatillness is mainly due to the direct damage to cells by hyperthermia (above 42 ℃). At different temperatures, the changes of cell adaptation, injury or death can lead to enzyme denaturation, mitochondrial dysfunction, loss of cell membrane stability and interruption of aerobic metabolic pathways, resulting in multiple organ dysfunction or failure. In addition, the high temperature environment and exercise make the cardiovascular blood be more distributed to the extremities, which reduces the blood flow of the gastrointestinal and other visceral organs to ischemia, and due to endotoxin reaction and oxidative stress. The reduction of brain blood flow makes metabolism and coagulation disorder, which results in central nervous system dysfunction.

The pathogenesis of heat cramps happens when people stay in high temperature environment, the way of human heat dissipation depends mainly on sweating. It is generally believed that the maximum physiological limit sweating per day is 6 liters, but in a high temperature environment, the sweating capacity of workers can be above 10 liters. The sweat contains sodium chloride 0.3% –0.5%. Therefore, excessive sweating makes water and sodium salt lost too much, causing muscle cramp and pain.

The pathogenesis of heat exhaustion is mainly due to the non-adaptation of the human body to the heat environment, which causes the dilatation of the peripheral blood vessels, the insufficiency of circulation blood, and the excess sweating, water loss and salt loss.

48.2   Diagnosis

48.2.1   Clinical manifestation

48.2.1.1   Premonitory heatillness

The symptoms such as dizziness, headache, sweat, thirst, exhaustion, heat palpitations, impaired concentration, disharmony of the movement after a certain period of working in a high temperature environment appear. The body temperature is normal or slightly elevated. If transferred to a cool and ventilated place in a timely manner to rest quietly, and replenished water and salt, patients will recover within a short time.

48.2.1.2   Mild heat illness

In addition to the aggravation of the above symptoms, the body temperature rises above 38 ℃, and symptoms such as the appearance of face flush, a large amount of sweating, burning skin, or the appearance of pale skin, wet cold of the extremities, descent of blood pressure and increasing pulse appear. If handled in a timely and effective manner, patients will restore within a few hours.

48.2.1.3   Severe heat illness

There are three types including heat cramps, heat exhaustion, and heatstroke.

(1) Heat cramps

It often occurs after strong physical labor under high temperature environment. As a result of excessive sweat, a large amount of drinking water and the lack of salt so that the concentration of sodium chloride in the blood drops significantly, which causes the cramps of the extremities, most often in the gastrocnemius muscles of the lower limbs, often accompanied by muscle pain, abdominal colic and hiccup. Most of the body temperature is normal. Laboratory tests show that sodium and chloride are decreased and creatinine is increased. It can be an early manifestation of heatstroke.

(2) Heat exhaustion

It often occurs in the elderly, children, patients with chronic diseases and those who have not adapted to the high temperature environment for a period of time. In severe heat stress, the patient has headache, dizziness, nausea and dizziness, paleness, cold sweating, weak or slow pulse, and low blood pressure due to the excessive loss of circulating blood volume caused by excessive loss of body fluid and body sodium. Symptoms such as syncope and hands or feet convulsions can occur. The body temperature can be slightly elevated. The severe patients have peripheral circulation failure. Laboratory tests show elevated hematocrit, hypernatremia, mild azemia and liver dysfunction. Heat exhaustion can be an intermediate process of heat cramp and heatstroke. If untreated, it will develop into heatstroke.

(3) Heatstroke

A fatal life-threatening emergency occurring when the thermoregulatory mechanisms fail. The failure of the thermoregulatory mechanisms causes extremely elevated body temperature, usually exceeding 40.5 ℃, resulting in multiple system tissue damage and organ failure. According to the status and pathogenesis of the patients at the onset of disease, it is divided into two types: exertional heatstroke and classic heatstroke, and the exertional heatstroke is mainly caused by the endogenous heat production in the high temperature environment; the classic heatstroke is mainly caused by the dysfunction of thermoregulatory mechanisms in the high temperature environment, which causes the decrease of heat dissipation.

1) Exertional heatstroke: it often occurs in the weather with high temperature, high humidity and wind free. Most of the patients are healthy young people who engaged in heavy manual labor or severe exercise in the high temperature environment after several hours. About 50% patients appear symptoms such as excessive sweating, a racing heat rate which ups to 160-180 bpm, and increasing pulse pressure. Rhabdomyolysis, acute renal failure, liver failure, DIC or MODS can appear and lead high mortality.

2) Classic heatstroke: under high temperature environment, it is common in crowded or poorly ventilated environment. Other high-risk groups include schizophrenia, Parkinson's disease, chronic alcoholism, hemiplegia or paraplegia, and those taking diuretics. The patients' skin is dry, hot and reddish. 84% - 100% cases do not sweat. The rectal temperature is usually above 41 ℃, up to 46.5 ℃. Early symptoms of abnormal behavior or epileptic seizures, followed by delirium, coma, severe cases of hypotension, shock, arrhythmia and heat failure, pulmonary edema and brain edema. Acute renal failure occurs in about 5% cases, usually accompanied with DIC, often ts develops into death about 24 hours after the onset of the disease.

48.2.2 Laboratory examination

According to the degree of illness, there can be the increasing of leukocytes and neutrophils numbers, AST, ALT, creatinine, urea, LDH and CK. In addiction, following manifestations such as thrombocytopenia, abnormal coagulation function, urine protein, tube type, blood concentration, electrolyte disorder, respiratory and metabolic acidosis, and cardiographic examination of arrhythmia or cardiac damage are also very comman. Evidence of dysfunction of vital organs should be detected as early as possible. When cranial hemorrhage or infection is suspected, cranial CT and cerebrospinal fluid examination should be done. Note that liver damage is the inherent characteristic of heatstroke. If the patient has no liver damage, he should be excluded from heatstroke.

48.3　Therapeutics

48.3.1　Premonitory heatillness and mild heatillness

Patients should be evacuated from the high temperature environment immediately, and have a rest in the cool place. Meanwhile, refreshing and salty drinks should be added. If there is a tendency of circulatory failure, glucose saline can be injected intravenously. Physical cooling should be used in time when the body temperature increases.

48.3.2　Heat cramps

Patients should be quickly transferred to a cool and ventilated place to rest. Patients with no dehydrated symptoms should be treated with 0.1%–0.2% saline and cool salt drink. Severe cases should be intravenously supplemented with saline or 5% glucose saline, by which patients usually can be recovered for 30 minutes to several hours after treatment.

48.3.3　Heat exhaustion

Quickly transfer the patient to a cool and ventilated place to rest. The basic feature of heat exhaustion is reduced blood volume. Patients usually recover quickly after receiving fluid. The amount of fluid or electrolyte should be determined according to the measurement of serum electrolyte. Patients with severe reduction of blood volume and electrolyte disorders usually need intravenous fluids. If symptoms are related to body position, adequate saline should be supplemented until hemodynamic stability is maintained. Water shortage can be slowly replenished within 48 hours, and plasma osmotic pressure should not fall faster than 2 mOsm/h. Excessive correction of hypernatremia can cause brain edema.

48.3.4　Heat stroke

Rapid cooling is the basis of treatment. Mortality is often associated with body temperature and organ dysfunction. If anuria, coma or heat failure occurs, the risk of death will increase. The temperature of the rectum should be reduced to less than 38.5 ℃ within one hour.

48.3.4.1　In vitro cooling methods

Transfering patients to a well ventilated and low temperature environment, remove their clothes, massage their limbs and skin, which expand skin blood vessels, accelerate blood circulation and promote heat dissipation. For patients without circulatory collapse, cold water can be used to bathe or immerse the body in water at 27–30 ℃. The patients with circulation deficiency can be cooled by evaporation, such as wiping the skin repeatedly with cold water at 15 ℃, or using an electric fan or air conditioner at the same time, or placing ice bags in the head, axillary and groin, all of which accelerate the heat dissipation. Without mentioned above conditions, patients who are in rural areas can be scrubbed with well water or spring water to promote evaporation and cooling.

48.3.4.2　Cooling methods in the body

If in vitro cooling methods are ineffective, we can use ice saline for gastric or rectal lavage, or use 5% glucose saline 1,000–2,000 mL for intravenous drip(the drop speed should be controlled at 30–40 drops/minute at the beginning), and saline at 20 ℃ or 9 ℃ also can be used for hemodialysis or peritoneal dialysis. Furthermore, the autotransfusion of autologous blood after cooling in vitro is also effective on cooling.

48.3.4.3　Drug cooling methods

Chlorpromazine is used commonly. Usage: dilute chlorpromazine 25–50 mg in 500 mL glucose saline or physiological saline for intravenous drip in 1 to 2 hours. When the condition is urgent, chlorpromazine and promethazine 25 mg can be diluted in the 5% glucose solution 100–200 mL and finished in 10–20 minutes. If the body temperature is still not descended within 1 hour, it can be repeated once. When the anal temperature drops to about 38 ℃, it should be suspended. If the body temperature rises, it can be repeatedly applied. Patients with the history of cardiovascular disease should be given carefully use of chlorpromazine and promethazine.

48.3.4.4 Brain edema and seizure preventing

Mannitol can be used. To a certain extent, glucocorticoids can cool, improve the body's responsiveness and reduce intracranial pressure. Albumin can also be used as appropriate. An irritable or convulsive patient can be given intramuscular injection of diazepam 10 mg or phenobarbital sodium 0. 1–0. 2 g/times.

48.3.4.5 Comprehensive and symptomatic treatment

It is necessary to keep the patient's respiratory tract unobstructed and give them oxygen. When coma or respiratory failure occurs, the patient should be intubated and mechanically ventilated. Besides, sodium and fluid should be replenished to maintain balance between water and electrolyte and acidosis should be corrected. Furthermore, when hypotension occurs, isotonic crystalloid solution should be applied in time to supplement blood volume, and effective blood volume should be assessed by monitoring urine volume. Vasoactive agents such as dopamine should be used if necessary.

Patients who has pulmonary edema can be given Lanatoside C, furosemide, glucocorticoid, and sedative. If there is an occurrence of rhabdomyolysis, the amount of urine should be maintained at least 2 mL/(kg · h). Persistent anuria, uremia and hyperkalemia are the indications for hemodialysis. Don't use antipyretic drugs and sedatives that can cause liver damage. B vitamins, vitamin C and brain cell activators can be used. It is important to prevent and treat heart, liver, kidney and respiratory insufficiency. When necessary, antibiotics should be used to prevent infection.

Wang Lin

Section 5

Disaster Medicine

Chapter 49

Disaster Medicine

Disasters occur in all areas of the world and cause harm to people, property, infrastructures, economies and the environment. Harm to people includes death, injury, disease, malnutrition, and psychological stress. Recent catastrophes include earthquakes in China(2008) and Haiti (2010), devastating tsunamis in the Indian Ocean(2004) and Japan (2011), massive hurricanes in the southern United States (2005), severe flooding in Australia (2011), and unusual weather conditions producing record snowfalls in the United States and Europe (2011). Increasing population density in floodplains and in earthquake and hurricane-prone areas may be a herald of future catastrophic disasters with large numbers of casualties.

Factors that indicate an increasing probability of mass casualty incidents include terrorist activity; increasing population density in floodplains, seismic zones and areas susceptible to hurricanes; production and transportation of thousands of toxic and hazardous materials; risks associated with fixed-site nuclear and chemical facilities; the possibility of catastrophic fires and explosions as well as global warming. For example, the U. S. Geological Survey has identified volcanoes in the western United States and Alaska that are likely to erupt in the future, including Mt. Hood, Mt. Shasta, and the volcano underlying Mammoth Lakes in California. Because of the rising population density in these areas, hazards from volcanic activity are increasing.

Given this probability and the increasing role of emergency medicine in disaster preparation, mitigation, response and recovery, this chapter discusses disaster planning and operations with emphasis on the role of the emergency physician. The emergency physician has extensive responsibilities for community disaster preparedness and disaster medical services, including response to terrorism. In position and policy documents, the American College of Emergency Physicians outlines the scope of emergency medicine's involvement in preparedness and response to disaster and terrorism, stating that "emergency physicians should assume a primary role in the medical aspects of disaster planning, management, and patient care" and that "emergency department personnel will become the first responders to a covert biological attack".

A committed emergency department alone is insufficient to provide hospitals with a successful disaster preparedness program. Institutional commitment by every hospital department and the administration is necessary to coordinate effectively with system-wide resources for disaster management.

Yang Yuxia, Zhu Changju

Chapter 50

The Principle of Group Injury Treatment

50.1 Perspective

The science of injury management is based on the concept that trauma in the disaster is like a disease rather than just the consequence of fate or random occurrences. The principle of managing a disease as widespread and multifactorial as injury can occur only through broad interdisciplinary effort, including that of medicine, public health, policy makers, law enforcement, educated citizens and others.

50.2 Principles

The major causes of group injury include earthquakes, tsunamis, hurricanes, flooding, car crashes, gunshots, drownings, and poisonings. Similar to other disease models, injury occurs from the interaction of agent and host through a vector and an environment that is conducive to exposure. Injury is a harmful event caused by the acute transfer of energy to a person that results in tissue and/or organ damage. Energy is the agent that is delivered to the host by a vector in an environment with variable risk.

The goal of injury control, similar to other forms of disease control, is to prevent or decrease the transfer of energy to the host by separating the host from the agent through modification of the environment, equipping the host with protection against the agent, or eliminating or modifying the vector that transmits the energy.

50.3 Injury control in medical practice

Emergency physicians play an important role in risk assessment, counseling, and referral of patients in high-risk groups for injury, such as with domestic violence patients. Emergency care providers are pivotal in the recording and accumulation of data about the injury event, which is useful for surveillance and epidemiologic analysis. Injury control techniques can be incorporated easily into emergency medicine practice as well. A rational approach to improve injury care in a community requires that emergency physicians, surgeons, pediatricians, and psychiatrists assume specific roles and activities in promoting injury control. This role for emergency physicians in injury control has been advocated by the Chinese College of Emergency Physicians. Documentation of injury information in the medical record, assessing risk factors in individual patients, counseling and referral, provision of systematized acute trauma, and public health advocacy are all important.

Yang Yuxia, Zhu Changju

Chapter 51

Traffic Crash

51.1 Introduction

A traffic crash, also called a motor vehicle collision (MVC) among other terms, occurs when a vehicle collides with another vehicle, pedestrian, animal, road debris, or other stationary obstruction, such as a tree, pole or building. Traffic crash is usually classified into vehicle accidents, motorcycle accidents, bicycle accidents and pedestrian accidents. A wide range of traffic crash also includes train accidents. Traffic crashes often result in injury, death, and property damage.

51.2 Characteristics of the hazards

51.2.1 Characteristics of the disaster

51.2.1.1 High incidence, mortality and disability

Every year the lives of more than 1.25 million people are cut short as a result of a road traffic crash. Between 20 and 50 millions people suffer non-fatal injuries, with many incurring a disability as a result of their injury. Road traffic injuries cause considerable economic losses to individuals, their families, and to nations as a whole.

51.2.1.2 Drivers, vehicles and road environment factors

Driver factors include fatigue or sleep deprivation, motor vehicle speed, driving under the influence of alcohol or other psychoactive substances, nonuse of motorcycle helmets, seat-belts and child restraints, distracted driving and so on. Vehicle factors mainly include mechanical failure and design defects. Road or environmental factors include road design and construction defects, icy road and visibility reduction etc.

51.2.1.3 The disaster prevention

Governments need to take action to address road safety in a holistic manner. This requires involvement from multiple sectors such as transport, police, health, education, and actions that address the safety of roads, vehicles, and road users. Effective interventions include designing safer infrastructure and incorporating road safety features into land-use and transport planning, improving the safety features of vehicles, improving post-crash care for victims of road crashes, setting and enforcing laws relating to key risks, and raising public awareness.

51.2.2　Types of traffic injury

51.2.2.1　Collision injury

The body collides with vehicles or other blunt objects, resulting in injury.

51.2.2.2　Mangled injury

The body is damaged by rolling and extrusion of vehicle tires.

51.2.2.3　Cutting or stabbing injury

The human body is cut and pierced by sharp objects such as glass and metal.

51.2.2.4　Fall injury

Traffic crash causes the human body flying outside or outside the car, and then falling down or falling behind, and cause injury by hitting the ground or other objects.

51.2.2.5　Whiplash injury

In car crash or emergency braking, the cervical spine and cervical spinal cord injury are caused by excessive neck extension or excessive anterior curvature.

51.2.2.6　Safety belt injury

In traffic crash, drivers and occupants are injured when using seat belts.

51.2.2.7　Steering wheel injury

When the vehicle impacts, the driver hits the steering wheel, causing the injury of the upper abdomen and the lower chest.

51.2.2.8　Burn or explosive injury

It is caused by fire and explosion after vehicle impact.

51.2.3　Characteristics of injury

51.2.3.1　Many injury factors and complicated mechanism of injury

In the process of traffic crash, there are many factors causing injury and complicated injury mechanism. Multiple injuries can occur at the same time. The same kind of injuries may occur in multiple body parts and systems.

51.2.3.2　Serious injury and high mortality

Due to the complicated injury mechanism of traffic injury, complicated injuries are easily caused by a series of complex systemic stress reactions, The incidence of multiple injuries, complex injuries and shock is high.

51.2.3.3　Difficulty in diagnosis and treatment

Closed and open injuries are very common in traffic injuries. There are multiple sites and multiple system damage at the same time. It is very difficult to make timely, accurate and complete diagnosis and treatment of multiple traffic injuries.

51.3 Rescue of traffic crash

51.3.1 Environmental assessment and self-protection

It is important to ensure the safety of the wounded and the rescuers on the spot. The risk factors after traffic crash include vehicle, dangerous substance, fire, dust and blood and body fluid of the wounded. Rescuers should have self-protection awareness, correctly assess the potential or ongoing risks, take effective measures to avoid hurting themselves and other personnel. The most common, simple and effective methods are to set up reminder signs, use lights and reflective vests to prevent other traffic injuries. At the same time, we should also pay attention to whether the vehicle will burn or explode, whether there is danger of falling rocks or collapsing.

51.3.2 Assessment of the type of accident and the sorting of the wounded

The number and severity of the wounded, if necessary, need to be assessed from Emergency Medical Services (EMS) system, fire protection, police and other support. Ask for help before the rescue begins. A large number of wounded may occur in traffic crash. Conventionally the wounded are divided into four classifications, marked by corresponding colors: red, yellow, green and black. According to a brief history of medical history and physical examination, a preliminary assessment of the wounded is made to determine the type of rescue required for the wounded, to shorten the first aid time, and to give priority to the wounded who need the most emergency rescue. The correct on-the-spot treatment of traffic injuries is the key and foundation for successful treatment. It mainly included maintaining respiratory and circulatory functions, hemostasis, oxygen supply, resuscitation, fracture fixation, protecting wounds and reducing pollution.

51.3.3 Cooperation of emergency-related organizations

To transport critically injured patients to emergency facilities quickly and smoothly, the police, firefighters, medical rescuers and other rescuers should take their responsibilities and coordinate with each other. Therefore, establishing a regional emergency plan in advance is very important. In this plan, a person (generally as the chief leader of the police or the fire department) should be identified as commander in chief, and he is fully responsible for the unified command and coordination at the scene of the accident.

51.3.4 Medical evacuation

According to the principle of serious patient's priority, the wounded are transported quickly and safely in batches. Before evacuation, the wounded should be checked and classified again. For those with active bleeding or life-threatening injuries on the way, they should be rescued first, and then be transferred after the condition is stable or intensive care should be taken in transit. During transportation, we should handle the wounded correctly and avoid the second injury. At the same time, we must closely observe the changes of injuries, conscientiously fill in the medical records and transfer cards and submit them to the medical institutions receiving them.

Zhang Rui, Zhu Changju

Chapter 52

Cardiopulmonary Resuscitation

Cardiopulmonary resuscitation is a lifesaving technique for victims of sudden cardiac arrest. In 2015, the American Heart Association (AHA) published the"lines Update for Cardiopulmonary Resuscitation and Emergency Cardiovascular Care", including recommendations for adult basic life support (BLS) and CPR quality.

52.1 Epidemiology

In Beijing, China, 0.18% of hospitalized patients had cardiopulmonary arrest during their hospitalization. Of these, 86.6% of patients underwent CPR. The most common causes of cardiopulmonary arrest were the diseases of respiratory system (29.3%) and circulatory system (19.0%). The most common initial rhythm was bradycardia (72.4%). About 62.1% had ROSC. About 28.2% patients survived to hospital discharge, 14.5% survived 6 months post discharge, and 12.1% survived 1 year post discharge. The rate of in-hospital CPR in the U.S. increased, and CPR recipients had become younger and sicker over time. It is estimated that between 236,000 and 325,000 patients are treated for out-of-hospital cardiac arrest each year in the United States. Survival to discharge has improved by 41.3%. Functional outcomes after in-hospital CPR appear to have worsened, with considerable clinical and economic implications. Between 2000 and 2009, CPR incidence was increased by 33.7%, from 1 case per 453 to 1 case per 339 in-hospital patients. Compared to CPR recipients in 2000—2001, those in 2008—2009 were more often younger and higher comorbidity scores. Adjusted rate of survival to discharge was increased by 41.3%. Compared to survivors in 2000, those discharged in 2009 were more often discharged to hospice; a 35% decrease in discharge to home was noted. Mean cost of hospitalization per day was increased for both survivors and decedents.

52.2 Etiology

Understanding the causes of cardiac arrest directs therapy and diagnostic testing during resuscitation and in the immediate postarrest period (Table 52-1).

52.2.1 Angiocardiopathy

Cardiac arrest from a primary cardiac origin typically presents as ventricular fibrillation (VF) or less often as pulseless ventricular tachycardia (VT). Coronary artery disease is the most common pathologic condition found in patients who die suddenly from VF. Autopsy studies show a 75% incidence of previous myocardial infarction (MI) and a 20%–30% incidence of acute MI. Other anatomic abnormalities associated with sudden cardiac arrest caused by VF or VT include myocardial hypertrophy, cardiomyopathy, and specifc structural abnormalities. Pulseless electrical activity (PEA) and asystole are less common initial presenting rhythms in patients with cardic arrest. These rhythms most often occur as a deterioration of VF or VT or develop in response to resuscitation treatments, such as central nervous system(CNS), chronic obstructive pulmonary disease(COPD). Primary respiratory failure generally causes initial hypertension and tachycardia, followed by hypotension and bradycardia and progressing to PEA, VF, or asystole. Circulatory obstruction (e. g. , tension pneumothorax, pericardial tamponade) and hypovolemia generally present with initial tachycardia and hypotension, progressing through bradycardia to PEA, but also may deteriorate to VF or asystole.

Table 52-1   Common Causes of Nontraumatic Cardiac Arrest

General	Specific	Disease/Agent
Cardiac		Coronary artery disease
		Cardiomyopathies
		Structural abnormalities
		Valve dysfunction
Respiratory	Hypoventilation	CNS dysfunction
		Neuromuscular disease
		Toxic and metabolic encephalopathies
	Upper airway obstruction	CNS dysfunction
		Foreign body
		Infection
		Trauma
		Neoplasm
	Pulmonary dysfunction	Asthma, COPD
		Pulmonary edema
		Pulmonary embolus
		Pneumonia
Circulatory	Mechanical obstruction	Tension pneumothorax
		Pericardial tamponade
		Pulmonary embolus
	Hypovolemia	Hemorrhage
	Vascular tone	Sepsis
		Neurogenic
Metabolic	Electrolyte abnormalities	Hypokalemia or hyperkalemia
		Hypermagnesemia
		Hypomagnesemia
		Hypocalcemia

Continue to Table 52-1

General	Specific	Disease/Agent
Toxic	Prescription medications	Antidysrhythmics
		Digitalis beta-blockers
		Calcium channel blockers
		Tricyclic antidepressants
	Drugs of abuse	Cocaine
		Heroin
	Toxins	Carbon monoxide
		Cyanide
Environmental		Lightning
		Electrocution
		Hypothermia or hyperthermia
		Drowning/near-drowning

52.2.2   Hyperkalemia

The most common metabolic cause of cardiac arrest is *hyperkalemia*, which is seen most frequently in patients with renal failure. Hyperkalemia results in progressive widening of the QRS complex, which can deteriorate to VT, VF, asystole, or PEA. Other electrolyte abnormalities (e. g. , hypomagnesemia, hypermagnesemia, hypokalemia) may lead to signifcant arrhythmia, but the frequency with which they cause cardiac arrest is not documented.

52.2.3   Drug toxicity

Cardiac arrest caused by drug toxicity has specifc characteristics depending on the drug involved. Specifc therapy directed at drug toxicity is essential but may not be immediately effective. Prolonged resuscitation efforts may be needed using a method that provides adequate perfusion.

52.2.4   Electrocution

Electrocution causes cardiac arrest through primary arrhythmia or apnea. Alternating current in the range of 100 mA to 1 A generally causes VF, whereas currents greater than 10 A can cause ventricular asystole. Lightning produces a massive direct current electrocution that can result in asystole and prolonged apnea.

52.2.5   Hypothermia

Hypothermia-induced cardiac arrest can present with any electrocardiogram (ECG) rhythm disorder, and successful resuscitation depends on rapid rewarming, which often requires aggressive and invasive measures [e. g. , peritoneal lavage, cardiopulmonary bypass (CPB), open-chest cardiac massage (OCCM)].

52.2.6   Drowning

Drowning is a form of asphyxia usually resulting in bradyasystolic arrest. Because drowning is often accompanied by hypothermia, the victim may beneft from prolonged resuscitation efforts similar to resuscitation efforts for hypothermia.

52.3   Early access: emergency medical dispatch

The first contact with emergency medical services (EMS) is usually via 1-2-0(China),9-1-1(U. S. A) or 1-1-2(EV) emergency call. The correct and timely identification of cardiac arrest is critical to ensuring the followings: the appropriate dispatch of a high-priority response, the provision of telephone CPR instructions, and the activation of community first responders carrying AEDs. In an observational study in the Netherlands, cases of cardiac arrestis were missed at initial telephone triage had much worse outcomes, 5% survival versus 14%. Optimizing EMS dispatch is likely to be one of the most cost-effective solutions to improve outcomes from cardiac arrest. Thus, optimizing the ability of dispatchers to identify cardiac arrest and deliver telephone CPR instructions are critical to improving outcomes.

52.4   Clinical features and management

Most cardiac arrest cases managed in the emergency department (ED) initially occur out-of-hospital. An increasing number of first responders, nontraditional providers, and public venues are being equipped with automated defibrillators. Dramatic resuscitation rates have been achieved when these programs enable providers to deliver counter shock within less than 4-5 minutes of arrest onset. Programs that fail to enable a significant number of patients to be defibrillated within this critical time window have limited or no effect on survival.

Advanced life support (ALS) units staffed by paramedics often have standing orders to follow advanced protocols. Because quality of CPR and time to defibrillation are the two most important determinants of outcome, there is no evidence to support interrupting properly performed advanced measures to transport a patient who is still in cardiac arrest. In cases of cardiac arrest refractory to properly performed advanced measures, the patient may be pronounced dead at the scene if appropriate protocols have been outlined within the system.

52.4.1   History

Historical information from the family, bystanders, and EMS personnel provides key information regarding cause and prognosis. Information surrounding the event includes whether the arrest was witnessed, the time of arrest, what the patient was doing (e. g. , eating, exercising, trauma), the possibility of drug ingestion, time of initial CPR, initial ECG rhythm, and interventions by EMS providers. Important past medical history includes baseline health and mental status; previous heart, lung, renal, or malignant disease; hemorrhage; infection; and risk factors for coronary artery disease and pulmonary embolism. The patient's current medications and allergies also should be obtained, if it is possible.

52.4.2   Physical examination

Physical examination of a cardiac arrest patient is necessarily focused on a few key goals: ensureting adequacy of airway maintenance and ventilation, confirming the diagnosis of cardiac arrest, finding evidence of cause, and monitoring for complications of therapeutic interventions. This examination must occur in descending order of importance, simultaneous with therapeutic interventions, and must be repeated frequently to assess for the response to therapy and occurrence of complications (Table 52–2).

Table 52–2 Potential cause of cardiac arrest and complications of therapy

Physical examination	Abnormalities	Potential causes
General	Pallor	Hemorrhage
	Cold	Hypothermia
Airway	Secretions, vomitus, or blood	Aspiration
		Airway obstruction
	Resistance to positive – pressure ventilation	Tension pneumothorax
		Airway obstruction
		Bronchospasm
Neck	Jugular venous distention	Tension pneumothorax
		Cardiac tamponade
		Pulmonary embolus
	Tracheal deviation	Tension pneumothorax
Chest	Median sternotomy scar	Underlying cardiac disease
Lungs	Unilateral breath sounds	Tension pneumothorax
		Right main stem intubation
		Aspiration
	Distant or no breath sounds or no chest expansion	Esophageal intubation
		Airway obstruction
		Severe bronchospasm
	Wheezing	Aspiration
		Bronchospasm
		Pulmonary edema
	Rales	Aspiration
		Pulmonary edema
		Pneumonia
Heart	Audible heart tones	Hypovolemia
		Cardiac tamponade
		Tension pneumothorax
		Pulmonary embolus
Abdomen	Distended and dull	Ruptured abdominal aortic aneurysm or ruptured ectopic pregnancy
	Distended, tympanitic	Esophageal intubation
		Gastric insufflation
Rectal	Blood, melena	Gastrointestinal hemorrhage
Extremities	Asymmetrical pulses	Aortic dissection
	Arteriovenous shunt or fistula	Hyperkalemia
Skin	Needle tracks or abscesses	Intravenous drug abuse
	Burns	Smoke inhalation
		Electrocution

Cardiopulmonary arrest is defined by the triad of unconsciousness, apnea, and pulselessness. The pulse must be palpated for in a large artery (carotid or femoral). If any question exists as to the diagnosis of pulselessness, CPR should be initiated and pulselessness confirmed by such methods as handheld vascular Doppler ultrasound or end-tidal carbon dioxide monitoring. Rapid bedside ultrasound may confirm loss of cardiac activity, but CPR should not be interrupted to determine this, except in the very late phases of the resuscitation, when termination of resuscitative efforts is contemplated. With sudden onset of circulatory arrest, as in VF, loss of consciousness occurs within 15 seconds, although agonal gasping respirations may persist for several minutes. A brief seizure may result from cessation of cerebral blood flow. Primary respiratory arrest results in transient tachycardia and hypertension that progress to loss of consciousness, bradycardia, and pulselessness, usually within 5 minutes.

After the initial minutes of cardiac arrest, physical examination may provide little evidence of the duration of arrest. Pupils dilate within 1 minute but constrict if CPR is initiated immediately and performed effectively. Dependent lividity and rigor mortis develop after hours of cardiac arrest. Temperature is an unreliable predictor of duration of cardiac arrest because it does not decrease significantly during the first hour of arrest. Moderate to severe hypothermia may cause cardiac arrest or may be caused by prolonged arrest, with opposite prognostic implications.

52.4.3 Monitoring

Traditional monitoring during CPR has relied on evaluation of the ECG in one or more leads and palpation of carotid or femoral artery pulse. Although the lack of a palpable pulse during CPR may indicate inadequate forward flow, the degree of forward flow can not be estimated accurately in the presence of a palpable pulse because pressures generated during CPR may be transmitted equally to the venous and the arterial vasculatures. In addition, myocardial blood flow does not depend on the palpated arterial systolic pressure, but rather on the difference between aortic diastolic pressure and right atrial diastolic pressure (coronary perfusion pressure). ECG monitoring during cardiac arrest indicates the presence or absence of electrical but not mechanical activity. Although these two monitoring modalities may be the best attainable incertain circumstances, they do not provide reliable information regarding the effectiveness of CPR and interventions or prognosis.

Unfortunately, no ideal monitoring technique provides all the information that might be desired during resuscitation, and even the modalities discussed next are often diffcult or impossible to establish or interpret during CPR. A brief overview is provided of coronary perfusion pressure (CPP), end-tidal carbon dioxide (ET_{CO2}), and central venous oxygen saturation (S_{CVO2}) monitoring, of which can be used to detect inadequate CPR with high specifcity (Table 52-3). In addition, several of these techniques are useful in the immediate postarrest period.

Table 52-3　Inadequate blood flow during cardiopulmonary resuscitation

Monitoring technique	Indicator
Carotid or femoral pulse	Not palpable
CPP	<15 mmHg
ET_{CO2}	<10 mmHg (before vasopressor)
S_{CVO2}	<40%

52.4.4　Resuscitation

Restoration of adequate cardiac function is the defining factor of Return of Spontaneous Cridulation (ROSC), restoration of normal brain function is the defining factor of successful resuscitation. The likelihood of achieving both of these goals decreases with every minute which the patient remains in cardiac arrest.

Early high-quality CPR saves lives. Important quality performance measures include compression rate (100-120 per minute), compression depth (>5 cm), duty cycle (at least 60% of time in compression), full relaxation, and minimum pauses especially before and after defibrillation. Furthermore hyperventilation has been shown to be common and reduces cardiac output during CPR. A 30 : 2 compression-to-ventilation ratio is currently recommended for health care professionals in all adult resuscitation scenarios, and with continued emphasis on the simplified universal Adult Basic Life Support (BLS) Algorithm. It may be reasonable for EMS providers to use a rate of 10 breaths per minute (1 breath every 6 seconds) to provide asynchronous ventilation during continuous chest compressions before placement of an advanced airway. The single rescuer is to initiate chest compression before giving rescue breaths (C-A-B rather than A-B-C) to reduce delay to first compressions. Although recent evidence suggests that chest-compression-only CPR is effective when performed by bystanders in the out-of-hospital setting, there is inadequate evidence to recommend this as an alternative strategy for heath care professionals, except when inadequate personnel are present to provide compressions, ventilation, and other resuscitative activites. Intubation should be performed only when capable personnel are available and without interruption of chest compressions. Use of supraglottic airway adjuncts such as the esophageal tracheal combitube and laryngeal mask airways may be good alternatives for airway management in the out-of-hospital phase of resuscitation with the main disadvantage being the inability to use the trachea as a route of drug administration. In addition to monitoring specific CPR performance parameters, physiologic monitoring, if available, can help optimize CPR quality for the individual patient (Table 52-3). Table 52-4 is an algorithm for management of cardiac arrest, lists the key elements of adult, child, and infant CPR.

Table 52-4　Summary of high-quality CPR components for BLS providers

Component	Adults	Children	Infants
Scene safety	Make sure the environment is safe for rescuers and victim		
Recognition of cardiac arrest	Check for responsiveness No breathing or only gasping (ie, no normal breathing) No definite pulse felt within 10 seconds (Breathing and pulse check can be performed simultaneously in less than 10 seconds)		
Activation of emergency response system	If you are alone with no mobile phone, leave the victim to activate the emergency response system and get the AED before beginning CPR Otherwise, send someone and begin CPR immediately; use the AED as soon as it is available	Witnessed collapse Follow steps for adults and adolescents on the left Unwitnessed collapse Give 2 minutes of CPR Leave the victim to activate the emergency response system and get the AED Return to the child or infant and resume CPR; use the AED as soon as it is available	

Continue to Table 52-4

Component	Adults	Children	Infants
Compression ventilation ratio without advanced airway	1 or 2 rescuers 30 : 2	1 rescuer 30 : 2 2 or more rescuers 15 : 2	
Compression ventilation ratio with advanced airway	Continuous compressions at a rate of 100-120/min Give 1 breath every 6 seconds (10 breaths/min)		
Compression rate	100-120/min		
Compression depth	At least 2 inches (5 cm)	At least one third AP diameter of chest About 2 inches (5 cm)	At least one third AP diameter of chest About 1 inches (4 cm)
Hand placement	2 hands on the lower half of the breastbone (sternum)	2 hands or 1 hand (optional for very small child) on the lower half of the breastbone (sternum)	1 rescuer 2 fingers in the center of the chest, just below the nipple line 2 or more rescuers 2 thumb-encircling hands in the center of the chest, just below the nipple line
Chest recoil	Allow full recoil of chest after each compression; do not lean on the chest after each compression		
Minimizing interruptions	Limit interruptions in chest compressions to less than 10 seconds		

52.4.4.1　Chains of survival

Separate Chains of Survival (Figure 52-1) have been recommended that identify the different pathways of care for patients who experience cardiac arrest in the hospital as distinct from out-of-hospital settings. The care for all post-cardiac arrest patients, regardless of where their arrests occur, converges in the hospital, generally in an intensive care unit where post-cardiac arrest care is provided. The elements of structure and process that are required before that convergence are very different for the 2 settings. Patients who have an out-of-hospital cardiac arrest(OHCA) depend on their community for support. Rescuers must recognize the arrest, call for help, and initiate CPR and provide defibrillation [i. e. , public-access defibrillation (PAD)] until a team of professionally trained emergency medical service (EMS) providers assumes responsibility and then transports the patient to an emergency department and/or cardiac catheterization lab. The patient is ultimately transferred to a critical care unit for continued care. In contrast, patients who have an in-of-hospital cardiac arrest(IHCA) depend on a system of appropriate surveillance (e. g. , rapid response or early warning system) to prevent cardiac arrest. If cardiac arrest occurs, patients depend on the smooth interaction of the institution's various departments and services and on a multidisciplinary team of professional providers, including physicians, nurses, respiratory therapists, and others.

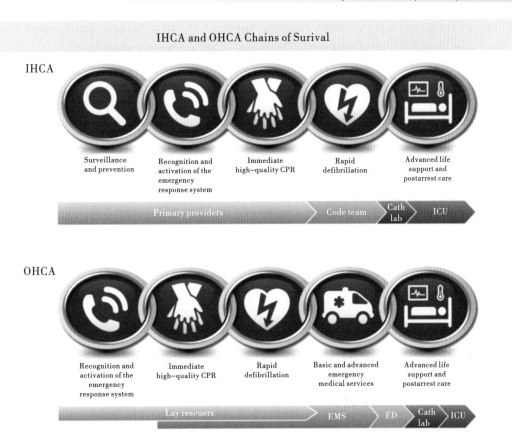

Figure 52-1   IHCA and OHCA chains of survival

52.4.4.2   Use of social media to summon rescuers

It may be reasonable for communities to incorporate social media technologies that summon rescuers who are in close proximity to a victim of suspected OHCA and are willing and able to perform CPR. There is limited evidence to support the use of social media by dispatchers to notify potential rescuers of a possible cardiac arrest nearby, and activation of social media has not been shown to improve survival from OHCA. However, in a recent study in Sweden, there was a significant increase in the rate of bystander-initiated CPR when a mobile-phone dispatch system was used. Given the low harm and the potential benefit, as well as the ubiquitous presence of digital devices, municipalities could consider incorporating these technologies into their OHCA systems of care.

52.4.4.3   Team resuscitation

For adult patients, rapid response team (RRT) or medical emergency team (MET) systems can be effective in reducing the incidence of cardiac arrest, particularly in the general care wards. RRTs or METs were established to provide early intervention for patients with clinical deterioration, with the goal of preventing IHCA. Teams can be composed of varying combinations of physicians, nurses, and respiratory therapists. These teams are usually summoned to a patient bedside when acute deterioration is identified by hospital staff. The team typically brings emergency monitoring and resuscitation equipment and drugs. Although the evidence is still evolving, there is face validity in the concept of having teams trained in the complex choreography of resuscitation.

52.4.4.4   Dispatcher identification of agonal gasps

Cardiac arrest victims sometimes present with seizure-like activity or agonal gasps that can confuse potential rescuers. Dispatchers should be specifically trained to identify these presentations of cardiac arrest to enable prompt recognition and immediate dispatcher–guided CPR. To help bystanders recognize cardiac arrest, dispatchers should inquire about a victim's absence of responsiveness and quality of breathing (normal versus not normal). If the victim is unresponsive with absent or abnormal breathing, the rescuer and the dispatcher should assume that the victim is in cardiac arrest. Dispatchers should be educated to identify unresponsiveness with abnormal and agonal gasps across a range of clinical presentations and descriptions.

52.4.4.5　Chest compressions

Untrained lay rescuers should provide compression–only (hands–only) CPR, with or without dispatcher guidance, for adult victims of cardiac arrest. The rescuer should continue compression–only CPR until the arrival of an AED or rescuers with additional training. All lay rescuers should, at a minimum, provide chest compressions for victims of cardiac arrest. In addition, if the trained lay rescuer is able to perform rescue breaths, he or she should add rescue breaths in a ratio of 30 compressions to 2 breaths. The rescuer should continue CPR until an AED arrives and is ready for use, EMS providers take over care of the victim, or the victim starts to move. Compression–only CPR is easy for an untrained rescuer to perform and can be more effectively guided by dispatchers over the telephone. Moreover, survival rates from adult cardiac arrests of cardiac etiology are similar with either compression–only CPR or CPR with both compressions and rescue breaths when provided before EMS arrival. However, for the trained lay rescuer who is able, the recommendation remains for the rescuer to perform both compressions and breaths.

52.4.4.6　Chest compression rate

In adult victims of cardiac arrest, it is reasonable for rescuers to perform chest compressions at a rate of 100–120/min.

52.4.4.7　Chest compression depth

During manual CPR, rescuers should perform chest compressions to a depth of at least 2 inches (5 cm) for an average adult, while avoiding excessive chest compression depths [greater than 2.4 inches (6 cm)]. Compressions create blood flow primarily by increasing intrathoracic pressure and directly compressing the heart, which in turn results in critical blood flow and oxygen delivery to the heart and brain. Rescuers often do not compress the chest deeply enough despite the recommendation to "push hard". While a compression depth of at least 2 inches (5 cm) is recommended.

52.5　Post–cardiac arrest

Resuscitation of a cardiac arrest victim does not end with ROSC. Management includes rapid diagnosis and treatment of the disorders that caused the arrest and the complications of prolonged global ischemia. Simultaneous management of these two entities makes caring for a post–cardiac arrest patient particularly challenging. Table 52–5 listed the goals for management, and Figure 52–2 provided a goal–directed guide for care of the post–cardiac arrest patient. There are 3 major aspects that require consideration in the management of the post cardiac arrest patient. After resuscitation, a decision must be made in relation to the appropriate triage of the OHCA patient. The next phase of management concerns the in–hospital treatment, which must address each component of the post–cardiac arrest syndrome as appropriate for the individual patient. Finally, there are issues relating to prognostication and the deployment of various secondary prevention measures.

Table 52-5 Post-cardiac arrest goals

Parameter	Goal
MAP	70-90 mmHg
CVP/PCWP	(10-15)/(15-18) mmHg
Hemoglobin	$\geqslant$10 g/dL
Lactate	<2.0 mm
Body temperature	32-34 ℃ for 12-24 hours then 36-37 ℃
SaO_2	94%-98%
$S_{cv}O_2/S_vO_2$	65%-75%
DO_2	400-500 mL/(min · m^2)
VO_2	>90 mL/(min · m^2)
	Avoid flow-dependent consumption

Induction of prolonged therapeutic hypothermia in comatose survivors of cardiac arrest has been shown to improve survival and functional outcome. Hypothermia was maintained for 12-24 hours followed by gradual rewarming over 12-24 hours. Although there are no absolute contraindications, relative contraindications include severe cardiogenic shock, life threatening arrhythmias, uncontrolled bleeding, preexisting coagulopathy, pregnancy, another obvious reason for coma (i. e. , drug overdose or status epilepticus), known end-stage terminal illness, and a preexisting do-not-resuscitate status. Thrombolytic therapy does not preclude the use of hypothermia. Finally, although the current data are limited to patients with witnessed VF out-of-hospital cardiac arrest, induced post-cardiac arrest hypothermia potentially should be effective in patients with other presenting rhythms disorder and cardiac arrest presentations.

When the decision is made to treat the patient with therapeutic hypothermia, cooling efforts should be initiated as soon as possible. Target core body temperature should be 32-34 ℃ and is best monitored by an indwelling temperature-sensitive bladder catheter or esophageal temperature probe. A simultaneous immediate concern in a comatose cardiac arrest survivor is whether the patient has an acute coronary syndrome. Diagnosing acute coronary syndrome in an unconscious patient after cardiac arrest presents a unique challenge. A standard 12-lead ECG should be obtained as soon as feasible after ROSC, with a right-sided 12-lead ECG, as indicated. Immediate percutaneous coronary intervention (PCI) is indicated in patients with ST segment elevation myocardial infarction or new left bundle branch block (LBBB) and can be performed during therapeutic hypothermia.

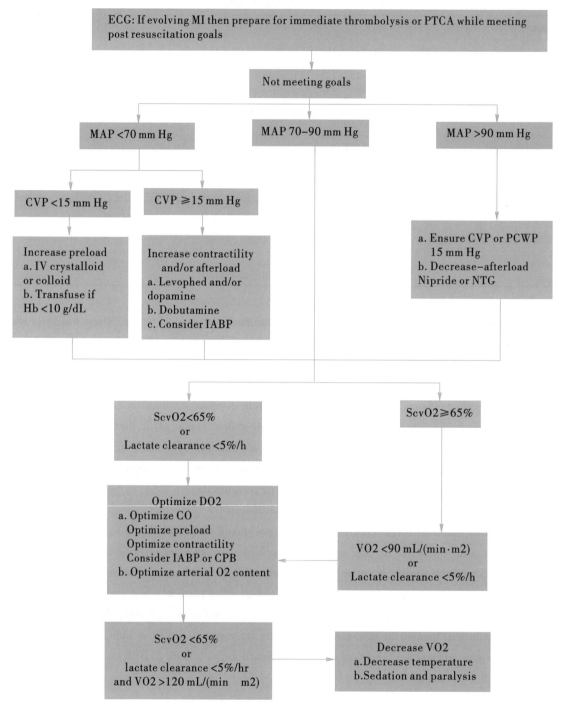

Figure 52–2   Goal–directed postarrest treatment algorithm

Gao Yulei

Chapter 53

Electrical and Temporary Pacing

The function of the human heart requires rhythmic beatings occurring between 60 and 100 times per minute. The close to 3 billion contractions of the cardiac musculature that must occur without fail are coordinated by an intricate network of specialized electrically active cells that are integrated with the myocytes that comprise the predominant mass of the heart. Any loss of electrical activity, even for a few seconds, results in syncope; loss of electrical activity for a few minutes may end in death. Cardiac cells are capable of being depolarized by an external stimulus such as an electrical pulse. Such depolarization will occur only if the external stimulus has sufficient strength to reach the threshold for stimulation and provided that the stimulus is not delivered while the cell is in a refractory period. Electrical cardioversion in severe arrhythmia, with extra high energy pulse current through the heart, so that all or most of the myocardial cells in an instant and depolarization caused by the electrical activity of the heart, short stop, and then by the supreme autonomic pacemaker treatment process of re-leading heart rhythm. Cardioversion is also commonly referred to as electrical defibrillation during ventricular fibrillation. Temporary pacemakers are used in a variety of critical care settings, which can provide clinicians with the ability to alter the electromechanical conductance of the heart in the emergency room, intensive care unit (ICU), or in the operating room.

53.1 Epidemiology

The International Classification of Diseases, the Tenth Revision, defines Sudden cardiac death (SCD) as death due to any cardiac disease that occurs out of hospital, in an emergency department, or in an individual reported dead on arrival at a hospital. In addition, death must have occurred within 1 hour after the onset of symptoms. SCD may be due to VT/VF, asystole, or nonarrhythmic causes. The annual incidence of sudden arrhythmic deaths has been estimated between 184,000 and 462,000. Sustained ventricular arrhythmias are usually caused by underlying structural heart disease, and the prevalence of arrhythmias increases with the severity of the heart disease. Ventricular arrhythmias are responsible for most of the 150,000–350,000 sudden deaths that occur annually in the United States and account for approximately 13% of all mortality. VF due to acute myocardial ischemia in the setting of coronary artery disease is the most common cause. The annual incidence of out of hospital VF is approximately 8 per 100,000. A 24-hour ECG recording will show premature ventricular beats and nonsustained VT in more than half of patients with advanced heart failure. In the heart failure population, sustained VT or VF develops at a rate of approximately 2% per year or less when the left ventricular ejection fraction is above about 30%, but the rate doubles for patients with worse ventricular function. The American Heart Association has promoted the concept of the "chain of survival", which includes early access to medical care, early cardiopulmonary resuscitation, early defibrillation, and early advanced care. Electrical cardiac pacing for the management of bradyarrhythmias was first described in 1952, and permanent transvenous pacing devices were introduced into clinical practice in the early 1960s. The first devices for endocardial defibrillation were implanted in surviving victims of SCD in 1980. A total of 3081 patients were admitted during the 1-year study period in which 348 consecutive patients (10.5%) had documented AF. Atrial fibrillation was of new onset in 139 patients (4.5%) and preexisting in 186 patients (6.0%). Electrical conversion was successful in 7 (27%) of 26 and 0 (0%) of 5 of patients with new-onset AF and patients with preexisting AF, respectively. Atrial fibrillation is common but transient in most ICU patients. Electrical cardioversion is often unsuccessful, and pharmacologic rhythm conversion is often only transiently effective. Modifiable risk factors are common among these patients.

53.2 Etiology

53.2.1 Cardiac arrest and life-threatening arrhythmias

Cardiac arrest is characterized by an abrupt loss of consciousness, if not treated promptly, it will lead to central nervous system injury or death within minutes. Cardiac arrest is often forewarned by a change in cardiovascular status, as indicated by the appearance or worsening of symptoms related to transient arrhythmias, such as palpitations, lightheadedness, or near-syncope or syncope. Other forewarnings may include new or worsening chest pain, dyspnea, or weakness. These warning symptoms, however, are limited by their sensitivity and predictive power in individual patients. Moreover, cardiac arrest may occur unexpectedly as a first cardiac event in an apparently healthy individual, in a patient with known previous cardiac disease, or as the final event in any fatal disease. The most common electrical mechanisms of cardiac arrest are the ventricular tachyarrhythmias-VF/VT. In a substantial minority of cardiac arrests, severe bradyarrhythmia, asystole, or pulseless electrical activity is the first rhythm abnormality noted. The later may be the primary mechanism of the cardiac arrest or a result of deterioration of VT/VF. Pulseless electrical activity or asystole may also be seen after termination of VT/VF by cardioversion. Pulseless electrical activity is defined as secondary when it occurs in the setting of predisposing factors, such as hypoxia or other metabolic disorders, and primary when it is the initial rhythm noted in patients with predisposing cardiac disorders. The probability of survival after intervention is far better for ventricular tachyarrhythmias than for bradyarrhythmic or asystolic mechanisms. The interval between cardiac arrest and the initiation of resuscitation and cardioversion is the major determinant of survival.

53.2.2 Supraventricular arrhythmias

The normal cardiac impulse begins in the sinus node complex, which is located at the junction of the right atrium and the superior vena cava. It then travels through the right atrium and primarily activates the left atrium through the coronary sinus. Supraventricular arrhythmias are divided into bradyarrhythmias and tachyarrhythmias.

Bradyarrhythmias may be caused by sinus node, AV node, or His-Purkinje dysfunction (Table 53-1).

Sinusbradycardia (Figure 53−1) is generally defined as a sinus rate of less than 60 b/min. It should be noted, however, that sinus rates as low as 45−50 b/min, particularly at rest, can be physiologically normal. Sinus node dysfunction encompasses a group of disorders including sinus bradycardia, sinoatrial (SA) exit block (Figure 53−2), sinus arrest (pause of>2−3 seconds) during sinus rhythm, chronotropic incompetence, and tachycardiabradycardia (tachy−brady) syndrome (Figure 53−3).

Table 53−1   The cases of bradyarrhythmias

Location	Characteristic
Sinus node	Sinus bradycardia < 45 b/min
	Sinoatrial exit block
	First−degree
	Second−degree
	Third−degree
	Sinus arrest
	Bradycardia−tachycardia syndrome
Atrioventricular node	First−degree
	Second−degree
	Mobitz type I (Wenckebach phenomenon)
	Mobitz type II
	Higher degree (e. g. ,2 : 1,3 : 1)
	Third−degree
	Atrioventricular node
	His−Purkinje system

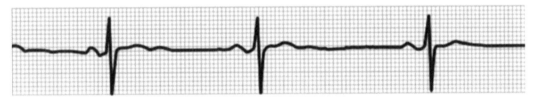

Figure 53−1   Sinus bradycardia

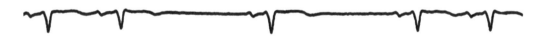

Figure 53−2   Sinoatrial block

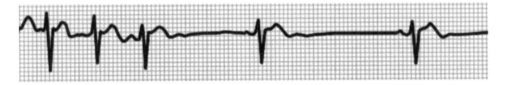

Figure 53−3   Electrocardiographic evidence of tachy−brady syndrome

AV conduction disturbances refer to abnormal conduction in the AV node or in the His−Purkinje system (HPS) below the AV node. Electrical transmission through the AV conduction system is primarily limited by the AV node, which conducts in a decremental fashion to prevent excessively rapid conduction to the ventricles. The AV blocks are classified as first, second, high, and third degree. First degree AV block is a misnomer because nothing is actually blocked, there is delay, usually in the AV node, manifest by a pro-longed PR interval (Figure 53–4). Second degree AV block is divided into Mobitz type I (Wenckebach) or Mobitz type II. High degree or advanced AV block, which is a form of second degree block with multiple or successive nonconducted P waves, or both (Figure 53–5), frequently recurs or persists. Third degree heart block can be seen with sinus rhythm or any atrial tachyarrhythmia with a regular escape rhythm in the AV junction or below (Figure 53–6).

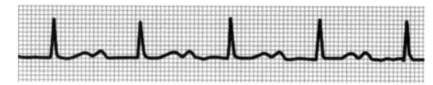

Figure 53–4   **First-degree AV block**

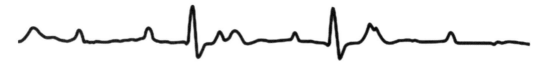

Figure 53–5   **High-degree AV block**

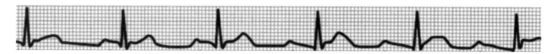

Figure 53–6   **Third-degree AV block**

53.2.3   Ventricular arrhythmias

Ventricular arrhythmias originate below the AV node in the ventricular myocardium or His–Purkinje system. These include premature ventricular beats, ventricular couplets, nonsustained and sustained ventric-ular tachycardias (VTs), and VF.

A single beat is referred to as a premature ventricular beat (Figure 53–7). Two consecutive beats are ventricular couplets. Three or more consecutive beats at a rate faster than 100 beats/min are VT (Figure 53–7 B and C). VT that terminates spontaneously within 30 seconds is nonsustained (Figure 53–7 B), whereas sustained VT persists longer than 30 seconds. A continually changing activation sequence produces polymorphic VT with a changing QRS morphology (Figure 53–8A). VF has continuous irregular activation with no discrete QRS complexes (Figure 53–8D). Although underlying structural heart disease is usually present, these arrhythmias do not require a fixed structural substrate. Arrhythmias that originate from the right ventricle or septum result in late activation of much of the left ventricle, thereby producing a prominent S wave in V_1, referred to as a left bundle branch block–like configuration (Figure 53–9). Arrhythmias that originate from the free wall of the left ventricle have a prominent positive deflection in V1, thereby produ-cing a right bundle branch block–like morphology (Figure 53–10). A frontal plane axis that is directed in-feriorly, as indicated by dominant R waves in leads II, III, and aVF, suggests initial activation of the cranial portion of the ventricle, whereas a frontal plane axis that is directed superiorly (dominant S waves in II, III, and aVF) suggests initial activation at the inferior wall.

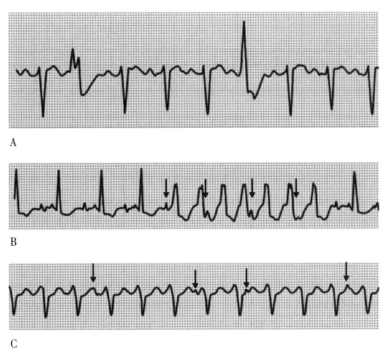

A

B

C

Figure 53-7   **Ventricular arrhythmias**

A. Multifocal premature ventricular beats; B. Nonsustained monomorphic ventricular tachycardia. Note dissociated P waves indicated by arrows; C. Sustained monomorphic ventricular tachycardia. Dissociated P waves are indicated by arrows.

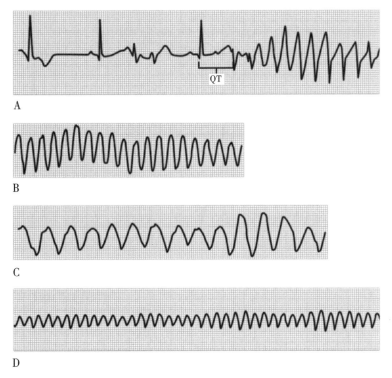

A

B

C

D

Figure 53-8   **Ventricular arrhythmias**

A. Polymorphic ventricular tachycardia associated with QT prolongation. Sinus rhythm, with a couplet of premature ventricular contractions, is followed by a sinus beat, and then by a polymorphic ventricular tachycardia. The QT interval of the sinus beats is markedly prolonged, exceeding 0. 56 second; B. Rapid sinusoidal ventricular tachycardia with a rate approximating 250 b/min; C. Sinusoidal ventricular tachycardia owing to hyperkalemia. The rate is slower than 150 b/min, but the QRS duration exceeds 200 msec, thereby creating the sinusoidal appearance; D. Ventricular fibrillation.

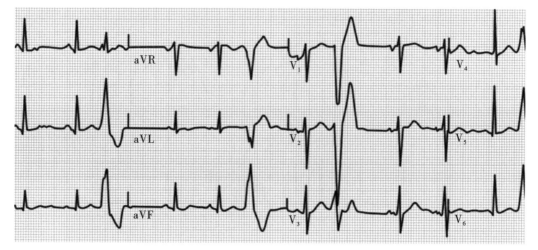

Figure 53-9   Twelve-lead electrocardiogram with simultaneous two-lead rhythm strip (V$_2$ and V$_5$) showing premature ventricular beats that originated from the right ventricular outflow tract

Sinus rhythm and frequent premature ventricular beats are present. The premature ventricular contractions all have the same morphology, best appreciated in the bottom two continuous leads, with a left bundle branch block-like configuration in V$_1$ consistent with an origin in the right ventricle or septum. The frontal plane axis is directed inferiorly, indicating initial depolarization from the cranial aspect of the ventricle.

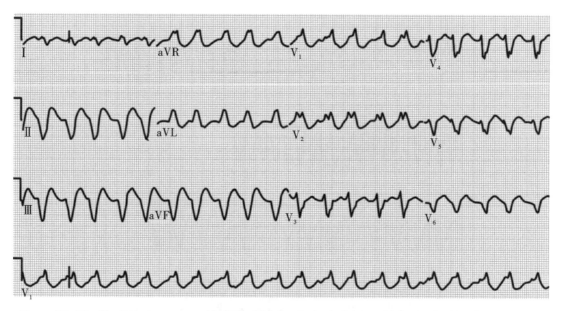

Figure 53-10   Sustained monomorphic VT originating from an infarcted left ventricular infarct region

VT has a right bundle branch block-like configuration in V$_1$, consistent with an origin in the left ventricle. The frontal plane axis is directed superiorly and consistent with initial depolarization of the inferior wall of the left ventricle.

53.3 Cardioversion

The general principle of cardioversion is that electrical cardioversion should be considered in cases where rapid arrhythmias lead to hemodynamic disturbances, or induce and increase focal angina, and are ineffective against arrhythmic drugs. If severe arrhythmias such as ventricular fibrillation are present, immediate defibrillation should be called for an emergency cardioversion. Whereas chronic rapid arrhythmia should be performed on the basis of preoperative preparation, elective cardioversion should be performed, which is called selective cardioversion.

53.3.1 Transthoracic cardioversion and defibrillation

A nonsynchronized shock that is delivered coincident with the T wave during supraventricular tachycardia (SVT) or VT may precipitate VF. Cardioversion refers to the termination of SVT or VT by delivery of a shock in synchrony with the QRS complex. When shocks are delivered to terminate VF, synchronization to the QRS complex is not necessary, and this process is referred to as defbrillation.

53.3.1.1 Technique

Whenever cardioversion or defbrillation is performed on an elective basis, the patient should be in a fasting state. Intravenous access to a peripheral vein should be established, and oxygen, suction, and equipment needed for airway management should be readily available. Transthoracic cardioversion and defibrillation are painful, and drugs are commonly used for anesthesia or amnesia such as methohexital and midazolam.

In the anteroapical configuration, one electrode is positioned to the right of the sternum at the level of the second intercostal space, and the second electrode is positioned at the midaxillary line, lateral to the apical impulse (Figure 53-11). In the anteroposterior configuration, an electrode is placed to the left of the sternum at the fourth intercostal space, and the second electrode is positioned posteriorly, to the left of the spine, at the same level as the anterior electrode. These two-electrode configurations result in similar success rates of cardioversion and defbrillation.

Variables are the shock waveform and shock strength, which affecting the success of cardioversion and defibrillation. Other technique-dependent variables that maximize delivery of energy to the heart include firm paddle pressure, delivery of the shock during expiration, and repetitive shocks. Patient-related variables that may decrease the probability of successful cardioversion and defibrillation include metabolic disturbances, long arrhythmia duration, some antiarrhythmic drugs such as amiodarone, and body weight in excess of 80 kg.

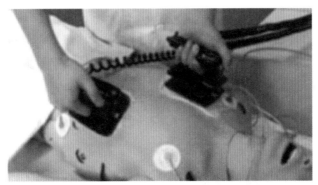

Figure 53-11 The site of electrode in the anteroapical configuration

Anticoagulation with warfarin is generally necessary for 3 weeks before cardioversion and for one month after cardioversion whenever atrial fibrillation has been present for 48 hours or longer up to cardioversion of atrial fibrillation may be complicated by thromboembolism. The 3-week anticoagulation before cardioversion can be eliminated if no atrial thrombi are seen on a transesophageal echocardiogram, but anticoagulation for one month after cardioversion is still necessary to prevent thrombus formation secondary to transient, post-conversion atrial stunning.

53.3.1.2 Indications

The most common arrhythmias treated by cardioversion and defibrillation are VF, VT, atrial fibrillation, and atrial flutter. Asynchronous shocks may precipitate VF. Rarely, VF may occur even when shocks are synchronized to the QRS complex. Treatment of VF should be as quickly as possible, and a 200 J shock is delivered, followed by one or more 360 J shocks if necessary in emergency department. Depending on the patients' hemodynamics, cardioversion of VT may be performed on an emergency basis. An initial shock strength of 50 J is appropriate, followed by higher energy levels if additional shocks are needed. An initial energy level of 50 J is appropriate for cardioversion of atrial flutter. In atrial fibrillation, an initial shock of 100–200 J is appropriate, depending on the patients' body weight, shocks of 300–360 J are then used if necessary. If atrial fibrillation must be treated on an urgent basis, such as in a patient with Wolff–Parkinson–White syndrome who has a very rapid ventricular rate and hemodynamic compromise, an initial shock of 200 J should be followed by 360 J shocks, as needed. Because the defibrillation energy requirement is a probability function, subsequent shocks may be effective for cardioversion and defibrillation even when the first 360 J shock is ineffective.

53.3.1.3 Complications

Cardioversion in patients with digitalis toxicity should be avoided because of the risk for post-shock ventricular arrhythmias is increased in the presence of a supratherapeutic plasma concentration of digitalis. Transient ST segment elevation may occur after cardioversion. Mild myocardial necrosis may occasionally occur if a total energy exceeding 425 J is delivered in a short period. Another rare complication of cardioversion is pulmonary edema, which may be due to transient left ventricular dysfunction. Post-shock bradycardia or asystole may occur because of vagal discharge or an underlying sick sinus syndrome. At times, atropine or emergency transcutaneous pacing may be necessary. In patients who have a pacemaker or implantable cardioverter–defibrillator (ICD), the shocking electrodes should be positioned as far away from the generator as possible, and the generator and pacing threshold should be checked afterward.

53.3.2 Implantable cardioverter–defibrilators

ICDs that deliver shocks to terminate atrial fibrillation, as well as VT and VF, are clinically available. Biventricular ICDs are available for patients who need an ICD and have advanced (class III or IV) heart failure and a bundle branch block.

53.3.2.1 Indications

ICDs have become first-line therapy in patients who have survived an episode of VF not associated with acute myocardial infarction (AMI) or who have had an episode of hemodynamically significant sustained VT.

ICDs are also implanted in individuals at high risk for cardiac arrest, including patients with idiopathic, dilated cardiomyopathy and unexplained syncope or patients with coronary artery disease (CAD), an ejection fraction of less than 35%, spontaneous episodes of nonsustained VT, and inducible sustained VT in the electrophysiology laboratory. Patients with a previous myocardial infarction and an ejection fraction of 30% or less, as well as patients with dilated cardiomyopathy (ischemic or nonischemic), an ejection fraction of 35% or less, and class II or III heart failure are usually as the indications for implantation of an ICD.

53.3.2.2   Programming

Testing is performed at the time of implantation to determine the energy requirement for defibrillation. A safety margin of at least 10 J should be present; for example, if the maximum output of the pulse generator is 32 J, successful defibrillation should be achieved with shocks of 22 J or less in strength. If the patient has had episodes of VT, antitachycardia pacing can be evaluated and programmed as needed to terminate the VT.

With ICDs that are tiered-therapy devices, as many as two VT zones and one VF zone are available to provide individualized therapy for ventricular arrhythmias that have different rates. The rate threshold and various sequences of antitachycardia pacing and low-or high-energy shocks can be programmed for each of the two VT zones. The VF zone is a high-rate zone in which high-energy shocks are delivered. Optimal programming is important for many reasons, including minimizing patient discomfort, reducing the chance of syncope with an arrhythmia episode, maximizing the battery life of the pulse generator, and preventing inappropriate shocks.

Patients who have an ICD do not require evaluation every time that they experience a device discharge. However, urgent evaluation is necessary if the patient experiences flurries of discharges.

53.3.2.3   Complications

Pneumothorax, myocardial perforation, and infection are the complications related to the implantation procedure, which have an incidence of less than 1%. Complications associated with the subcutaneous or submuscular pocket into which the device is placed include hematoma formation and erosion of the pocket. The endocardial leads that are used in the ICD system occasionally become dislodged shortly afer implantation, thus necessitating a second procedure to reposition the leads. Other complications include fracture or breakdown of the insulation, either of which may result in failure to defibrillate. Fracture of a lead may also result in an artifact that mimics VF and triggers inappropriate shocks. The frequent shocks may be appropriate shocks triggered by flurries of VT or VF; if a correctable cause such as a metabolic defect or proarrhythmic drug can not be identified, antiarrhythmic drug therapy or catheter ablation, or both, should be used to eliminate these arrhythmia flurries. Flurries of shocks may be triggered by atrial fibrillation with a rapid ventricular response, in which case aggressive management of the atrial fibrillation is indicated. In addition, flurries of shocks may be a manifestation of a lead fracture, in which case lead replacement is necessary.

53.4   Temporary pacing

Paul Zoll first applied clinically effective temporary pacing in 1952 using a pulsating current applied through two electrodes attached via hypodermic needles to the chest wall in two patients with ventricular standstill. Temporary pacemaker leads are generally inserted percutaneously into an internal jugular or subclavian vein or by cut-down into a brachial vein and then positioned under fluoroscopic guidance in the right ventricular apex and attached to an external generator. Temporary pacing is used to stabilize patients awaiting permanent pacemaker implantation, to correct a transient symptomatic bradycardia caused by drug toxicity or a metabolic defect, or to suppress torsades de pointes by maintaining a rate of 85-100 beats/min until the causative factor has been eliminated. Temporary pacing may also be used in prophylactic fashion in patients at risk for symptomatic bradycardia during a surgical procedure or high−degree AV block in the setting of an AMI. The most common complication of temporary pacemakers is infection; this risk is minimized by limiting the use of a pacemaker lead to 48 hours. In emergency situations, ventricular pacing can be instituted immediately by transcutaneous pacing with electrode pads applied to the chest wall.

53. 4. 1　Indications

The indications for temporary pacing can be considered in two broad categories; emergency or elective. For many patients presenting with bradycardia, conservative therapy and treatment of the underlying problem is the most appropriate management strategy. As a general rule, patients who may need to go on to permanent pacing should only have a temporary pacing if they have suffered syncope at rest, are hemodynamically compromised by the bradycardia or have ventricular tachyarrhythmias in response to bradycardia. Patients with sinus node disease rarely need temporary pacing, and compromise of subsequent venous access for permanent pacing usually outweigh because of the risks of infection. In patients requiring permanent pacing, prompt transfer for the procedure is appropriate but consideration of rate support to cover transfer to another hospital may occasionally require provision for temporary pacing.

Any patient with acute hemodynamic compromise caused by bradycardia and/or episodes of asystole should be considered for temporary cardiac pacing. For the majority of patients, this is likely to occur in the setting of AMI; complete heart block with anterior infarction usually indicates a poor prognosis and a need for pacing whereas complete heart block with inferior infarction is usually reversible, associated with a narrow QRS, and responds to atropine. The ACC/AHA guidelines for the management of AMI provide indications graded according to weight of evidence for benefit of pacing rather than site of infarction (Table 53−2). Although temporary pacing is clearly indicated in patients suffering episodes of asystole, there is little evidence for hemodynamic benefit of temporary ventricular pacing over spontaneous rhythm in patients with bradycardia following AMI, although temporary dual chamber (atrioventricular synchronous) pacing has been shown to be beneficial.

53. 4. 2　Approaches to temporary pacing

53. 4. 2. 1　Transvenous, endocardial pacing

As this procedure is often performed in emergency/acute situations by relatively junior staff, the choice of route is often dictated by individual experience. Other considerations should include length of time that the temporary wire is anticipated to need to stay in situ; femoral placement probably offers the least stable wire position and limits patient mobility more than other routes. Current guidelines from the British Cardiac Society recommend the right internal jugular route as most suitable for the inexperienced operator; this offers the most direct route to the right ventricle, and is associated with the highest success rate and fewest complications. This was also the recommendation of Hynes and colleagues as a result of five years of temporary pacing experience in a coronary care unit setting. In patients receiving or likely to receive thrombolytic treatment, the femoral, brachial or external jugular are the routes of choice. It is also generally best to avoid the left subclavian approach if permanent pacing may be required, as this is the most common site for permanent pacing. Some permanent implanters prefer the right side, however, and establishing a relationship with the physician or surgeon who is responsible for permanent pacing is important. Many implanters also prefer to use the non−dominant side; assessing the patient's dominant hand is, therefore, appropriate.

Table 53-2　ACC/AHA classification of indications for pacing

Class	Indications
Class I	Conditions for which there is evidence and/or general agreement that a given procedure or treatment is beneficial, useful and effective
Class II	Conditions for which there is conflicting evidence and/or a divergence of opinion about the usefulness/efficacy of a procedure or treatment
Class II a	Weight of evidence/opinion is in favour of usefulness/efficacy
Class II b	Usefulness/efficacy is less well established by evidence/opinion
Class III	Conditions for which there is evidence and/or general agreement that a procedure/treatment is not useful/effective and in some cases may be harmful

Temporary transvenous ventricular pacing must be advanced to the right atrium and then crossed the tricuspid valve. With a temporary wire, crossing the tricuspid valve is often performed most easily by pointing the lead tip downwards and towards to the left cardiac border and advancing across the valve. The lead is then advanced to a position at the right ventricular apex. If difficulty is experienced with this technique, an alternative is to create a loop in the right atrium by pointing the lead tip to the right cardiac border and then prolapsing the loop across the valve by rotating the lead. The lead tip may then require manipulation to the apex; this is often performed most easily by passing the lead tip to the right ventricular outflow tract, gently withdrawing the lead, and allowing the tip to drop down into the apex.

Temporary atrial pacing leads have a preshaped J curve to enable positioning in the right atrial appendage. This necessitates approach from a superior vein and positioning is greatly assisted by a lateral screening facility on fluoroscopy. The tip of the lead should point forward with the J shape slightly opened out when slight traction is applied; unless this is achieved it is unlikely that the lead will be stable.

Both leads must be secured to the skin to prevent displacement by movement or traction. The majority of current temporary transvenous electrodes have a smooth, isodiametric profile with no fixation mechanism; this is to enable easy removal but does tend to make displacement more likely. Newer active fixation temporary leads are available with a fixation screw; these are small diameter (3.5 French), catheter delivered leads which remain easy to remove after 1–2 weeks. The active fixation mechanism improves lead stability and may improve the ease and acceptability of more physiological atrial based pacing in the temporary setting.

53.4.2.2　Epicardial pacing

This route is used following cardiac surgical procedures as it requires direct access to the external surface of the myocardium. Fine wire electrodes are placed within the myocardium from the epicardial surface and the connectors emerge through the skin. These electrodes can be removed with gentle traction when no longer required; their electrical performance tends to deteriorate quite rapidly with time, however, and reliable sensing/pacing capability is often lost within 5–10 days, especially when used in the atrium.

53.4.2.3　External (transcutaneous) pacing

External pacing has been refined to make it more clinically acceptable and easier to institute, should now be available in all coronary care units and accident and emergency units. Clinical studies have demonstrated the efficacy of the Zoll type noninvasive temporary pacemaker for periods of up to 14 hours of continuous pacing with success rates of 78% –94%, although many patients require sedation if conscious. This approach certainly offers a "bridge" to transvenous approach for circumstances where the patient can not be moved or staff with transvenous pacing experience are not immediately available. Positioning of the transcutaneous pacing electrodes is usually in an anteroposterior configuration, but if this is unsuccessful, if external defibrillation is likely to be needed or if electrodes are placed during a cardiac arrest situation, the anterior —lateral configuration should be considered.

53.4.2.4 Transoesophageal pacing

The oesophageal or gastro—oesophageal approach has been advocated for emergency ventricular pacing as it may be better tolerated than external pacing in the conscious patient. Success rates of around 90% are claimed for ventricular stimulation using a flexible electrode positioned in the fundus of the stomach and pacing through the diaphragm. Transoesophageal atrial pacing (performed by placing the electrode in the mid to lower oesophagus to obtain atrial capture) is also well described, but this approach is rarely used in the acute setting as electrode stability can be difficult to achieve and there is no protection against atrioventricular conduction disturbance.

53.4.3 Complications

Complications may relate to the venous access, mechanical effects of the lead within the heart, the electrical performance of the pacemaker lead, or infection or thromboembolism caused by the presence of a foreign body. Complications can be expected in around 14% –20% of patients and the majority of these will be manifest as development of a pericardial rub, ventricular arrhythmias produced during electrode positioning, or infection.

Gao Yulei

Chapter 54

Establishment and Management of Artificial Airway

54.1　Introduction

What is artificial airway and what is the indication of artificial airway?

An artificial airway is a gas passage that is inserted directly into the trachea or through the upper airway into the trachea. As the means of rescue, the establishment of artificial airway is conducive to sputum drainage. although the establishment of artificial airway makes the patient lose the function of heating, humidifying and filtering of upper respiratory tract, weakens the ability of removing foreign body in respiratory tract, is not convenient for pronunciation, reduces the quality of life of patients, increases the probability of nosocomial infection, To improve the effectiveness of ventilation, the existence of catheter balloon can prevent aspiration, and can reduce air leakage, to ensure the effective implementation of positive pressure ventilation. The indications for artificial airway should be comprehensive consideration of circulatory, respiratory and central nervous system factors.

Generally speaking, the indications for establishing an artificial airway are as follows.

(1) Upper respiratory tract obstruction, nasal cavity and larynx soft tissue injury, foreign body or secretion retention can cause upper respiratory tract obstruction, threatening the lives of patients. Timely establishment of artificial airway ensures upper airway patency.

(2) When the protective mechanism of the airway is impaired, the pharynx, larynx, vocal cords, airway and protuberance play a protective role on the respiratory tract through physiological reflexes (mainly vagus nerve emission). There are pharyngeal reflex (nausea and deglutition reflex), laryngeal reflex (glottis closed and epiglottis covered glottis), tracheal reflex (foreign body or secretion stimulates the airway in turn. Causing cough) and protuberance reflex (a strong cough caused by stimulation of the carina). Patients with changes in consciousness (especially coma) and under anesthesia, normal physiological reflexes are inhibited, resulting in impaired airway protective mechanisms, susceptible to aspiration and secretion retention, may lead to serious pulmonary infection. Therefore, for patients with impaired airway protective mechanisms, it is necessary to establish artificial airway to prevent aspiration and secretion retention.

(3) When airway secretions are normally retained, airway secretions reach the airway through mucocili-

ary movement, and cough reflex occurs after the airway is stimulated. When the normal cough reflex is impaired, it can cause secretions to be trapped in the airway, which can easily lead to pulmonary infection and respiratory obstruction. Although the suction tube can be inserted into the pharynx and airway through the nasal cavity or oral cavity, but often the effect is very poor, and the stimulation is greater, patients are not easy to cooperate, serious cases can also cause nasopharyngeal bleeding and induce serious arrhythmia. Therefore, it is necessary to establish artificial airway in time to remove airway secretions.

(4) Patients who need mechanical ventilation should first be established an artificial airway which provides access to the ventilator. Of course, positive pressure ventilation can be carried out in a short time, and sometimes mask can be connected with ventilator to achieve non-invasive ventilation. However, when long-term mechanical ventilation or noninvasive ventilation is required, artificial airways must be established, such as respiratory and cardiac arrest, complicated with other important organ failure (severe encephalopathy, severe upper gastrointestinal bleeding, hemodynamic instability or severe arrhythmia), facial surgery or traumatic deformities, and loss of airway protective mechanisms. Loss of expectoration, severe hypoxemia or acidosis, and recent upper abdominal surgery.

54.2   The indication of emergency endotracheal intubation

Artificial airway needs to be established urgently in the following circumstances.
(1) Airway integrity is destroyed or obstructed in a short time.
(2) Respiratory failure requires ventilator-assisted breathing.
(3) Airway protection is needed to prevent predictable factors affecting airway patency.

Common critical conditions requiring the establishment of an emergency artificial airway include deep coma, respiratory failure or respiratory arrest, cardiac arrest, severe airway spasm, airway foreign body obstruction, sedative or anesthetic effects, craniocerebral and cervical trauma, accidental extubation, and uncontrollable risk of aspiration (such as massive upper gastrointestinal bleeding). Upper respiratory tract hemorrhage and acute upper respiratory tract obstruction.

54.3   Indication and contraindication of orotracheal intubation

The orotracheal intubation is easy to operate, the intubation diameter is relatively large and facilitats the clearance of airway secretion, but affects epiglottic function, patients are poorly tolerant.

Indications for orotracheal intubation include: ①severe hypoxemia or hypercapnia, or other causes requiring prolonged mechanical ventilation without considering tracheotomy; ②inability to remove upper respiratory tract secretions, gastric reflux or bleeding independently, and the risk of aspiration; ③excessive or bleeding secretions of the lower respiratory tract, and poor autonomous clearance; ④inability to remove tracheotomy. There are upper respiratory tract injury, stenosis, obstruction, tracheoesophageal flaccidity and so on, seriously affecting normal respiration; Patients with sudden respiratory arrest, need to establish an emergency artificial airway for mechanical ventilation. The key to orotracheal intubation is to expose the glottis, which is prone to failure or complications when the glottis is not exposed.

Contraindication or relative contraindication include: ①difficulty in opening mouth or small oral space, unable to intubate through mouth;②neck can not be back (if suspected of cervical spine fracture).

54.4   The indications and contraindications of nasotracheal intubation

Nasotracheal intubation is easier to fix and more comfortable than orotracheal intubation. Patients are more tolerant, but the diameter of the intubation is smaller, which leads to increased respiratory work and is not conducive to the drainage of airway and sinus secretions.

Indications for naso tracheal intubation are all performed with orally tracheal intubation except for e-mergency rescue.

Contraindications for nasotracheal intubation include:

(1) Emergency rescue, especially the hospital.

(2) Severe traumatic nasal or maxillofacial fractures.

(3) Coagulation dysfunction.

(4) Nasal or nasopharyngeal obstruction, such as nasal septum deviation, polyps, cysts, abscess, edema, foreign bodies, hematoma and so on.

(5) Skull base fracture.

The incidence of nosocomial sinusitis is closely related to the pathogenesis of ventilator – associated pneumonia. Therefore, oral tracheal intubation should be preferred for patients who can be discharged from ventilator in the near future. However, transnasal tracheal intubation may be considered prior to nasotracheal intubation when the technique is skilled or the patient is not suitable for transoral tracheal intubation.

54.5   The main points of orotracheal intubation

Endotracheal intubation through mouth is the most common way to establish artificial airway, and is also cardiopulmonary resuscitation. Therefore, it is necessary to quickly and accurately insert endotracheal intubation. It is very necessary to rescue patients.

Main points:

(1) Prepare appropriate laryngoscope. According to the shape of the lenses, divect laryngosuope is divided into straight laryngoscope and curved laryngoscope, the use of the two methods are different; straight laryngoscope is inserted under the epiglottis upward and can expose the glottis; curved laryngoscope is inserted between the epiglottis and the root of the tongue, upward and forward, the epiglottis indirectly pulled up, thereby exposing the glottis. Otolaryngologists usually use straight laryngoscope for full exposure in order to perform biopsy, while anesthesiologists mainly use curved laryngoscope for intubation. As a critical medical practitioner, it is necessary to adapt to all kinds of emergency environment. Two kinds of laryngoscope should be mastered.

(2) Prepare different types of catheters for use in reserve and check if the catheter balloon leaks. The air bag can be immersed in normal saline and injected into the gas to check whether it leaks or not and then completely extract the gas. The smear of wax oil on the distal 1/3 of the endotracheal tube will help to insert glottis and reduce trauma. If the guide wire is used, the guide wire is inserted into the catheter, and the catheter is shaped by the guide wire.

(3) Proper head and neck position is the main guarantee for successful intubation. Shoulder back pad height is about 10 cm, head back, neck in the overextension position, so that the mouth, glottis and trachea in a straight line, in order to facilitate the intubation. Even in emergencies, it is necessary to adjust the patient's position for a moment.

(4) Preoxygenation, artificial ventilation and vital signs monitoring should be done while preparing for intubation. Pure oxygen is inhaled with a mask and a manual ventilator or anesthesia machine, while artificial ventilation is given to avoid hypoxia and carbon dioxide retention. When transcutaneous oxygen saturation is above 90% (preferably over 90%), intubation can only begin. If the intubation is not successful, or the percutaneous oxygen saturation is less than 90%, especially less than 85%, who should immediately stop the operation, re-through the mask oxygen, until oxygen saturation recovery. Electrocardiogram and transdermal oxygen saturation should be monitored closely before, during and after intubation.

(5) Inserting a laryngoscope, observing and cleaning the upper respiratory tract, the operator stands on the patient's head, holds the laryngoscope with the left hand, inserts the laryngoscope from the right side of the patient's mouth, pushes the tongue to the left. The laryngoscope should be placed in the middle of the mouth to observe the oropharynx. If there is secretion, it is necessary to fully suck, so as not to affect the visual field of intubation.

(6) The anatomical markers of glottis. Epiglottis and arytenoid cartilage are the anatomical markers of glottis. The epiglottis is located above the glottis (anterior), and the arytenoid cartilage is located below the glottis (posterior). The operators insert the laryngoscope between the epiglottis and the root of the tongue or under the epiglottis, they will be tired of protruding. Generally, the operators will see the arytenoid cartilage first, then the vocal cords. When tracheal intubation is not necessarily to see the vocal cords, as long as the arytenoid cartilage, or even see the arytenoid cartilage below (behind) the esophagus, they can determine the position of the glottis.

(7) After inserting the tracheal catheter and adjusting the depth of the catheter to observe the anatomical markers of glottis or glottis, the right hand tracheal holds catheter and insert into the glottis. Adjust the depth of catheter, avoid inserting deeply into the main bronchus, and pay attention to the symmetry of bilateral breathing sounds. In general, male patients are inserted at depths ranging from incisor 24-26 cm to female 20-22 cm. Immediately inflate the balloon, connect the tracheal tube to a ventilator or anesthesia machine, perform mechanical ventilation, and inhale pure oxygen. If using the guide wire, after the tracheal catheter was inserted into the glottis, the guide wire is removed.

(8) To confirm that the catheter is inserted into the trachea mainly through the following means: ①Stethoscope is used to listen to the breathing sounds of the chest and abdomen, and the breathing sounds of the chest are stronger than those of the abdomen. ②Monitoring the concentration of exhaled carbon dioxide in patients, such as the trachea, can see the square wave of carbon dioxide when exhaling. ③For patients with. Spontaneous breathing, the contraction of the amesthesia machine balloon can be confirmed the catheter was inserted into the trachea.

(9) Fixing the tracheal tube and inserting the dental pad into the mouth cavity, then the laryngoscope can be removed and the tracheal tube and the dental pad can be fixed together in the cheek and mandible with butterfly tape.

(10) The distance between the distal end of the tracheal tube and the protuberance should be 2-4 cm by taking X-ray film of the chest and further adjusting the position of the tracheal tube. Adjust the depth of the catheter according to the chest X-ray. At the same time, we observed lung condition and pneumothorax.

Zhu Zhiqiang

Chapter 55

Central Venous Catheterization

55.1 Introduction

Central venous pressure monitoring should be carried out after heart failure, shock, severe trauma and major operation. Patients who need complete parenteral nutrition such as patients after major gastrointestinal surgery, short bowel syndrome, high intestinal fistula, gastrointestinal obstruction for a long time. Long term intravenous infusion and peripheral blood vessels collapse, hardened, delicate and vulnerable to puncture. When the peripheral vein collapses, the internal jugular and subclavian veins can be used to give hypertonic or irritant solution.

55.2 Contraindications

(1) Patients with coagulopathy or systemic heparin.

(2) Patients who are easy to occur pneumothorax with chest deformity, unclear anatomical markers or severe emphysema and high pulmonary apex.

(3) Restless and unrestrained.

(4) Patients who are not able to take the body position with high shoulder low head and ecphysesis should avoid subclavian vein puncture.

(5) The venipuncture should be avoided in those who have undergone neck surgery, have significant anatomical changes and have local infection.

55.3 Operation methods and procedures

55.3.1 Subclavian vein catheterization

(1) Supraclavicular puncture: the patient should be the position with head low and shoulder height or

supine position (shoulder pillow), head turns to the opposite side (generally choose the right neck needle), reveal the shape of sternocleidomastoid muscle. The angle between the lateral edge of the clavicular head and the superior edge of the clavicle is drawn with methyl violet. The puncture point is at the top of the bisector or about 0. 5 cm behind it. Routine skin disinfection, laying aseptic hole towel. At the pre-marked needle point, 2% lidocaine is sucked with a syringe for intradermal and subcutaneous infiltration anesthesia. The needle point is pointed at the sternoclavicular joint, and the needle angle is 30-40 degrees. Generally, the insertion of 2. 5-4 cm means subclavian vein. The assistant sucks the normal saline with the syringe in advance, put one end of the expanded silicone tube into the syringe tube, and the other end penetrats through the orifice of the syringe and inserts into the cavity of the puncture needle. The puncture needle and the syringe are linked. According to the direction and angle of the puncture, the puncture needle quickly passes through the skin, punctures the subclavian vein, and promptly pushes the silica gel after the blood is returned. Tube, silica gel tube with liquid into the blood vessels. Press the finger at the top of the puncture needle, exit the needle, and insert the silicone tube into the needle.

(2) Subclavian puncture: position and preparation for supraclavicular puncture and intubation. Take the subclavian edge of the medial 1-2 cm of the midpoint of the clavicle (or between the midpoint of the clavicle and the inner 1/3) as the puncture point. Local infiltration of 2% lidocaine anesthesia, in the selected puncture point, the needle points to the head, with the sternum longitudinal axis at 45 degrees, and chest wall plane at 15 degrees, to just across the clavicle and the first rib space as the standard. In general, 3-5 cm can be seen in the adult, and it can be placed and fixed by supraclavicular puncture and catheterization.

55. 3. 2   Internal jugular vein catheterization

Lying prone, head 20-30 degrees low angle or take shoulder pillow overextension, head to the opposite side (usually take the right side puncture). Find out the triangle area formed by clavicle head, sternum head and clavicle of sternocleidomastoid muscle. The top of the triangle area is the puncture point, or take the intersection point of 3 cm above clavicle and 3 cm beyond the median line as the puncture point. Routine skin disinfection, laying aseptic hole towel, 2% lidocaine local infiltration anesthesia, the direction of puncture parallel to the sagittal plane, and the coronal plane with a 30 degree angle down and slightly outward to the sternoclavicular joint below the rear. The catheterization is performed by supraclavicular puncture and catheterization.

55. 3. 3   Femoral vein catheterization

Skin preparation, disinfection and towel spreading. Determine the position of femoral vein by pulsatile Doppler ultrasound or midpoint of anterior superior iliac spine and pubic symphysis. For conscious patients, lidocaine is used for local skin infiltration anesthesia. The puncture needle is connected with a 5 mL or 10 mL syringe and punctured at the medial part of the femoral artery at the 2 transverse fingers below the inguinal ligament at an angle of 45 degrees (or 90 degrees) with the skin or coronal plane until the puncture needle can't go any further. The puncture needle is drawn back and drawn back until the syringe draws blood. Lower the tail of the needle parallel to the coronal plane and keep it fixed, place a guide wire and put the catheter into (the cannula device outside the needle) or remove the syringe into the catheter (the cannula device inside the needle). The catheter should be sutured by suture.

55.4   Matters needing attention

In strict accordance with the operating procedures, the tail end of the guide wire must go beyond the tail of the catheter and be fixed outside the patient to prevent the guide wire from slipping into the catheter and entering the blood circulation.

Strict aseptic operation to prevent infection. The catheter should be treated with iodine tincture and ethanol for 1 times every 1 – 2 days, and dressing should be replaced with adhesive tape. When connecting the infusion tube, gas embolism should be prevented. Properly fix venous catheter to prevent falling off. Keep the lumen unobstructed and rinse regularly with 1,000 U/mL heparin saline. Replace the infusion catheter daily. Do not use central venous catheter for blood transfusion, chemotherapy and other uses.

Zhu Zhiqiang

Chapter 56

Emergency Renal Replacement Technology

56.1 Prospect

Reanal replacement refers a group of treatment technologies that use a purification device through an extracorporeal circulation to remove abnormal plasma components, drugs or accumulated toxic substances and toxic products such as metabolites in order to correct disturblance and restore the stability of internal environmental in the body of critical ill patients. Renal replacement includes hemodialysis, hemofiltration, hemoperfusion, plasma exchange, and immunoadsorption. Hemodialysis, hemofiltration and hemodiafiltration are most commonly used renal replacement techniques.

56.2 Indication for renal replacement

Hyperkalemia (K>6.5 mmol/L).

Progressive acidosis with blood pH<7.20.

Diuretic resistant fluid overload with pulmonary edema.

Acute kidney injury, uremia.

Congestive cardiac failure.

Acute liver failure.

Severe acute pancreatitis.

Severe sepsis and septic shock.

Drug and toxin removal.

56.3 Contraindication for renal replacement

Allergy to blood purification related materials. There are no absolute contraindications to the rest. However, physician should be aware to patients with active bleeding, hemodynamic instability, serious arrhythmia, thrombocytopenia, abnormal coagulation function, and accidents. For end-stage patients, it is necessary to estimate the advantages and disadvantages of Renal Rreplacement Technology(RRT).

56.4   Mode of renal replacement technology

Hemodialysis (HD) :in hemodialysis (HD),the exchange of material between blood and dialysate is mainly done on both sides of the filtration membrane. Diffusion is the main mechanism of solute transport. The removal efficiency of HD is high for small molecules,including urea nitrogen,creatinine,potassium and sodium,but poor clearance of large molecular substances such as inflammatory mediators.

Hemofiltration (HF):the principle of glomerular filtration and renal tubular reabsorption is similared in normal people,and excessive water and uremic toxins are eliminated by convection. Compared with hemodialysis,hemofiltration has the advantages of less impact on hemodynamics and higher clearance of intermediate molecules.

Hemodiafiltration (HDF):hemodiafiltration is developed on the basis of HF. The solute transport mechanism increases dispersion on the basis of convection,which can not only effectively remove the medium molecular solute,but also make up for the low efficiency of HF in solute removal. It is a combination of hemodialysis and hemofiltration. With the advantages of two treatment modes,Solutes can be removed by diffusion and convection. More small and medium−sized molecular substances are eliminated in a unit time than hemodialysis or hemofiltration alone.

Plasma exchange (PE) is a blood purification method used to remove macromolecules in the blood. The basic process is to pump the patient's blood through the blood pump and separate the plasma and cellular components through a plasma separator. Removal of pathogenic plasma or certain pathogenic factors in the plasma,then the cellular components,the purified plasma and the replacement fluid required for replacement are returned to the body.

Blood perfusion(BP) is the introduction of blood from the body into the extracorporeal circulation system. Non−specific absorption of poisons,drugs,and metabolites by the adsorbent in the perfusor achieves a blood purification treatment method or means for removing these substances. Combined with other blood purification methods can form different hybrid blood purification therapies.

Hemoperfusion (HP):HP is the simplest method of adsorption. It refers to take the patient's blood from the body and removing the poison,drug or metabolite directly through the perfusion device. In general it is used for barbiturates,non−barbiturate sedatives,organophosphorus poisoning,etc. The indications of hemoperfusion has been extended to hepatic encephalopathy,uremia,sepsis and severe pancreatitis and other diseases.

56.5   Complication

Vascular access complliactions:local bleeding,hematoma,thrombosis,distal limb ischemia,aneurysm or nerve injury,blood pneumothorax at the puncture site,etc.

Cardiovascular complications:hemodynamic instability,arrhythmia,cardiac arrests.

Hypoxemia Respiratory failure.

Dialysis imbalance syndrome,severe hypertension and cerebrovascular accidents.

Bleeding,hemolysis,air embolism,dialyzer response,sepsis.

Zhang Guoxiu

Chapter 57

Emergency Bedside-echocardiography

57.1 Introduction

Emergency ultrasound (EUS) is the medical use of ultrasound technology for the bedside evaluation of emergency medical conditions and diagnoses, resuscitation of the acutely ill, critically ill or injured, guidance of high risk or difficult procedures, monitoring of certain pathologic states and as an adjunct to therapy. Typically, emergency ultrasound examination, performed and interpreted by emergency physician or those under the supervision of emergency physician, is a goal-directed focused ultrasound examination that answers emergent and important clinical questions. Emergency ultrasound is synonymous with the terms 'bedside' 'point-of-care' 'focused' 'clinical and physician performed'.

57.2 Ultrasound physics and definitions

Multiple modes of ultrasound imaging are used to enhance image acquisition. B-mode or brightness mode is the default mode of most ultrasound machines, and is most commonly used imaging modality in the bedside diagnostic ultrasound imaging. M-mode or motion mode is frequently used to evaluate the dimensions of cavities or movement of structures over time, such as cardiac valves, cardiac chamber and vessel walls, by emitting a steered line within the 2-D image and gathering data on movement of all tissues along that line. Doppler ultrasound can show the direction of moving structures relative to the transducer and the velocity of these structures based on the principle of Doppler/frequency shift. In general, color flow Doppler shows the direction by color, where blue represents blood flow away from the transducer and red represents blood flow toward the transducer, and shows the velocity by the degrees of brightness of the color, where brighter represents higher velocity.

57.3　Equipment and safety

Ultrasound imaging is a very safe imaging modality, but limitations must be considered. When applied to tissues, intense ultrasound beams can potentially cause two types of injuries: thermal (heat generation) and nonthermal (cavitation) from contrast-enhanced ultrasound. Because of this theoretical risk, societies advocate the As Low As Reasonably Achievable (ALARA) principle, producing satisfactory imaging with minimization of duration of exposure at a single point being the most important modifiable risk factor. Doppler modes should be minimized over sensitive tissue, including early gestation, germinal tissue, and mucosal or neural tissue. The thermal index (TI) should be kept below 2.0, and the mechanical index (MI) should be kept below 1.9.

57.4　Applications and categorization

Grouping of these US applications into categories of resuscitative, diagnostic, symptom or sign based, procedural guidance, and monitoring and therapeutic helps describe the relationship between the uses of US in emergency medicine (Table 57-1). The most common applications of emergency US include: cardiac, thoracic (pleura and lung), traumatic, vascular, pelvic, procedural auxiliary diagnosis.

Table 57-1　Classification of emergency ultrasound applications

Resuscitative	Diagnostic	Symptom or sign based	Procedural guidance	Monitoring and therapeutic
Cardiac	Cardiac	Hypotension	Any emergency	Central vein size
Trauma	FAST	Dyspnea	Medicine procedure	Fluid collections
Abdominal aorta	Pregnancy	Chest pain		Cardiac contractility
Pregnancy	AAA	Abdominal pain		Fetal heart rate
Thoracic	DVT	Extremity pain		Low-frequency clot
Procedural	Thoracic			Dissolution
	Advanced uses			
	New uses			

AAA = Abdominal aortic aneurysm; DVT = Deep venous thrombosis. Accessed from Marx J A, Hockberger R S, Walls R M, et al. Rosen's emergency medicine : concepts and clinical practice[J]. Emergency Medicine, 2013, 15(2):196-196.

57.4.1　Focused cardiac ultrasound

Focused cardiac ultrasound (FOCUS) is one of the most important and frequently used applications of ultrasonography in emergency setting. It is used more often in a variety of diagnostic and symptom and sign-based clinical presentations through the rapid assessment of cardiac size, structure, function, and hemodynamics. Indications include undifferentiated hypotension/shock, dyspnea, chest pain, suspected pericardial effusion, trauma and cardiopulmonary arrest. Many algorithms and protocols have been developed incorporating FCOUS to address specific questions, such as RUSH for shock, FAST for trauma.

The four typical cardiac views can be obtained to assess the heart at the bedside through the transthoracic and transabdominal windows with use of small curvilinear or phased array probes, and involve the parasternal long-axis view (PLAX), parasternal short-axis view (mid-ventricular level) (PSAX), apical 4-chamber view (A4C), and subcostal 4-chamber view (S4C). The specific cardiac views and images acquisition differ depending on clinical need. The PLAX view and the S4C view are two views most frequently used to evaluate for contractility and pericardial effusion. Note that only the subcostal and apical views allow for four-chamber visualization and comparison of right and left ventricles. The PLAX view is used primarily to assess left ventricular size and function, the aortic and mitral valves, and left atrial size (Figure 57-1A). The PSAX view gives an excellent circumferential view of the left ventricle and is often used for assessment of contractility and segmental wall motion abnormalities (Figure 57-1B). A4C view allows assessment of RV systolic function and size relative to the LV and evaluation of pericardial effusion (Figure 57-1C). The S4C view gives a good view of the right ventricle and detection for a pericardial effusion (Figure 57-1D). It is also the standard view for cardiac evaluation during the FAST exam.

Detection of pericardial effusion in patients at risk is one of the most well-established uses of FOCUS. Studies have shown a high degree of sensitivity and specificity in the detection of pericardial effusions in both medical and trauma patients using FOCUS. As previously stated, imaging in the PLAX and S4C view can provide accurate detection of pericardial effusion when looking for circumferential black or anechoic fluid surrounding the heart within the pericardium. Suspicion of a cardiac tamponade must be raised in any hemodynamically unstable patient with pericardial effusion, but diagnosis must be made in conjunction with clinical signs including hypotension, tachycardia, pulsus paradoxus, and distended neck veins.

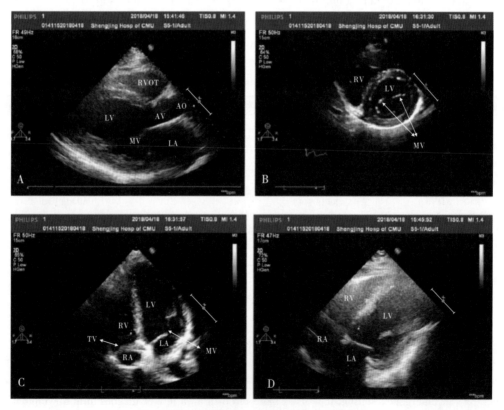

Figure 57-1　The four typical cardiac views

A. PLAX view; B. PSAX view; C. A4C view; D. S4C view. LV=left ventricle; RV= right ventricle; LA=left atrium; RA =right atrium; AO=aorta; AV=aortic valve; RVOT=right ventricular outflow tract; MV=mitral valve; TV=tricuspid valve.

Evaluation of the RV is essential in diagnosis and management of shock and respiratory failure in acutely ill patients. Among several important and common causes for RV enlargement and dysfunction, the presence of massive or submassive pulmonary embolus is prognostically critical and associated with significantly higher in-hospital mortality. FOCUS can be used to identify hemodynamically significant pulmonary emboli by observing right ventricular dilatation (>1 : 1 RV/LV ratio) , right ventricular hypokinesis, septal flattening or paradoxical motion, or a hyperdynamic LV with a full IVC, or occasionally by visualizing free-floating thrombus. The PSAX view and the A4C view can offer good chances to compare chamber sizes and evaluate the septum.

Rapid assessment of systolic LV function is frequent in ED and indications include, but are not limited, to the following: periarrest, unidentified hypotension, shock states, dyspnea, chest pain and suspicion of cardiac failure. It is important to note that the goal of such assessment is primarily to differentiates patients into "normal" or function impaired ("depressed") and to facilitate clinical decision-making. To estimate LV function, a minimum of 4 views (PSLA, PSSA, A4C, and S4C) should be obtained.

The goal of FOCUS in the setting of cardiac arrest is to improve the outcome of cardiopulmonary resuscitation by identifying organized cardiac contractility to help the clinician distinguish among asystole, pulseless electrical activity (PEA) , and pseudo-PEA (visualization of ventricular contractility by FOCUS in patients without palpable pulses) ; determine reversible etiologies of arrest such as pericardial tamponade, pulmonary embolism, and hypovolemia; and guide lifesaving procedures at the bedside.

For patients presenting with undifferentiated hypotension/shock, the primary advantage of FOCUS is in allowing providers to rapidly differentiate the etiology of shock at the bedside and monitor response to therapies, which is extremely important in consideration that early intervention to prevent organ from inadequate tissue perfusion. The FOCUS exam, as previously stated, should evaluate for the presence of pericardial effusion, global cardiac function, right ventricular size, and IVC size/collapsibility as a marker of central venous pressure. Various protocols have been published to describe FOCUS approach in shock, and one easily learned and quickly performed shock ultrasound protocol, the RUSH exam (Rapid Ultrasound in Shock) , is shown in Table 57-2.

Table 57-2   The RUSH protocol to diagnose the type of shock

	Step No. 1	Step No. 2	Step No. 3
Pump	Pericardial effusion: (a) Effusion present? (b) Signs of tamponade? 　　Diastolic collapse of R Vent +/R Atrium?	Left ventricular contractility: (a) Hyperdynamic? (b) Normal? (c) Decreased?	Right ventricular strain: (a) Increased size of RV? (b) Septal displacement 　　from right to left?
Tank	Tank volume: (1)Inferior vena cava: 　　(a) Large size/small Insp collapse? 　　　　−CVP High− 　　(b) Small size/large Insp collapse? 　　　　−CVP Low− (2) Internal jugular veins: small or large?	Tank leakiness: (1)E-FAST exam: 　　(a) Free fluid Abd/Pelvis? 　　(b) Free fluid thoracic cavity? (2)Pulm edema: Lung rockets?	Tank compromise: Tension pneumothorax? (a) Absent lung sliding? (b) Absent comet tails?
Pipes	Abdominal aorta aneurysm: 　　Abd aorta>3 cm?	Thoracic aorta aneurysm/dissection: (a) Aortic root>3. 8 cm? (b) Intimal flap? (c) Thor aorta>5 cm?	(1)Femoral vein DVT? Noncompressible vessel? (2)Popliteal vein DVT? Noncompressible vessel?

Undifferentiated chest pain and dyspnea are frequently encountered in emergency setting, and patients commonly present with both symptoms. Ultrasonongraphy is helpful to differentiate the various causes of chest pain or dyspnea and rule out life threatening etiology. The RADiUS (rapid assessment of dyspnea with ultrasonograpgy) approach outlined by Manson and Hafez is a protocol to assess patients with dyspnea. Being the most important component of this protocol, FOCUS plays a role in search for pericardial effusion, identification of global LV systolic dysfunction, and assessment of the size of the right ventricle as a proxy for indicating the presence of a hemodynamically significant pulmonary embolus or not. The life-threatening chest pain syndromes where FOCUS may be helpful are to evaluate patients with a hemodynamically significant pulmonary embolus or screen patients with suspected aortic dissection. The following is a algorithmic sonographic approach for evaluation of patients with undifferentiated chest pain and dyspnea (Figure 57-2).

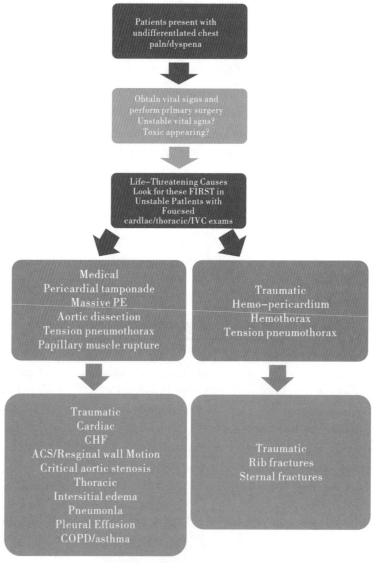

Figure 57-2　A suggested algorithmic sonographic approach to the patient with chest pain or dyspnea

Accessed from Meer J, Beck S, Ali K. Symptom-Based Ultrasonography[J]. Ultrasound Clinics, 2014, 9(2): 227-246.

57.4.2   Thoracic ultrasound

Thoracic ultrasound greatly relies on several important artifacts produced at the readily visualizable pleural line. These artifacts are few and discrete and intimately linked to pathologic processes. By interpreting these artifacts as well as relevant alternations emergency physicians can make important inferences about the underlying lung parenchyma. These diagnoses include pneumothorax, pulmonary edema, pneumonia and pleural effusions.

The fundamental and important artifact of thoracic ultrasound is "pleural line", which is the first horizontal, curvilinear, hyperechoic line and represents the apposition of the parietal and visceral pleural interface (Figure 57-3A). Typically, when seen in real-time scanning, the mobile visceral pleura move against the static parietal pleura and produce a back-and-forth movement that is synchronized with respiration. This sign is called lung sliding. If lung sliding is present that will present a 'seashore sign' on M-mode (Figure 57-3B), while the "bar code" or "stratosphere" sign on M-mode signifies absence of lung sliding. The 'seashore sign' is characterized by motionless parietal tissue over the pleural line and a homogenous granular pattern below it. A second important artifact is the A-lines, which are some hyperechoic, horizontal, equidistant lines arising from the pleural line. A-lines are reverberation artifacts created by repetitive reflection of ultrasound waves between the pleural line, a strong reflector, and the transducer. A-lines combined with lung sliding can be seen in a normal or excessive aerated lung, such as COPD, asthma, or pulmonary emboli. The third important artifact is the B-line, also known as comet tail artifact or lung rocket. It is a vertical narrow-based artifact that arises from pleural line, spreads out to the edge of the screen without fading and moves synchronously with lung sliding.

In ED, much of works in ultrasound focus on ruling out a pneumothorax (PNX). The presence of lung sliding has been reported to be highly sensitive and specific in ruling out a PNX when showed throughout the lung fields. Normal lung sliding and the presence of the sonographic B-lines can rule out pneumothorax with a 100% negative predictive value. Definitive diagnosis of a PNX is more difficult and is associated with the presence of a lung point (area where the PNX begins), absence of lung sliding, absence of comet-tail artifacts.

Interstitial syndrome, including acute pulmonary edema, interstitial pneumonia, acute respiratory distress syndrome (ARDS), and pulmonary fibrosis, can cause interloubular septa to widen with fluid accumulation, which permit propagation of ultrasound waves and generation of B-lines. However, one or two of these lines can be seen in 30% of normal people, particularly in gravity-dependent areas, such as lateral-basal area. Generally, three or more B-lines in an intercostal space are considered as a positive finding for pulmonary edema. Moreover, the number of B-lines may correspond to the severity of pulmonary edema. At follow-up US, resolution of B-lines also correlates with improvement of a patient's symptoms and radiographic findings.

Pleural effusion is the typical indication for thoracic ultrasonography and has the potential ability to identify, as well as characterize, quantify, and guide the drainage of fluid. US is far more sensitive than chest radiography for detection of pleural effusion, being able to depict as little as 5-20 mL of pleural fluid with an overall sensitivity of 89%-100% and specificity of 96%-100%. Simple pleural effusion is free of echoes and can be seen as anechoic space between the visceral and parietal pleura. Swirling hyperechoic debris secondary to cardiac or respiratory motion may be seen ("plankton sign"). It should be aware that transudative fluid is always anechoic, whereas exudative fluid can be either anechoic or hyperechoic.

An approach to thoracic ultrasound in the clinical evaluation of patients has been previously described

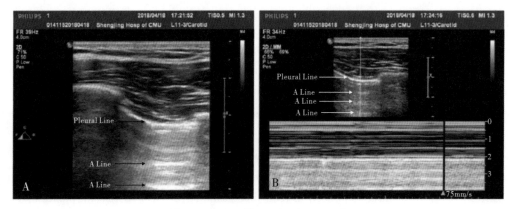

Figure 57-3　Thoracic ultrasound

A：Sonographic appearance of an aerated lung scan；B：Time-motion（M-）mode ultrasonography illustrating lung sliding by the presence of the 'seashore sign'.

in the BLUE protocol（Figure 57-4）. Systematically compiling lung ultrasound findings at these points allows for rapid identification of possible etiologies in acute dyspnea or respiratory failure. Following is an adapted algorithm that may be used for interpreting patterns found during a systematic thoracic ultrasound exam in the context of acute respiratory failure, remembering to always interpret ultrasound findings in the clinical context.

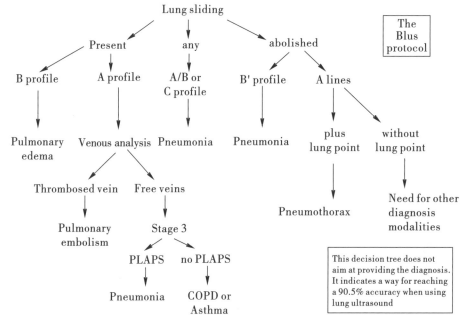

Figure 57-4　A decision tree utilizing lung ultrasonography to guide diagnosis of severe dyspnea and acute respiratory failure

Accessed from Lichtenstein D A, Mezière G A. Relevance of lung ultrasound in the diagnosis of acute respiratory failure：the BLUE protocol.［J］. Chest,2008,134（1）：117-125.

57.4.3　Trauma

Trauma is a leading cause of morbidity and mortality in adult patients in the ED, and prompt diagnosis and intervention are important to successfully manage trauma patients. Despite the availability of other modalities to evaluate trauma patients, such as computed tomography (CT) and diagnostic peritoneal lavage (DPL), ultrasound revolutionized the manegement of trauma patients with the introduction of the FAST (Focused Assessment with Sonography for Trauma) examination. The FAST examination is a rapid assessment of the hemodynamically unstable patient by ultrasound to identify the presence of peritoneal and/or pericardial free fluid. New version includes the evaluation of pneumothorax and hemothorax in pleural space, named the eFAST (extended FAST). The American College of Surgeons has adopted the FAST into the Advanced Trauma Life Support (ATLS) protocol.

As a non-invasive test, the FAST examination can be performed rapidly at the bedside to address a specific clinical question. The E-FAST allows the assessment of a hemothorax or pneumothorax, and has become an accepted standard of care in the resuscitation of the injured patient. The FAST protocol consists of the evaluation of four regions to detect hypoechoic images related to free pericardial and peritoneal fluids. Conventionally, a low-to middle-frequency (2-5 MHz) probe is used to evaluate all four regions. These four regions include:

(1) The left upper quadrant (RUQ) or hepatorenal fossa (Figure 57-5A), to detect fluid in the hepatorenal space (Morison's pouch).

(2) The sub-xyphoid view (Figure 57-5B), to detect pericardial fluid.

(3) The left upper quadrant (LUQ) or splenorenal recess (Figure 57-5C), to detect perisplenic fluid.

(4) The pelvis (Figure 57-5D), where fluid may accumulate in the retrouterine pouch (pouch of Douglas) or retrovesical pouch. The most sensitive view in the FAST examination for detecting peritoneal fluid is RUQ, and free fluid is often detected in the pelvic or Morison's pouch regardless of the site of the intra-abdominal injury.

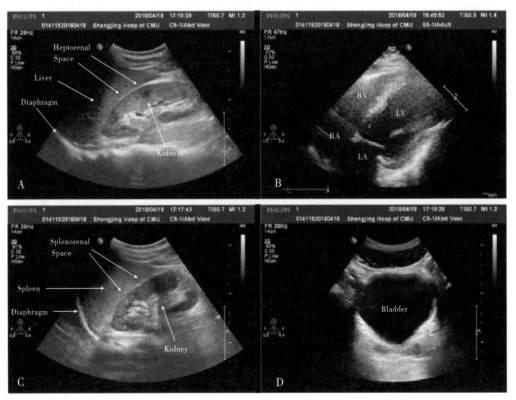

Figure 57-5   Normal B-mode images of four regions in FAST Protocol

A. RUQ view; B. the sub-xyphoid view; C. LUQ view; D. the pelvic view. LV = left ventricle; RV = right ventricle; LA = left atrium; RA = right atrium.

The FAST exam has been shown to be good to outstanding sensitivity in many studies (73% –99%). Its application has managed to reduce mortality from cardiac and abdominal trauma. Its extended application to the thorax (E–FAST) for detecting pneumothorax and hemothorax is very important. Firstly because it is more sensitive than radiography techniques for diagnosing pneumothorax (48% vs. 20%), a pathology that occurs to be occult in 5% of all traumas and in up to 55% of severe traumas. Secondly, sonography has a superior sensitivity and specificity to detect hemothorax than radiography given that ultrasound may detect fluid with a volume of 20 mL while radiography detects 200 mL. The following is a algorithm for unstable blunt trauma(Figure 57–6).

57.4.4 Vascular ultrasound

Change of right atrial pressures, representing central venous pressure (CVP), and volume status can be estimated by viewing the inferior vena cava (IVC) size and respiratory change from the subcostal cardiac window. Changes in intrathoracic pressure during spontaneous breathing are transmitted to the IVC and IVC shows respiratory variation, expanding with expiration (positive intrathoracic pressure) and contracting with inspiration (negative intrathoracic pressure) (Figure 57–7). This change is reversed in patients with mechanical ventilation and the IVC expanding with inspiration and contracting with expiration. Studies show that IVC ultrasound has good accuracy in assessment of blood loss, hypovolemia, and congestive heart failure. IVC evaluation in combination with BNP can be beneficial to guide fluid management of patients with heart failure.

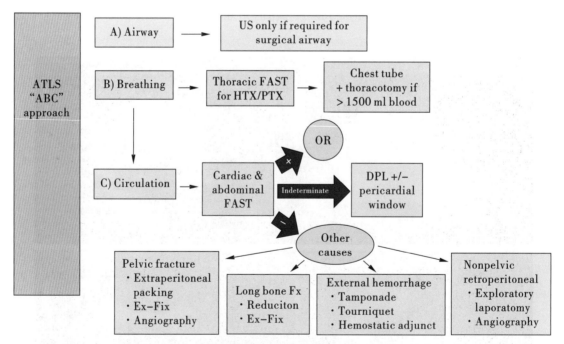

Figure 57–6 **Unstable blunt trauma algorithm**

(From) ATLS, advanced trauma life support; ABC, airway, breathing, circulation; US, ultrasound; FAST, focused assessment with sonography in trauma; HTX, hemothorax; PTX, pneumothorax; OR, operating room; DPL, diagnostic peritoneal lavage; Fx, fracture; Ex–Fix, external fixation. Accessed from Soni N J, Arntfield R, Kory P. Point–of–Care Ultrasound[M]. Point–of–care Ultrasound. 2014;77–81.

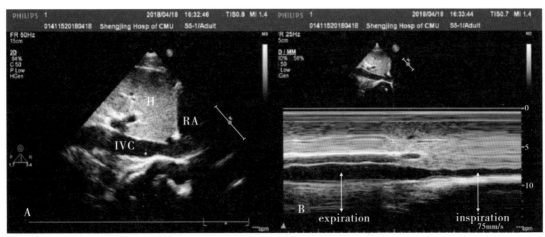

Figure 57-7   Inferior vena cava ultrasound

A. B-mode image of IVC; B. M-mode image of IVC showing normal respiratory change in a spontaneously breathing patient.

IVC = inferior vena cava; RA = right atrium; H = hepar.

Suspicion for aortic abnormality is indispensible in any patient presenting with abdominal discomfort, especially in patients with known risk factors and those that present with classic histories or exam findings (hypotension, back pain, palpable abdominal mass). Abdominal aortic aneurysms (AAA) are the most commonly identified aortic pathology. Ultrasonography can be a either diagnostic or screening tool to detect AAA and has demonstrated high sensitivity (97.5%-100%) and specificity (94.1%-100%) for detection of AAA. Sonographic visualization of the abdominal aorta is obtained from the subxiphoid space to the umbilicus in both transverse and longitudinal planes, and when suspicion of infrarenal aneurysms, the technique should visualize the aorta from the diaphragm to the aortic bifurcation. The aortic diameter should be measured from proximal outer wall to distal outer wall. Findings of abdominal aortic diameter greater than or equal to 3 cm or greater than or equal to 1.5 times the diameter of the more proximal aorta are considered to be positive. Perform a FAST examination in RUQ area to detect intraperitoneal fluid after an aneurysm is found.

Patients with symptomatic pulmonary embolism (PE) or with swollen and aching extremity need to be assess for deep venous thrombosis (DVT). Compression US is often the first choice of emergency physicians to rule out DVT. An inability to compress the vein with augmentation of the artery is concerning for a DVT. The "two-site" compression ultrasound exam involves visualization of the compressibility of the common femoral and popliteal veins. The three-dimensional technique adds the visualization of the superficial femoral vein (SFV), based on studies showing up to 22% of DVTs can be found in the SFV. Use of upper extremity veins is less common because Doppler US is needed for the subclavian vein, which is not compressible under the clavicle. The accuracy of this technique ranges from 70% to 99%, depending on experience of operator.

57.4.5   Pelvic ultrasound

Emergency physician-performed pelvic ultrasound allows for a rapid and safe diagnosis of a variety of pathologiesis in the first trimester of pregnancy. The most common and pressing application of pelvic ultrasound is to evaluate potential ectopic pregnancy. Suspicious symptoms and signs including, but not limited to, abdominal pain, pelvic pain, vaginal bleeding, syncope, abdominal distension, are amenable to evaluation for ectopic pregnancy with pelvic ultrasound regardless of β-hCG concentrations. Typically, pelvic ultrasound is performed to indirectly exclude an ectopic pregnancy based on visualizing an intrauterine pregnancy (IUP) or, less commonly, to identify an ectopic pregnancy by visualization. A recently published meta-analysis revealed a pooled sensitivity of 99.3% to rule out ectopic pregnancy by confirming intrauterine gestation. Other applications during pregnancy include detection of nonviable pregnancy, gestational tropho-blastic disease, spontaneous abortion. Additionally, pelvic ultrasound can be used to evaluate potential causes of abdominal pain in the nonpregnant patients including ovarian cysts, tubo-ovarian abscesses, ovarian torsion, masses, and hemoperitoneum in the hemodynamically unstable patient.

Pelvic US image acquisition involves transabdominal pelvic scanning (TAS) and transvaginal scanning (TVS) of pelvis. The TAS uses a curved-array transducer (2-5 MHz) placed over the lower abdomen above the pubic symphysis. A full bladder is preferred as it provides an acoustic window to visualize the uterus and adnexa, but this can be ignored if the uterus is large or the patient is thin. In the TVS, an intracavitary (5-8 MHz) probe is placed in the vagina. The patient should be placed in lithotomy position and optimally with an empty bladder. Both techniques have inherent advantages and are complementary. The advantage of TAS technique is that it can provide a wider and deeper field of view, beneficial to assessment of the spatial relationship of the pelvic organs to surrounding structures and detection of large pelvic masses. Alternatively, the utility of TVS lies in the ability to visualize intrauterine contents with high resolution. For example, TVS technique allows for earlier and more clearly detection of intrauterine yolk sacs and fetal poles within gestational sacs compared to TAS. Moreover, transvaginal ultrasound is sensitive to detect as little as 8mL of peritoneal fluid, making it a replacement of culdocentesis for detection of ruptured ectopic pregnancy in the hemodynamically compromised patient.

Definitive IUP on limited pelvic ultrasound examination is confirmed by visualization of a yolk sac, fetal pole or embryo within the fundus of the uterus. The yolk sac appears as an echogenic ring with an anechoic center located inside the gestational sac, which is the first definitive evidence of an IUP. Absence of cardiac movement in a fetal pole measuring greater than 5 mm or a gestational sac diameter of greater than 20 mm without an embryo indicates an embryonic or fetal demise. The sonographic finding of a "snowstorm" or "cluster of grapes" appearance in an echogenic, cystic uterus is highly predictive of a molar pregnancy, and decision-making should be combined with serum β-hCG levels. Sonographic features of ectopic pregnancy include the following with varying degrees of specificity: extra-uterine gestational sac containing yolk sac or embryo, extra-uterine fetal cardiac activity, tubal ring, complex adnexal mass, and free peritoneal fluid. Additionally, indeterminate scans occur frequently, haveing the proportion varying between 20% to 50% of ED pregnant patients undergoing pelvic ultrasound examinations. Point-of-care pelvic ultrasound has been shown having good value to evaluate the pelvic organs and pathologiesis in non-pregnant patients, but they do not often fall within the scope of emergency medicine.

57.4.6 Procedural ultrasound

Procedural guidance with ultrasound is also a common application in the emergency patient. The use of US for procedural guidance is aimed at not only improving the success rates of the procedure itself but also reducing adverse events and, thus, maximizing patient safety. Procedural guidance is commonly used more in vascular access, drainage of torso free fluid and less in the management of soft tissue inflammatory conditions, foreign body identification and removal.

Vascular access is one of the most basic skills required of emergency physician. Focused questions for vascular access involve location and patency of target vein. Procedural ultrasound has replaced surface anatomy and anatomic landmarks for more precise assessment of vein location, patency, and real-time visualization of venous cannulation. The most common venous cannulations assisted by ultrasound guidance are internal jugular, femoral vein, and peripheral venous cannulations. Generally, a high-frequency (5-10 MHz) linear transducer is used for vascular access, as it can generate higher-resolution imaging, and the linear image display makes needle guidance and identification somewhat more intuitive.

In the ED, US-guided internal jugular cannulation has been shown being useful to reduce time to flashback and improve success in the difficult-stick patient, improve overall success rate and first attempt and overall rates, reduce time to insertion, and reduce complication rate. The Valsalva maneuver and Trendelenburg position can make the internal jugular vein much easier to be visualized and increase the diameter improving the success rate of cannulation. Success rate of femoral vein cannulation can be improved by application of several techniques, including the reverse Trendelenburg position and putting pressure on the iliac vein close to the femoral vein. Ultrasound-guided peripheral venous cannulation can be used in any patient, but the technique is particularly useful in patients with nonpalpable or nonvisualizable peripheral veins. One study demonstrated a 36% increase in success of ultrasound-guided peripheral venous cannulation compared with usual methods.

Using techniques similar to those described earlier, ultrasound can facilitate an ever-growing number of common bedside aspiration procedures, including paracentesis, thoracentesis, and pericardiocentesis. These procedures are indicated for therapeutic drainage of a large symptomatic fluid collection, and may be performed for diagnostic purposes, such as cytology exam. Ultrasound is used to verify the presence of abnormal fluid, amount, and relative location with anatomic and sonographic windows. It can also locate anatomic structures that may be in the way or define structures for location of the space. Paracentesis including US-guided diagnostic peritoneal lavage has been described. Ultrasound assessment can identify as little as 250 mL of free intraperitoneal fluid and has a higher success rates when compared with landmark-based techniques (95% vs. 65%). Static or dynamic guidance may assist this procedure by localizing the largest collection of ascitic fluid and obstructing bowel loops. Thoracentesis is assisted by positive identification of the diaphragm plus liver or spleen to avoid puncture of these organs. A depth of at least 15 mm from the parietal to the visceral pleura throughout the respiratory cycle is advocated for a safe thoracentesis. Routine use of sonography has lowered the incidence of pneumothorax after thoracentesis to 1%-5% and in some studies the rate even decreased to near zero. Pericardiocentesis also can be facilitated by ultrasound through identifying the location of the best window and guiding needle insertion into the pericardial space. Ultrasound-assisted pericardiocentesis has proven to be an effective procedure with a success rate of 97% and an overall complication rate of 4.7%.

Bedside ultrasound is a useful tool to provide needle guidance for many emergent procedures. It increases the confidence of operator and helps to determine the ideal location for needle insertion. The use of ultrasound has been shown to increase success rates, decrease complication rates, and reduce health care costs. With practice, physicians can obtain the skills and competence required to incorporate ultrasound into their daily practice while performing procedures.

57.5   Integration into emergency medicine practice

Bedside ultrasound is a safe, effective, noninvasive, painless, repeatable and portable imaging technique, and has been integrated into emergency medicine practice for its numerous advantages. As technology available continues to develop and emergency physicians grow increasingly more comfortable with a wide variety of applications that can benefit their patients, predictably, the scope of emergency ultrasound will continue to expand, to fill multiple voids and needs. The emerging telesonography and three-dimensional ultrasound will further facilitate the diagnosis of emergent disease and management of critically ill patients.

Li Tiegang

References

[1]BOBROW B J,SPAITE D W,BERG R A,et al. Chest compression−only CPR by lay rescuers and survival from out−of−hospital cardiac arrest[J]. JAMA,2010,304(13):1447−1454.

[2]REA T D,FAHRENBRUCH C,CULLEY L,et al. CPR with chest compression alone or with rescue breathing[J]. N Engl J Med,2010,363(5):423−433.

[3]ABELLA B S. High−quality cardiopulmonary resuscitation:current and future directions[J]. Curr Opin Crit Care,2016,22(3):218−224.

[4]XU F,ZHANG Y,CHEN Y. Cardiopulmonary Resuscitation Training in China:Current Situation and Future Development[J]. JAMA Cardiol,2017,2(5):469−470.

[5]HASSAGER C,NAGAO K,HILDICK−SMITH D. Out−of−hospital cardiac arrest:in−hospital intervention strategies[J]. Lancet,2018,391(10124):989−998.

[6]KLEINMAN M E,GOLDBERGER Z D,REA T,et al. 2017 American Heart Association Focused Update on Adult Basic Life Support and Cardiopulmonary Resuscitation Quality:An Update to the American Heart Association Guidelines for Cardiopulmonary Resuscitation and Emergency Cardiovascular Care[J]. Circulation,2018,137(1):7−13.

[7]ASTIGIANO S,MORINI M,DAMONTE P,et al. Transgenic mice overexpressing arginase 1 in monocytic cell lineage are affected by lympho−myeloproliferative disorders and disseminated intravascular coagulation[J]. Carcinogenesis,2015,36(11):1354−1362.

[8]STENSBALLE J,HENRIKSEN H H,JOHANSSON P I. Early haemorrhage control and management of trauma−induced coagulopathy:the importance of goal−directed therapy[J]. Curr Opin Crit Care,2017, 23(6):503−510.

[9]MCCARTHY H J,TIZARD E J. Clinical practice:Diagnosis and management of Henoch−Schonlein purpura[J]. Eur J Pediatr,2010,169(6):643−650.

[10]ALALWANI M,BILLINGS S D,GOTA C E. Clinical significance of immunoglobulin deposition in leukocytoclastic vasculitis:a 5−year retrospective study of 88 patients at cleveland clinic[J]. Am J Dermatopathol,2014,36(9):723−729.

[11]CHEN S Y,CHANG K C,YU M C,et al. Pulmonary hemorrhage associated with Henoch−Schonlein purpura in pediatric patients:case report and review of the literature[J]. Semin Arthritis Rheum, 2011,41(2):305−312.

[12]FOWLKES J B. American Institute of Ultrasound in Medicine consensus report on potential bioeffects of diagnostic ultrasound:executive summary[J]. J Ultrasound Med,2008,27(4):503−515.

[13]TOOSI M S,MERLINO J D,LEEPER K V. Prognostic value of the shock index along with transthoracic echocardiography in risk stratification of patients with acute pulmonary embolism[J]. Am J Cardiol, 2008,101(5):700−705.

[14]GRIMBERG A,SHIGUEOKA D C,ATALLAH A N,et al. Diagnostic accuracy of sonography for pleural effusion:systematic review[J]. Sao Paulo Med J,2010,128(2):90−95.

[15]BALL C G,KIRKPATRICK A W,LAUPLAND K B,et al. Incidence,risk factors,and outcomes for occult pneumothoraces in victims of major trauma[J]. J Trauma,2005,59(4):917−924,924−925.

[16]STONE M B,MOON C,SUTIJONO D,et al. Needle tip visualization during ultrasound−guided vascular access:short−axis vs long−axis approach[J]. Am J Emerg Med,2010,28(3):343−347.

[17]WERNER S L,JONES R A,EMERMAN C L. Effect of hip abduction and external rotation on femoral vein exposure for possible cannulation[J]. J Emerg Med,2008,35(1):73-75.

[18]RHA J H,KWON S M,OH J R,et al. Snakebite in Korea:A guideline to primary surgical management [J]. Yonsei Med J,2015,56(5):1443-1448.

[19]SHIN J J,KIM S H,CHO Y E,et al. Primary surgical management by reduction and fixation of unstable hangman's fractures with discoligamentous instability or combined fractures:clinical article[J]. J Neurosurg Spine,2013,19(5):569-575.

[20]CORONADO V G,HAILEYESUS T,CHENG T A,et al. Trends in sports- and recreation-related traumatic brain injuries treated in US emergency departments:The National Electronic Injury Surveillance System-All Injury Program (NEISS-AIP) 2001-2012 [J]. Head Trauma Rehabil,2015,30 (3):185-197.

[21]GUPTA D,SHARMA D,KANNAN N,et al. Guideline Adherence and Outcomes in Severe Adult Traumatic Brain Injury for the CHIRAG (Collaborative Head Injury and Guidelines) Study[J]. World Neurosurgery,2016,89(6):169-179.

[22]AGHAKHANI K,HEIDARI M,YOUSEFINEJAD V,et al. Frequency of intracranial injury in cadavers with head trauma with and without scalp injury in Tehran[J]. Journal of Forensic & Legal Medicine, 2014,28(4):36-38.

[23]YEUNG C Y,HONG K T,CHIANG C P,et al. Anaplastic Lymphoma Kinase-Negative Anaplastic Large Cell Lymphoma Manifesting as a Scalp Hematoma After an Acute Head Injury—a Case Report and Literature Review[J]. World Neurosurgery,2016,88(10):13-16.

[24]ZHANG Y M,JIAN-MIN L I,JIANG X. Successful salvage in a scalp avulsion through unilateral microvascular anastomosis[J]. Chinese Medicine(English),2013,126(7):1386-1387.

[25]PRASAD G L,ANMOL N. Compound elevated skull fractures:Review of literature[J]. Brain Inj, 2017,31(4):1-6.

[26]MAROON J C,MATHYSSEK C,BOST J. Cerebral concussion:a historical perspective[J]. Progress in Neurological Surgery,2014,28(28):1.

[27]YANG G,SHAO G. Clinical effect of minimally invasive intracranial hematoma in treating hypertensive cerebral hemorrhage[J]. Pakistan Journal of Medical Sciences,2016,32(3):677-681.

[28]YE X,WANG H,HUANG Y,et al. Surgical treatment for ruptured dural arteriovenous fistula with large intracranial hematoma. [J]. Int J Clin Exp Med,2014,7(12):5244-5251.

[29]GHATAN S,ELLENBOGEN R G. Pediatric spine and spinal cord injury after inflicted trauma[J]. Neurosurgery Clinics of North America,2002,13(2):227-233.

[30]KREINEST M,SCHOLZ M,TRAFFORD P. On-scene treatment of spinal injuries in motor sports[J]. European Journal of Trauma & Emergency Surgery Official Publication of the European Trauma Society,2017,43(2):191-200.

[31]THOMSON C H,CHOUDRY M,WHITE C,et al. Multi-disciplinary management of complex pressure sore reconstruction:5-year review of experience in a spinal injuries centre[J]. Annals of the Royal College of Surgeons of England,2016,99(2):1.

[32]VALENZANO T J,WAITO A A,STEELE C M. A Review of Dysphagia Presentation and Intervention Following Traumatic Spinal Injury:An Understudied Population[J]. Dysphagia,2016,31(5):1-12.

[33]JÖRGENSEN S,IWARSSON S,NORIN L,et al. The Swedish Aging with Spinal Cord Injury Study (SASCIS):Methodology and initial results[J]. Pm & R,2016,8(7):667-677.

[34]BOGDAN Y,HELFET D L. Use of tourniquets in limb trauma surgery[J]. Orthopedic Clinics of North

America,2018,49(2):157.

[35]FARAHMAND S,HAMRAH H,ARBAB M,et al. Pain management of acute limb trauma patients with intravenous lidocaine in emergency department[J]. Am J Emerg Med,2018,36(7):1231-1235.

[36]SCERBO M H,HOLCOMB J B,TAUB E,et al. The trauma center is too late:Major limb trauma without a pre-hospital tourniquet has increased death from hemorrhagic shock[J]. Journal of Trauma & Acute Care Surgery,2017,83(6):1165.

[37]LIN Y K,CHEN C W,LEE W C,et al. Development and pilot testing of an informed consent video for patients with limb trauma prior to debridement surgery using a modified Delphi technique[J]. Bmc Medical Ethics,2017,18(1):67.

[38]CEBALLOS M,VALDERRAMA C O,OROZCO L E,et al. Cost-utility analysis of reconstruction compared with primary amputation for patients with severe lower limb trauma in colombia[J]. J Orthop Trauma,2017,31(9):288-294.

[39]RESNIK L,BORGIA M,SILVER B,et al. Systematic review of measures of impairment and activity limitation for persons with upper limb trauma and amputation[J]. Arch Phys Med Rehabil,2017,98 (9):1863-1892.

[40]BANSAL A,ARORA D,MEHTA Y. Fallacious fracture of clavicle after cardiac surgery[J]. Hsr Proceedings in Intensive Care & Cardiovascular Anesthesia,2012,4(1):51.

[41]HAENTJENS P,AUTIER P,COLLINS J,et al. Colles fracture,spine fracture,and subsequent risk of hip fracture in men and women. A meta-analysis[J]. Journal of Bone & Joint Surgery American Volume,2003,85(10):1936-1943.

[42]BARQUET A,GIANNOUDIS P V,GELINK A. Femoral neck fractures after removal of hardware in healed trochanteric fractures[J]. Injury-international Journal of the Care of the Injured,2017,48 (12):2619-2624.

[43]HORNER N S,KHANDUJA V,MACDONALD A E,et al. Femoral neck fractures as a complication of hip arthroscopy:a systematic review[J]. J Hip Preserv Surg,2017,4(1):9-17.

[44]HANI R,KHARMAZ M,BERRADA M S. Traumatic obturator dislocation of the hip joint:a case report and review of the literature[J]. Pan African Medical Journal,2015,21(6):356-358.

[45]SCHERMERHORN S M,AUCHINCLOSS P J,KRAFT K,et al. Patella Fracture in US servicemember in an austere location[J]. Journal of Special Operations Medicine A Peer Reviewed Journal for Sof Medical Professionals,2018,18(1):142.

[46]GHASSEMI K A,JENSEN D M. Lower GI bleeding:epidemiology and management[J]. Curr Gastroenterol Rep,2013,15(7):333.

[47]PANDEY V,INGLE M,PANDAV N,et al. The role of capsule endoscopy in etiological diagnosis and management of obscure gastrointestinal bleeding[J]. Intest Res,2016,14(1):69-74.

[48]WILKINS T,KHAN N,NABH A,et al. Diagnosis and management of upper gastrointestinal bleeding [J]. Am Fam Physician,2012,85(5):469-476.

[49]BAI Y,LI Z S. Guidelines for the diagnosis and treatment of acute non-variceal upper gastrointestinal bleeding (2015,Nanchang,China)[J]. J Dig Dis,2016,17(2):79-87.

[50]GARCIA-TSAO G,BOSCH J. Management of varices and variceal hemorrhage in cirrhosis[J]. N Engl J Med,2010,362(9):823-832.

[51]BAI Y,CHEN D F,WANG R Q,et al. Intravenous Esomeprazole for Prevention of Peptic Ulcer Rebleeding:A Randomized Trial in Chinese Patients[J]. Adv Ther,2015,32(11):1160-1176.

[52]FORTUNE B,GARCIA-TSAO G. Current Management Strategies for Acute Esophageal Variceal Hem-

orrhage[J]. Curr Hepatol Rep,2014,13(1):35-42.

[53]GARCIA-TSAO G,SANYAL A J,GRACE N D,et al. Prevention and management of gastroesophageal varices and variceal hemorrhage in cirrhosis[J]. Hepatology,2007,46(3):922-938.

[54]HOLSTER I L,KUIPERS E J,VAN BUUREN H R,et al. Self-expandable metal stents as definitive treatment for esophageal variceal bleeding[J]. Endoscopy,2013,45(6):485-488.

[55]INTAS G,STERGIANNIS P. Seat belt syndrome:a global issue[J]. Health Sci J,2010,4(4):202-209.

[56]HAMIDIAN JAHROMI A,SKWERES J,SANGSTER G,et al. What we know about management of traumatic abdominal wall hernia:review of the literature and case report[J]. Int Surg,2015,100(2):233-239.

[57]COMO J J,BOKHARI F,CHIU W C,et al. Practice management guidelines for selective nonoperative management of penetrating abdominal trauma[J]. J Trauma,2010,68(3):721-733.

[58]ISENHOUR J L,MARX J. Advances in abdominal trauma[J]. Emerg Med Clin North Am,2007,25(3):713-733.